Research Methodology and Project Management in Biotechnology

Authored By

Simmi Kharb

Department of Biochemistry
and Nodal Officer, Multidisciplinary Research Unit, Pt. B. D
Sharma Postgraduate Institute of Medical Sciences (PGIMS), Rohtak
Haryana 12400, India

Akshat Singh

Research Scholar, University Institute of Engineering
and Technology, MD University
Rohtak, India

Abhyuday Singh

Department of Computers, University of Southern California
LosAngeles, USA

&

Deepa Kharb

Faculty, Indian Law Institute
New Delhi, India

Research Methodology and Project Management in Biotechnology

Authors: Simmi Kharb, Akshat Singh, Abhyuday Singh and Deepa Kharb

ISBN (Online): 978-981-5080-74-2

ISBN (Print): 978-981-5080-75-9

ISBN (Paperback): 978-981-5080-76-6

First published in 2023.

Bentham Science Publishers Pte. Ltd.
80 Robinson Road #02-00
Singapore 068898
Singapore
Email: subscriptions@benthamscience.net

BENTHAM
SCIENCE

CONTENTS

PREFACE

The core concepts of biotechnology rely upon the application of a series of techniques now increasingly available to the researchers worldwide. The prelude to these techniques is essential for understanding their processes and possible applications leading to successful products & practices. A comprehensive textbook that encompasses the frontiers of technological advancements available in the field of biotechnology and integrates these concepts with the scientific method is hence a need of the day. This book will aim to reestablish and update the fundamental knowledge and understanding required for planning and executing fruitful projects for both students and faculty in biological sciences.

This book progresses with introducing the basic concepts of molecular biology techniques, genetic engineering, and bioinformatics, followed by scientific writing, project writing and funding opportunities available for entrepreneurs in biotechnology, guiding further regarding intellectual property rights and biotechnology regulations. The final chapters of the book are comprised of the modern knowledge and updates essential to every biological researcher on genomics, proteomics, and anti-sense technology, keeping in mind the practices of ethics in scientific research. The finale is focused on the applications of biotechnology in the area of molecular medicine.

Unique features of the book:

a. It is a textbook and not a reference book

b. It is comprehensive and includes various subjects and topics essential for biotechnology researchers

c. Each chapter will have learning objectives, self-assessment exercises, bullet points, tables and figures for better understanding and recollection of the subject/topics.

Simmi Kharb
Department of Biochemistry
and Nodal Officer, Multidisciplinary Research Unit, Pt. B. D
Sharma Postgraduate Institute of Medical Sciences (PGIMS), Rohtak
Haryana 12400, India

Akshat Singh
Research Scholar, University Institute of Engineering and Technology, MD University Rohtak, India

Abhyuday Singh
Department of Computers, University of Southern California LosAngeles, USA

&

Deepa Kharb
Faculty, Indian Law Institute New Delhi, India

CHAPTER 1

Techniques in Biotechnology

LEARNING OBJECTIVES

This chapter gives an overview of techniques used in biotechnology for the isolation of nucleic acid. Their handling, precautions in DNA mapping and automated DNA sequencing are discussed.

Abstract: Nucleic acid absorbs UV light maximally at 260 nm owing to its bases. Thus, DNA or RNA yield can be quantified based on this principle. Restriction endonucleases (type II) are one of the most important groups of enzymes for the manipulation of DNA. They are bacterial enzymes that can cut/split DNA of any source at specific sites and were first discovered in bacteria E. coli restricting the replication of bacteriophages, by cutting the viral DNA. This led to differences in the size of restriction fragments obtained due to digestion with specific restriction enzymes. A restriction map is formulated by comparing the fragment size produced in every single digestion with those from double digests. In target amplification, the nucleic acid region around the area of interest is copied many times by in vitro methods. Polymerase Chain Reaction (PCR) is the best-known and the most widely applied of the target amplification methods. Original sample DNA is digested by a restricted endonuclease, separated by agarose electrophoresis, and transferred by agarose electrophoresis, and transferred to a solid support (Nylon or Nitrocellulose membrane) followed by selective visualization of fragments using labeled hybrid

DNA sequence has now become a routine procedure. It is the process of determination of nucleotide or base sequence of a DNA molecule/fragment. A probe is a nucleic acid whose identity is known and is used to reveal the identity or abundance of a target or sample. They are simple to prepare and are labelled with nucleotides that are radioactive, or fluorescent or have attached affinity labels. Also, by using a biotin-labelled primer, single-stranded probes can be obtained. Microarrays represent high-density miniaturized arrays of molecular samples. The technology involves a series of probes immobilized on a glass slide as microdots, which are then hybridized with a mixture of test DNA sequences labelled with a fluorochrome.ization probes.

Keywords: Blotting, DNA chip, Haplotypes, Norther, Oligonucleotide, Polymerase chain reaction, RFLPs, Restriction enzymes, Recombinant DNA technology, SNPs.

Amazing developments in biotechnology in late twentieth century include: decoding of human genome, cloning, gene therapy, progress in stem cell research and RNA interference.

Simmi Kharb, Akshat Singh, Abhyuday Singh & Deepa Kharb (Eds.)

Many earlier landmark discoveries unveiled the mysteries of genetics and paved way for modern molecular biology. Beginning with the Mendel's experiments with garden peas published in 1866, the concept of genes as discrete units of heredity emerged. Morgan in 1910 revealed chromosomes as units of heredity and Avery in 1944 confirmed through bacterial studies that DNA carried genetic information and with Watson Crick's DNA double-helical model in 1953, Smith demonstrated that DNA can be cleared by restriction enzymes. This facilitated the subsequent development of Recombinant DNA Technologies (Fig. **1**).

With the construction of genetic map using restricting enzymes by Nathans, Southern blot was invented in 1975 to detect specific DNA sequences. This led to the development of DNA sequencing methodologies and the first complete DNA sequence of bacteriophage was discovered. PCR (polymerase chain reaction) was developed by Mullis and co-workers in 1985. Then, simultaneous interrogation of gene transcripts by DNA microarrays became a reality in 1996. The human genome sequence was completed in 2003.

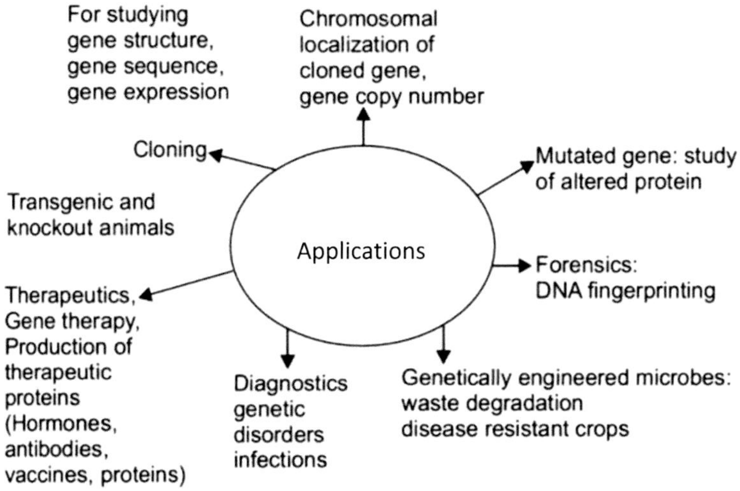

Fig. (1). Recombinant DNA technology applications.

ISOLATION AND SEPARATION OF NUCLEIC ACID

Almost all experiments dealing with gene manipulations require pure forms of DNA, RNA, or both. Thus, there is a need for reliable isolation techniques for nucleic acids (Fig. **2**).

Steps

1.Breaking of cells to expose nucleic acids
2.Separation of nucleic acid from other components
3.Recovery of nucleic acid

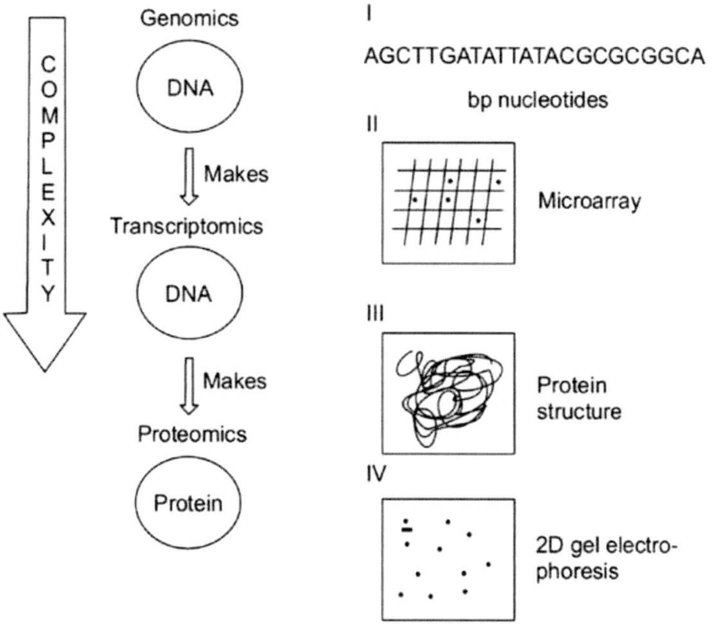

Fig. (2). Genomic data processing.

The study of purified nucleic acids have led to many key advances in the understanding DNA and RNA. Extraction and isolation of nucleic acid is a key step to subsequent molecular analysis (Fig. **3**).

Depending on the type of specimen, the required volume, yield, purity, the size of isolated nucleic acid, ease of operation, throughput, cost, the use of hazardous reagents, and the automation of the procedure, the most appropriate protocol is selected.

Whole blood, plasma, serum, tissue biopsies, cultured cells, buccal swabs, paraffin-embedded tissues, CSF, amniotic fluid, *etc*. are used. Protocols for DNA extraction can be classified as:

1.Liquid-phase extraction.
2.Solid-phase extraction.

1. **Liquid-phase extraction**— Useful when large quantity of DNA or large sample volumes are involved.

2. **Solid-phase extraction**— They are most used.

Advantage

— Easy to operate

— Large batches of specimen can be processed

— High reproducibility

— Can be automated.

1.First Step: *Cell lysis*—both cells and nuclear membrane envelopes are disrupted.
2.Next: *Removal of cell proteins*—by salt precipitation or degradation of cell proteins—by enzymes.
3.Additional Step: RNAase *digestion*—optional
4.Next: Precipitation of genomic DNA remaining in solution by alcohol.
5.Next: *Isolation and rehydration* of DNA precipitation DNA extract.

Solution is allowed to pass through silica-impregnated filter which binds and purifies DNA from other debris present in the alcohol solution or magnetic particles can be used instead of silica.

Or Centrifugation or vacuum manifolds can be used for filtration steps, the resultant DNA extract can be stored until the subsequent analysis.

Difference is:

1. In the separation of cellular and protein debris from soluble DNA by solvent extraction, *e.g.*, phenol-chloroform protocol (Fig. **4**).
2. After DNA is precipitated by alcohol, the DNA pellet is isolated by careful manual removal of excess alcohol and then air-dried to remove residual drops of alcohol (Fig. **5**).

3. Sample throughput is less because of the number of manual steps involved in the solution base methods.

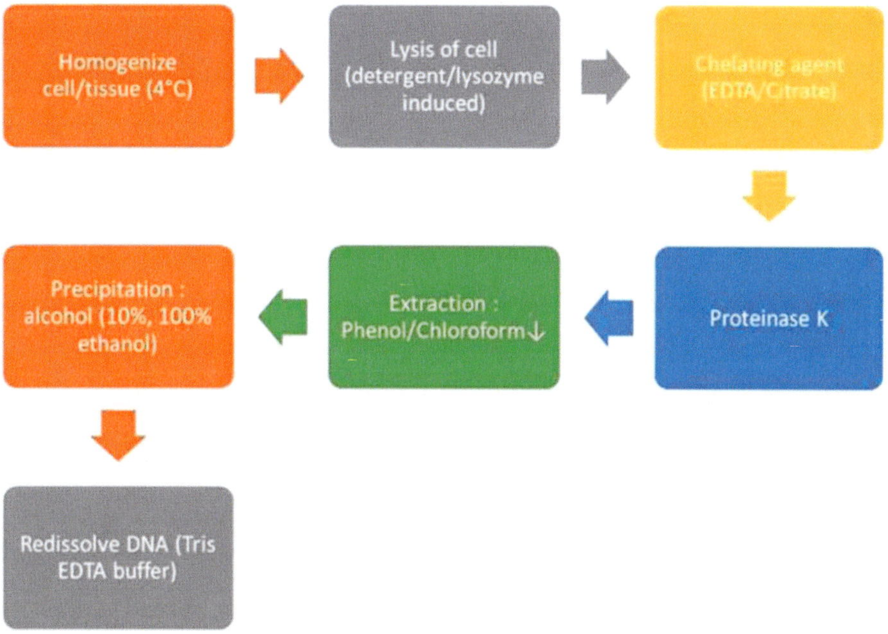

Fig. (3). Extraction of DNA from cells or tissues.

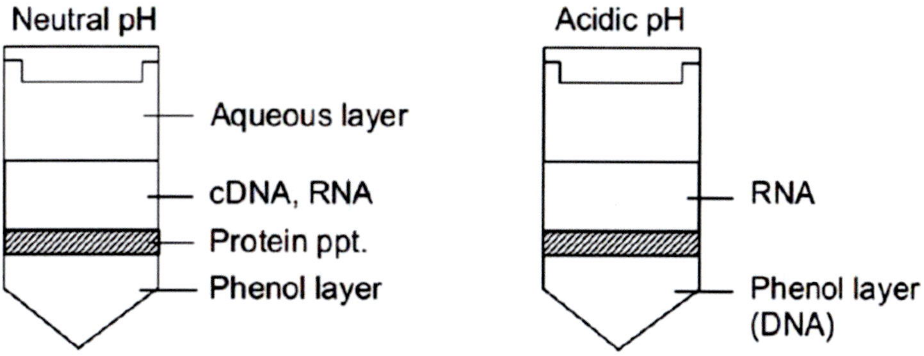

Fig. (4). Phenol extraction

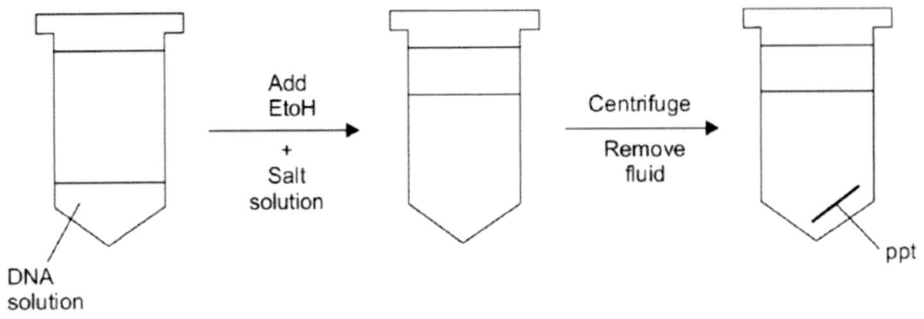

Fig. (5). Ethanol extraction.

Bound DNA is usually washed and eluted by using nuclease-free water or low ionic strength buffers. If magnetic particles are used, then DNA molecules coated with magnetic beads are retained by placing solution under the magnetic field. Magnetic beads are then removed from purified DNA.

1. The use of isolated columns: 96-well plate formats are available commercially.
2. Automated platforms.

RNA extraction and analysis are required for gene expression studies.

RNA: Less stable than DNA

•Not protected by double-helical conformation.
•Subject to alkaline hydrolysis *via* 2′ hydroxyl group of its ribose moiety.
•Degraded by RNA-specific Nuclease (RNAases).
•RNAases are ubiquitous, hence difficult to work with native RNA molecules in the lab.
•Thus, special attention is required while working with RNA.

1. Due to inherent instability, specimens intended for RNA analysis should be:

a. Processed promptly in a fresh state or
b. Preserved immediately by:
  i. Addition of preservation agents, *e.g.*, RNA later TM
  ii. Snap frozen by liquid nitrogen

2. The number of freeze-thaw cycles should be minimized.

3. Use RNAase-free-reagents and plastic ware to avoid RNAase contamination.
4. Clean or decontaminate the working surface and equipment with RNAase-free detergents or chemicals.
5. Use water-treated DEPC (Diethyl pyrocarbonate) for inactivation of RNAase.
6. Care should be taken to avoid DNA contamination. DNAase I treatment is commonly incorporated to digest DNA during RNA purification.

Identical to DNA extraction, RNA extraction is also solution-based and solid-phase extraction protocols (Fig. **6**).

1. First cell lysis—the RNA tissue specimens need to be ground thoroughly to a fine powder form before lysis. This procedure should be performed on either snap-frozen tissue or specimen preserved with RNA stabilizing agents to prevent RNA degradation to release RNA.

Treatment with RNAase inhibitors

(Diethyl pyrocarbonate, DEPC)

↓

Homogenize cells/Tissues

(4°C)

↓

Lyze cells

(detergents/lysozyme)

↓

RNA solvents

(Guanadinium thiocyanate)

↓

Proteinase K

(Fig. 6) contd.....

↓

Extraction

phenol/chloroform

↓

Precipitation: alcohol

(70%, 100% ethanol)

↓

Redissolve RNA

Fig. (6). Steps involved in extraction of RNA from cells or tissues.

Lysis buffers:

•Add phenol
•Sodium dodecyl sulphate
•Guanidinium salts
•Lyse the cells
•Inhibit the RNAase

2.Next: Isolation and purification of RNA from protein and lipids by:
i.Phenol-chloroform extraction
ii.Reversible binding to silica.

3.Next: Precipitation of RNA by alcohol.

Thus, with the above procedure, total RNA comprising mRNA, rRNA, snRNA and tRNA is isolated.

Polyadenylated tails on 3′ ends of mRNA by hybridization to cellulose-bound oligo

(Dt molecules).

Nucleic acids absorb UV light maximally at 260 nm owing to their bases. Thus, DNA or RNA yield can be quantified based on this principle.

1. Spectrophotometric methods—give purity of same.
2. The densitometric method—gives the size of isolated DNA or RNA—provides better precision.
3. Automated analyzers—using prefabricated chips and microfluidic channels are available which are both sensitive and precise.

RESTRICTION MAPPING OF DNA FRAGMENTS

Restriction mapping involves the size analysis produced by several restriction enzymes individually and in combination (Table **1**).

Table 1. Enzymes used in molecular biology.

Molecular Tools Enzymes
1. Restriction Endonuclease
2. DNA Ligase
3. Alkaline phosphatase (ALP)
4. DNA modifying enzyme:
i. Nucleases: Endonuclease Exonuclease:
a. DNA-dependent DNA polymerase
b. RNA-dependent DNA polymerase
c. DNA-dependent RNA polymerase
ii. Polymerase
iii. Enzyme modifying ends of DNA
a. ALP
b. Polynucleotide Kinase
c. Terminal (Deoxy nucleotide) transferase
iv. Others

Restriction endonucleases (type II) are one of the most important group of enzymes for manipulation of DNA. They are bacterial enzymes that can cut/split DNA of any source at specific sites. They were first discovered in bacteria E. coli restricting the replication of bacteriophages, by cutting the viral DNA. Thus, the enzymes that restrict viral replication are known as Restriction Enzymes or Restriction Endonucleases. Restriction enzymes cut DNA by cleaving the phosphodiester bond (in the sugar-phosphate backbone) that joins adjacent nucleotides in a DNA strand. Restriction enzymes are DNA-cutting enzymes and plasmid DNA is a circular form of self-replicating DNA that can be manipulated to carry other pieces of DNA (Table **2**).

Three different types of restriction enzymes are known.

Table 2. Types of Restriction endonucleases.

-	Type I	Type II	Type III
Methylase and Endonuclease Activity	Single bifunctional enzyme	Separate enzymes	Single bifunctional enzyme
Subunits	Three R2 M2 S1	Two One for Methylase One for endonuclease (Two copies)	Two
Recognition site	Bipartite asymmetric	4–6 bp often Palindromic sequence	5–7 bp Asymmetric sequence
Cleavage site	Non-specific	Within or close to recognition site	24–26 bp down stream of recognition site
ATP requirement for Restriction	Required	None	Required
Practical applications	–	Restriction mapping recombinant DNA) technology	–

Type II restriction endonucleases recognize certain DNA sequences, usually 4–6 bp in length and cleave them in a defined manner. The sequences recognized are palindromic or of an inverted repeat nature, (they read the same in both directions on each strand). When cleaved they leave blunt or sticky-ended fragments depending on the enzymes used.

Table 3. Recognition, sequences, and restriction enzymes from various sources.

Enzyme (source)	Recognition	Sequence	Products
Hla II (*H- Para influenzae*)	5′-CCGG-3′ 3′-GGCC-5′	5′-C 3′-GGC	CGG-3′ C-5′
Hae II (*H-Aegyptus*)	5′-GGCC-3′ 3′-CCGG-5′	5′-GG 3′-CC	CC-3′ GG-5′
Bam H1 (*Bacillus)* *acyloxies factions*)	5′-GGATCC-3′ 3′-CCTAGG-5′	5′-G 3′-CCTAG	GATCC-3′ G-5′
Eco RI (*E. coli*)	5′-GAATTC-3′ 3′-CTTAAG-G-5′	5′-G 3′-CTTAAG	AATTC-3′ G-5′
Hind III (*H. influenzae*)	5′-A-A-GCTT-3′ 3′-TTCGAA-5′	5′-A 3′-TTCGA	AGCTT-3′ A-5′

Approximately 500 restriction enzymes have been characterized and recognized around 100 different target sequences (Table **3**).

The nomenclature follows a general pattern:

1.1st letter indicates the genus name (in capital, italics)

2.Next two letters (in italics) indicate species.

3. Then comes the strain of the organism, *e.g.*, *Eco RI* is the form of *Escherichia (E) coli* (co), strain RY 13(R) and first endonuclease (I) to be discovered.

4. This is followed by a roman numeral, indicating the order of discovery.

The recognition sequences for type II restriction endonuclease are palindromes with rotational symmetry. *Palindromes*: the arrangement of nucleotides reads the same forward and backward on opposite strands of the DNA molecule. They are 4–6 bp, GC rich, *e.g.*, *Eco RI* recognition site (Fig. 7).

Most type II restriction endonucleases cleave DNA within their specific recognition sequences and these cut fragments may have sticky ends or cohesive ends. DNA fragments with sticky ends are particularly useful for recombinant DNA experiments.

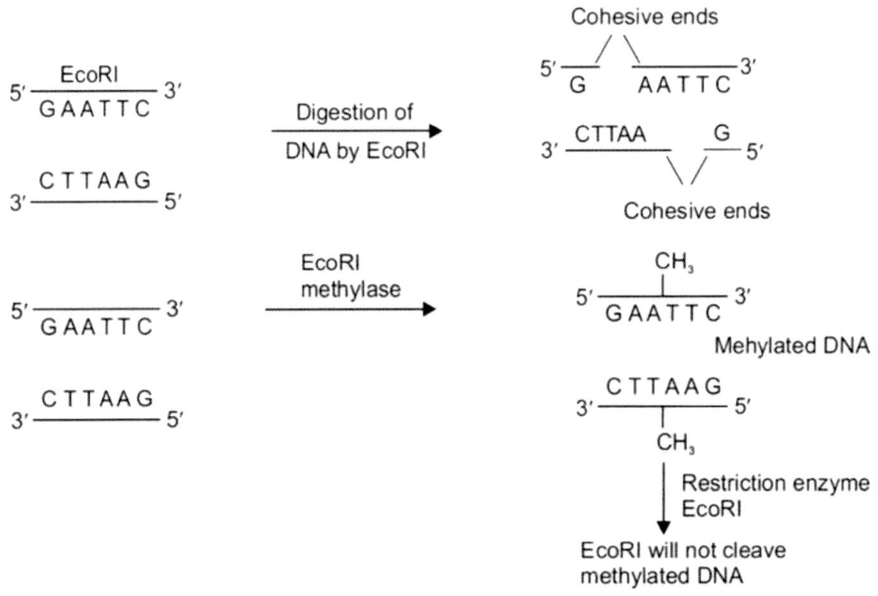

Fig. (7). Restriction enzyme: *Eco RI.*

Why do they not digest chromosome in bacterial cells? (Many bacteria and even certain bacteriophages have evolved to use methylation to protect their DNA from being destroyed by restriction enzymes).

Type II restriction endonucleases have target sites which are 4–8 bp in length. If all the bases are equally frequent in a DNA molecule, then a tetranucleotide is expected to occur on every 44 (*i.e.*, 256) nucleotide pairs in a long random DNA sequence.

Table 4. Expected number of DNA fragments produced by restriction enzymes from different genomes

Organism	Genome Size (Haploid, n)	Expected number of fragments		
		4 cutters ($4^4 = 256$)	6 cutters ($4^6 = 4096$)	8 cutters ($4^8 = 65536$)
E. coli	4.70×10^6 bp	18,359	1,147	72
Saccharomyces cerevisiae	1.35×10^7 bp	52,734	3,296	206
Drosophila melanogaster	1.80×10^8 bp	7,03,125	43,945	2,764
Homo sapiens	2.80×10^9 bp	10,93750	6,83593	42,274

Source: *Francisco Murillo Zebrinny, Fabio Nascimento da Silva, Gloria Patricia Castillo Urquizo, Marcos Fernando Basso, Chapter 8 - Transgenic Plants, Editor(s): Albizia Bore, Roberto Fritsche-Neto, Biotechnology and Plant Breeding, Academic Press, 2014, Pages 179-199,*

Sticky (staggered) ends are complementary and will strengthen each other. These pairings are transient owing to the weakness of hydrogen bonding between a few bases in the sticky ends, but they can be stabilized by the enzyme DNA ligase. Fragments are produced by cleavage with Bam HI (Fig. **8**).

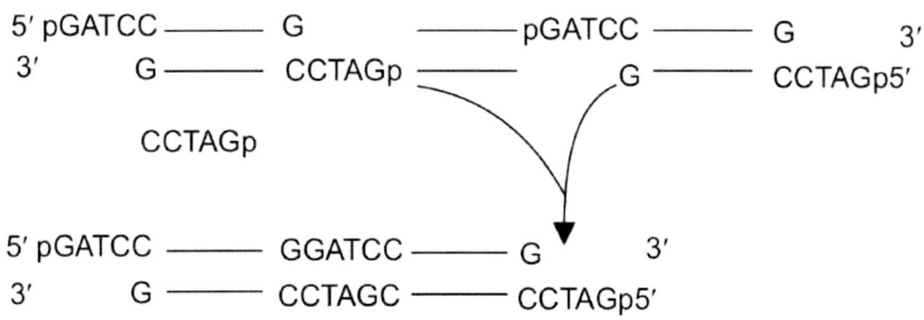

Fig. (8). Ligation molecules with cohesive (sticky) ends.

Complementary ends base-pair, to form a temporary link between two DNA fragments which is stabilized with $3' \rightarrow 5'$ phosphodiester linkages between these ends is catalyzed by DNA ligase.

This covalent joining of ends by DNA ligase enzyme is widely exploited in molecular biology to construct the recombinant DNA, *i.e.*, the joining of DNA fragments from different sources (Tables **4** and **5**).

Table 5. Other enzymes used in the manipulation of nucleic acids.

Enzymes	**Use**
1. Alkaline Phosphatase	Removes the phosphate group of prevent unwanted ligation of DNA (*i.e.*, prevent recirculation and DNA dimer formations). This allows the insertion of foreign DNA through DNA ligases.
2. DNA ligase	Joins DNA molecules by forming a 3′–5′ phosphodiester linkage.
3. DNA Polymerase I	Synthesizes complementary DNA
4. Taq DNA polymerase	Used in PCR
5. Nuclease i.DNAase I i.RNAase A i.SI nuclease	Non-specific endonucleases produce single-stranded nicks in DNA Cleaves and digests RNA. Used in mapping studies single-strand-specific nuclease (degrades single-stranded DNA and RNA)
6. Reverse transcriptase Polymerase (RNA-dependent DNA)	Synthesizes DNA from RNA used in the cDNA synthesis
7. Terminal transferases	Add a homopolymer tail (Nucleotides to 3′ end of DNA)

(Table 5) cont.....

8. Polynucleotide Kinase (PNK)	Transfers the terminal phosphate group from ATP to 5′-OH groups of DNA or RNA.
9. Methylase	Methylates specific residues and protects from cleavage by restriction enzymes.

Restriction mapping involves the size analysis of restriction fragments produced by several restriction enzymes individually and in combination (as discussed above).

Restriction enzymes recognize specific nucleotide sequences: recognition sequences in the DNA. Restriction sequences are usually 4, 5 or 6 nucleotides long and restriction enzymes can cut both strands of DNA at specific locations.

There are three ways in which DNA fragments can be cut (Fig. **9**):

i. Staggered cut to leave a 5′ overhang: a short single-stranded region of DNA is left that has a 5′ end and overhangs the end of the double-stranded DNA.
ii. Staggered cut to leave a 3′ overhang.
iii. Blunt end: a cut in the same place on both ends.

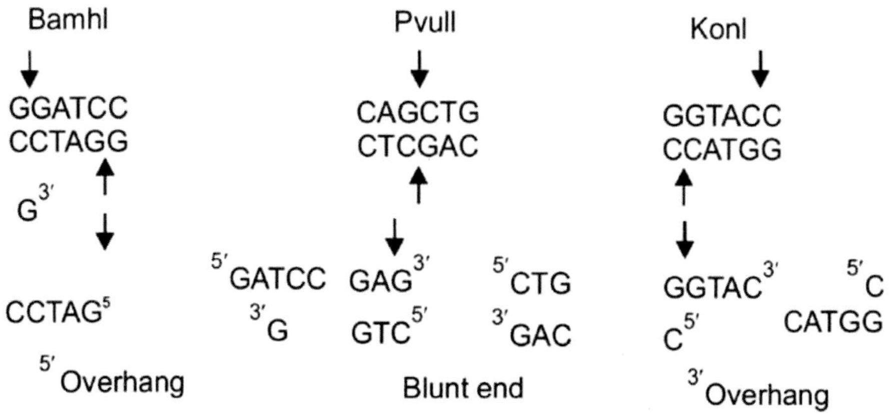

Fig. (9). Three ways in which DNA fragments can be cut.

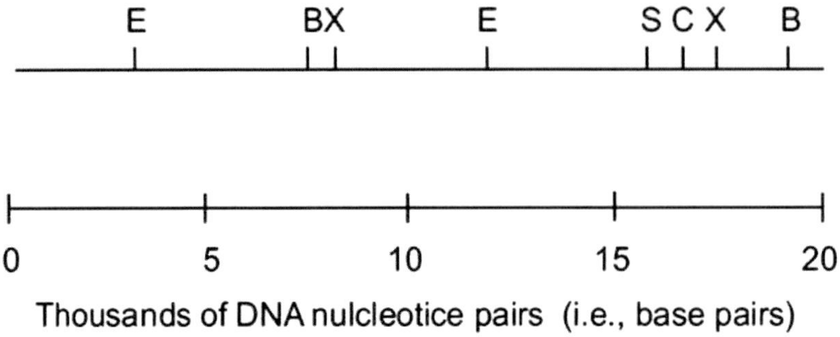

Fig. (10). Restriction map of a DNA molecule

Double-stranded DNA can be cut by various restriction enzymes having different recognition sequences. Using gel electrophoresis, the restriction fragments are separated, their sizes are measured and the deduction of the site of cut. A restriction map of the DNA molecule can be drawn showing the location of these cut sites termed as restriction sites (Fig. **10**). By using the restriction map, different DNA molecules can be compared (*e.g.*, examining evolutionary relationship between two species) without determining their nucleotide sequences (Table **6**).

Also, restriction maps are important experimentally in recombinant DNA work, for planning the desired cutting of the DNA molecule and for monitoring the progress of the experiment.

Taking the following example of mapping of DNA in which restriction sites of two enzymes A and B are mapped:

Cleavage of 9 kb molecule with A gives fragments 2 and 7 kb. So, a single A site can be positioned 2 kb from one end. Similarly, enzyme B gives fragments of 3 and 6 kb, *i.e.*, B has a single site 3 kb from one end. However, it is not possible at this state to predict whether it (B) is near to A site or at the opposite end of DNA.

Table 6. Restriction mapping.

Treatment	Fragment size (kb)	Interpretation
No digestion	9	
Enzyme A	2+7	

(Table 6) cont.....

<table>
<tr><td>Enzyme B</td><td>3+6 either

or</td><td rowspan="2">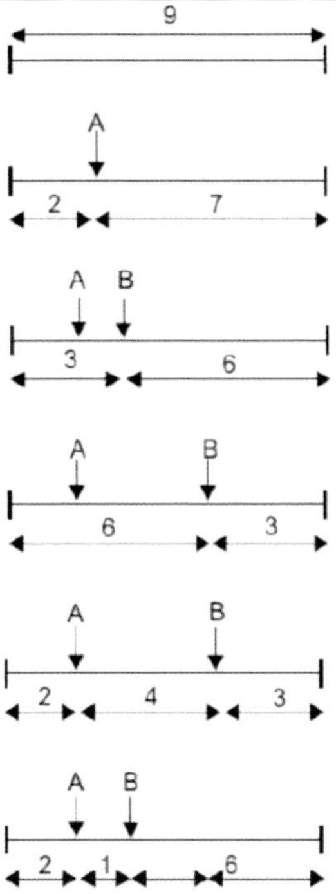
</td></tr>
<tr><td>Enzyme A + B</td><td>2,3+4

Alternative result
1, 2 + 6</td></tr>
</table>

RFLPs are based on polymorphisms due to base substitutions, insertions, deletions, and translocation that might have occurred in a specific region of genomic DNA. This led to differences in the size of restriction fragments obtained due to digestion with specific restriction enzymes (Fig. **11**).

RFLPs can be detected by the DNA probe, Southern blotting.

The value of RFLPs lies in their ability to be used as markers for human genetic diseases.

A restriction map is formulated by comparing the fragment size produced in every single digestion with those from double digests. Since each digestion produces three fragments from a linear DNA molecule, it is expected that the original piece of DNA must contain two sites for each restriction endonuclease.

The 300 bp fragment produced by single Eco RI digestion remains intact after the double digestion, whereas 850 and 500 bp Eco RI fragments are cleared.

This is resolved by double digestion and if the resultant fragments are 2, 3 and 4 kb, then A and B cut at opposite ends of the molecule and if they are 1, 2 and 6 kb, the sites are close to each other.

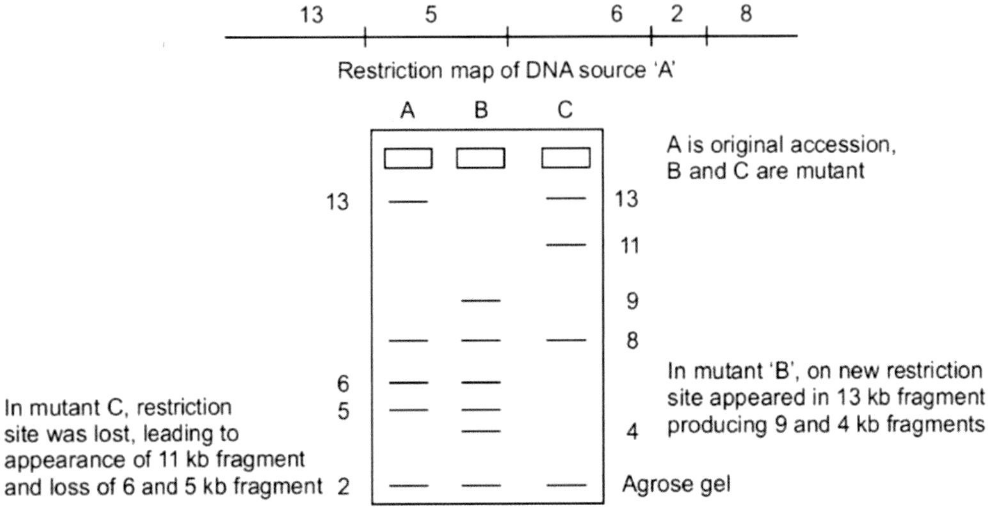

Fig. (11). Technique involved in detection of RFLPs

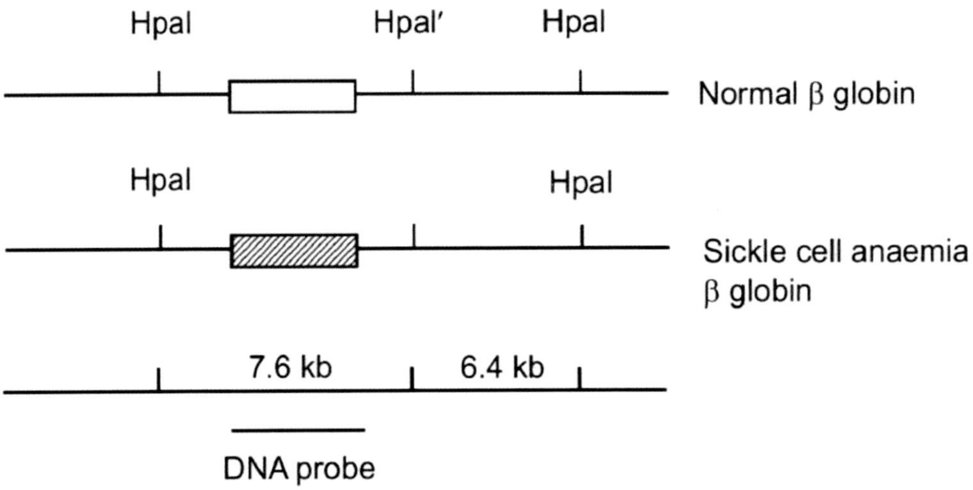

(a) Analysis for sickle cell anaemia β globin gene loss of HpaI' site

(Fig. 12) contd.....

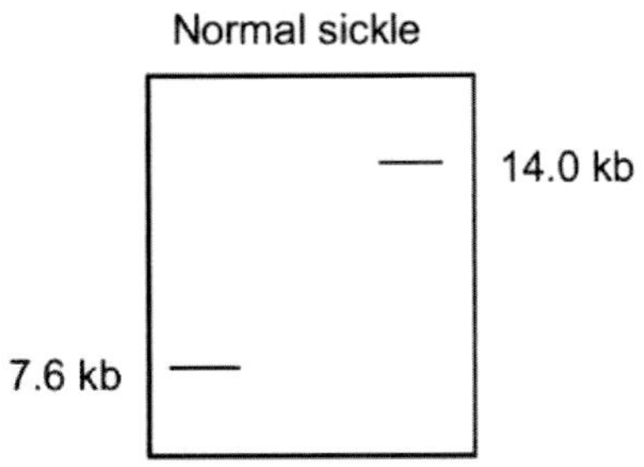

(b) Normal gene yield 7.6 kb fragment detected by DNA probe and sickle DNA 14.0 kb fragement due to loss of HpaI' site

Fig. (12). Analysis of genetic disease using RFLP

Thus, the mapping of molecules can be done following computer analysis of restriction fragment lengths to construct a map. Proper superimposition of the restriction map and the genetic map of a genomic region or whole genome allows locating genes in absolute physical terms (Fig. **13**).

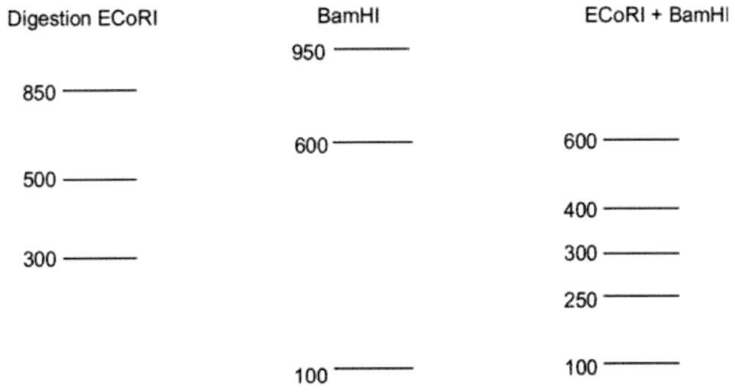

(a) Restriction enzyme digestion and electrophoretic mobility

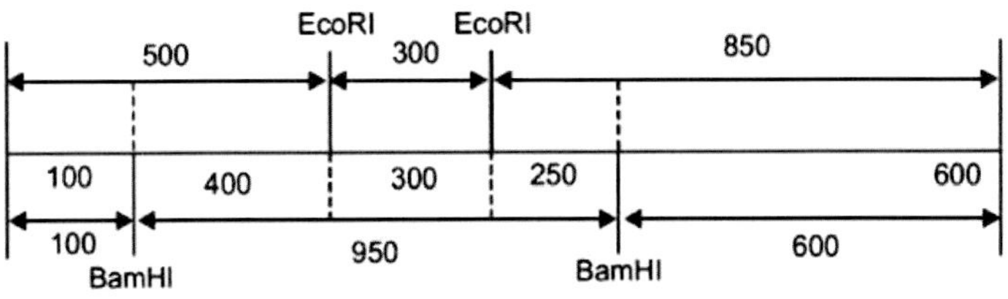

(b) Restriction endonuclease map derived from (a)

Fig. (13). Mapping of restriction endonuclease.

Achieving adequate detection limits is the main concern of nucleic acid analysis. Techniques that increase the amount of either the target, detection signal, or probe are known as methods for amplification of the target.

PCR

Amplification of target includes:

1.PCR
2.Ligase chain reaction (LCR)
3.Transcription-based amplification (TAS)
4.Transcription-mediated amplification (TMA)
5.Strand displacement amplification (SDA)
6.Line displacement amplification (LDA)
7.Whole genome amplification (WGA)
8.Anti-sense RNA amplification (RNA)

In target amplification, the nucleic acid region around the area of interest is copied many times by *in vitro* methods. Polymerase Chain Reaction (PCR) is the best-known and the most widely applied target amplification method (Fig. **14**).

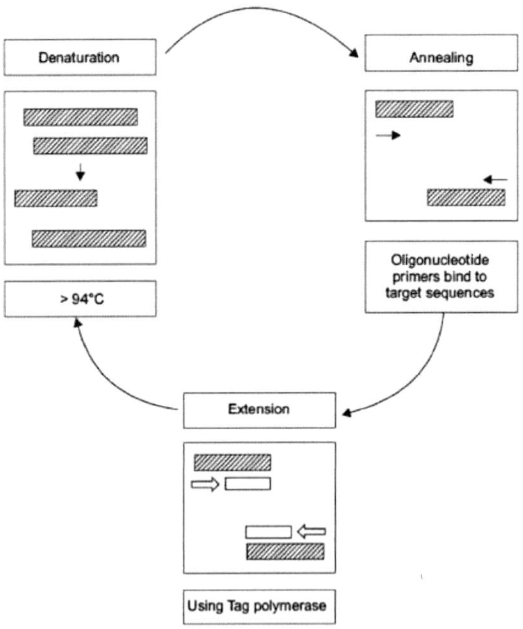

Fig. (14). Scheme: single PCR cycle.

It is the most widely adopted, and routinely used method in molecular biology labs (Fig. **15**).

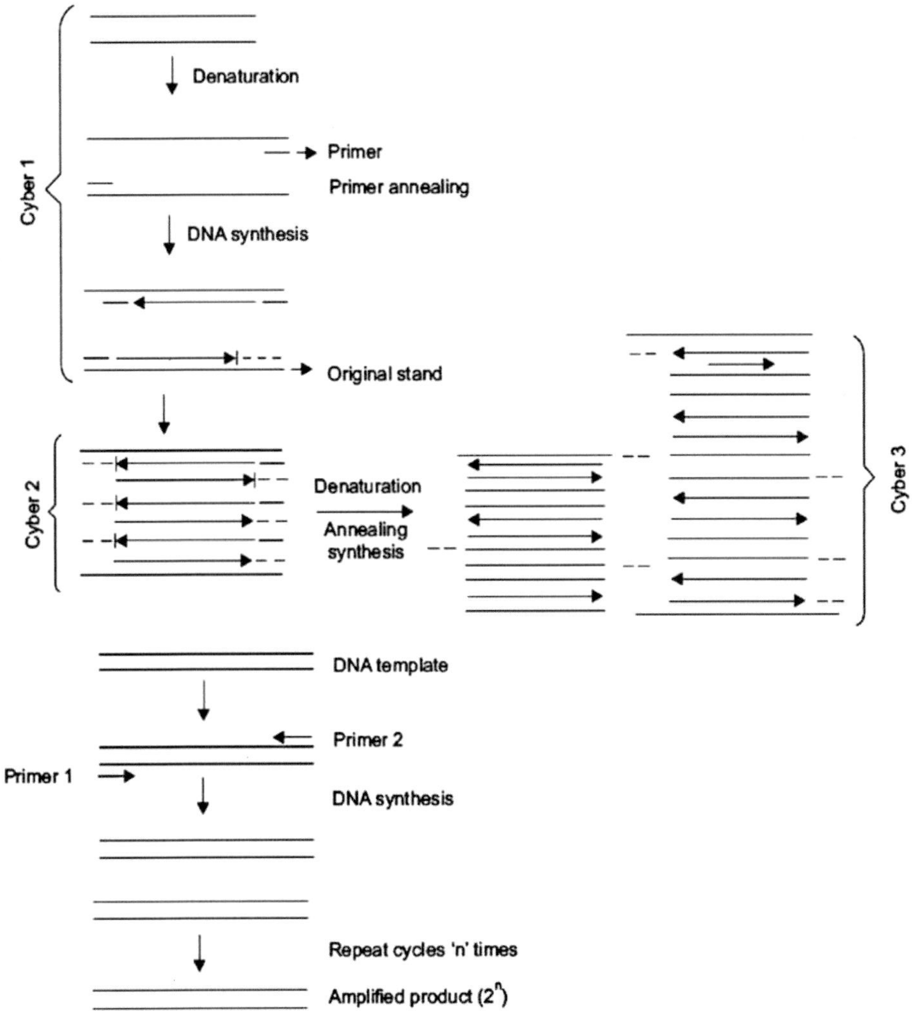

Fig. (15). PCR cycle.

–Thermostable DNA polymerase.
–Nucleotides of each base (d NTPs).
–Target sequence.
–Primer (Pair of oligonucleotides complementary to opposite strands flanking the sequence to be detected).

(i)1st step— the denaturation of target: target duplex is denatured into single strands by the head.

(ii)Annealing of primers: Cooling of mixture and introduction of primers to the solution to specifically anneal complementary sequences on the target.

(iii)Polymerization: Polymerase synthesizes two additional DNA strands containing the primers as 5′ ends and the cycle is completed.

(iv)Denaturation: The 2nd cycle also begins with denaturation. Now, there are twice as many strands available for primer annealing and subsequent polymerization.

1.High temperature: To denature the target sequence at (94°C).

2. Low temperature: Allows annealing of primers to target (55°C).

3. Optimal temperature: Polymerase extension (72°C).

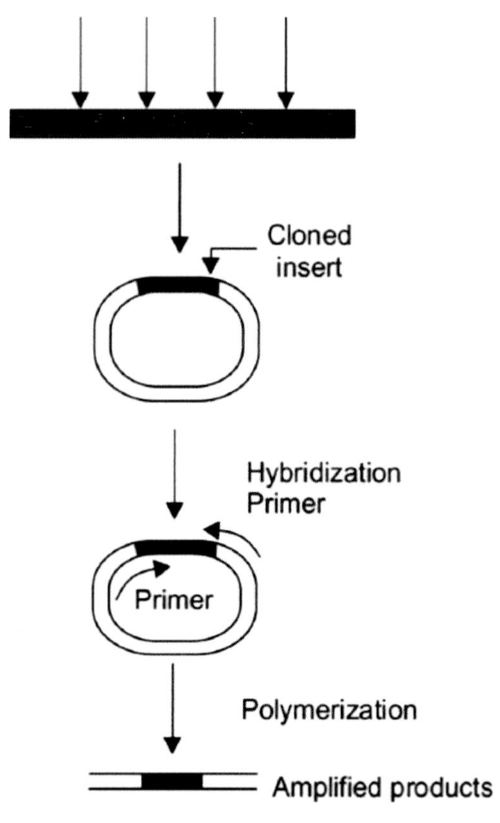

Fig. (16). Amplification of gene using flanking vector sequences as primers.

Thermocycler is an instrument that takes samples through multiple steps at varying temperature. Repetitive thermocycling results in the exponential accumulation of product.

$$N_t = N_o e^r$$

N_t = amount of DNA at time 't'

N_o = initial amount of DNA at time 't'

$r = 1.386\ mm^{-1}$ for PCR

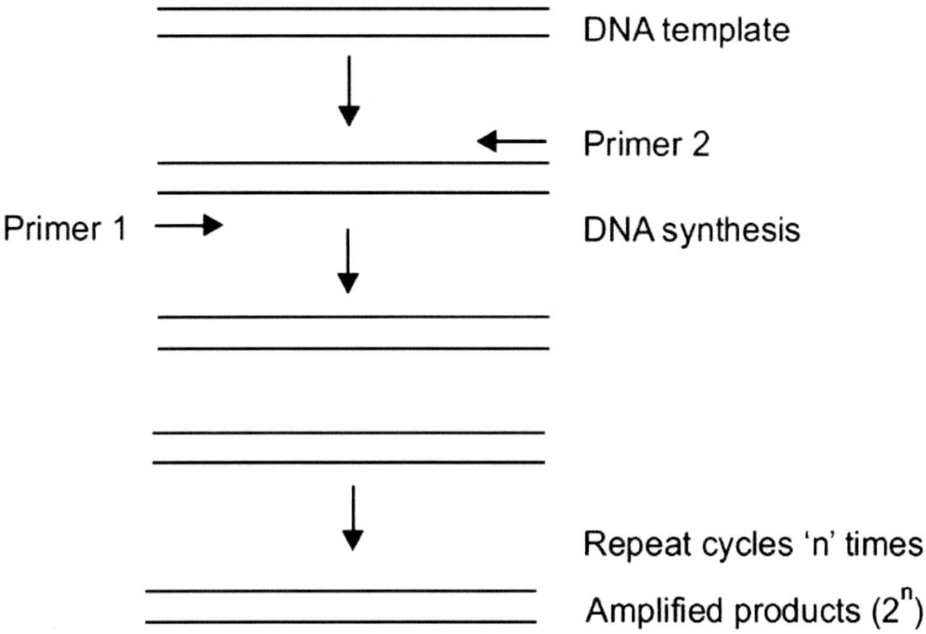

Fig. (17). PCR provides a large quantity of usable specific DNA fragment.

A doubling time of 30 sec is assumed for PCR and starting with only one target copy, it takes 23 min (46 cycles) to amplify the target to saturation. Thus, 0.5 µg of each primer gives 1011 copies µg in a typical PCR reaction (Figs. **16** and **17**).

If the efficiency of each cycle is optimal, the number of target sequences doubles each cycle (efficiency = 2.0)

• Primer

• Temperature—cycling conditions

• Presence or Absence of polymerase inhibitors

Efficiency fails due to

• Exhaustion of components.

• Competition between primer and product annealing.

RNA targets can also be successfully amplified into DNA copies.

It can be carried out by various methods:

1.Simple gel electrophoresis with ethidium bromide staining.

2.Fluorescently labelled primers. For DNA sequencing devices, (they form part of real-2time (PCR).

3.Hybridization assays.

4.Automated and closed-tube methods.

•Use physically separated areas for preamplification and post-amplification step.

•Use positive displacement pipettes to minimize aerosol contamination.

•Use pre-aliquoted reagent.

•Do not let the product out of the tube.

•Perform amplification, detection, and characterization in a closed tube. Otherwise, a minute aerosol droplet contains more than enough targets for robust amplification.

1.Inverse PCR (Fig. **18**).

2.Anchored PCR (Fig. **19**).

3.PCR for site-directed mutagenesis

4.Asymmetric PCR for DNA sequencing

5.Allele-specific PCR

6.PCR walking

7.RT (reverse transcribed)—PCR

In inverse PCR, the amplification of those DNA sequences takes place that are away from the primers and not those flanked by the primer, *e.g.*, if border sequences of a DNA segment are not known and those of the vector are known, then the sequence to be amplified may be cloned in the vector and border sequences of the vector may be used as primers in such a way that the polymerisation proceeds in the inverse direction.

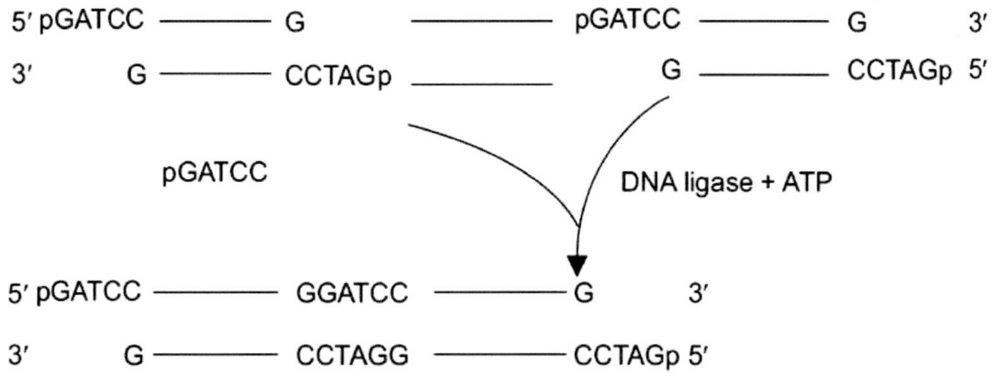

Fig. (18). Inverse PCR.

While the basic PCR and inverse PCR use two primers representing the sequences lying at the ends of sequences to be amplified. In anchored PCR, a single primer is utilised instead of two. So, only one strand is copied first after which a poly G tail is attached at the end of the newly synthesized strand. Then, this newly synthesized strand with a poly G tail becomes a template for daughter strand synthesis utilizing an anchor primer with which a poly C sequence is linked to complement the poly-G of the template. In the next cycle, both the original primer and anchored primers are used for gene amplification (Figs. **22** and **23**).

In this technique, mutations are introduced in a DNA sequence at desired places by altering the sequences of primers. These mutations are limited to the ends of the gene sequence because they are introduced through primers. To introduce mutations at any place of interest in the gene, a technique has been described having a primer at the end of the gene and the second one having an internally modified primer (desired mutation) with an overlap extension, where the gene of interest is amplified into two separate segments *i.e*, two separate PCR reactions.

The extension of these primers by Taq polymerase results in the formation of a complete gene with mutations incorporated at internal sites.

This enables preferential amplification of one genetic allele over another.

The 3′ end of one primer is placed at the polymorphic site and is extended only if it is completely complementary to the target.

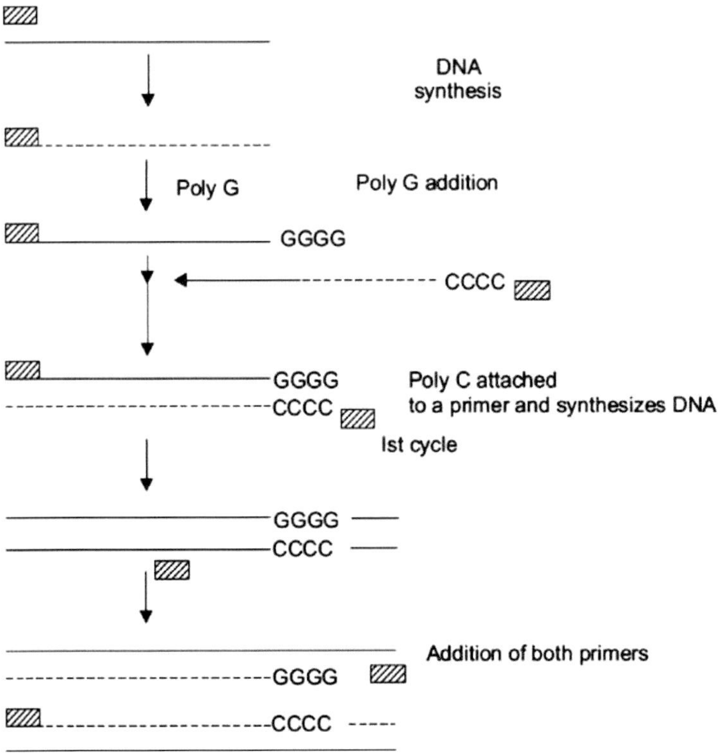

Fig. (19). Anchored PCR.

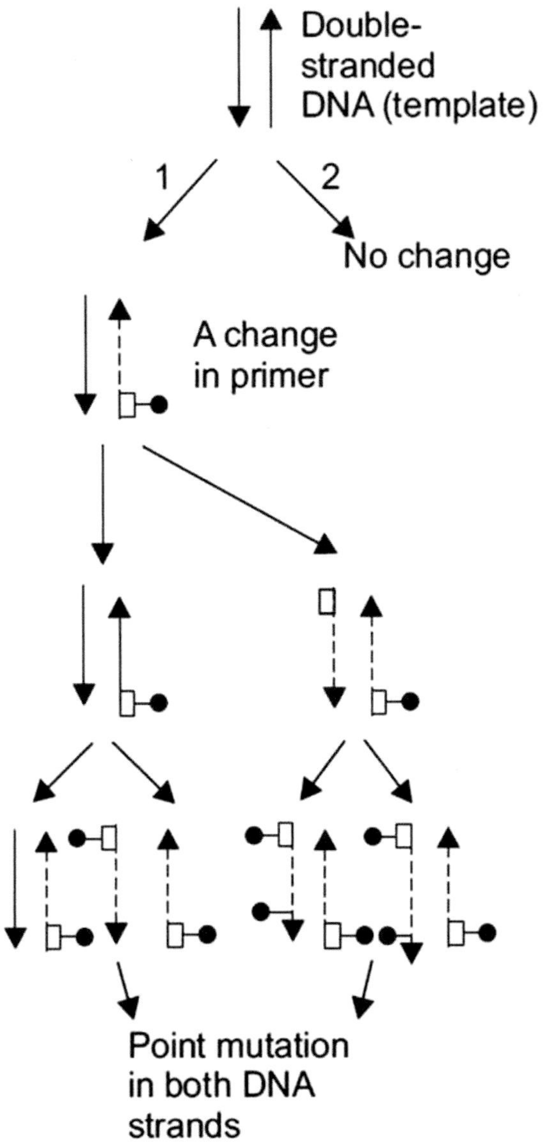

Fig. (20). Site- directed mutagenesis.

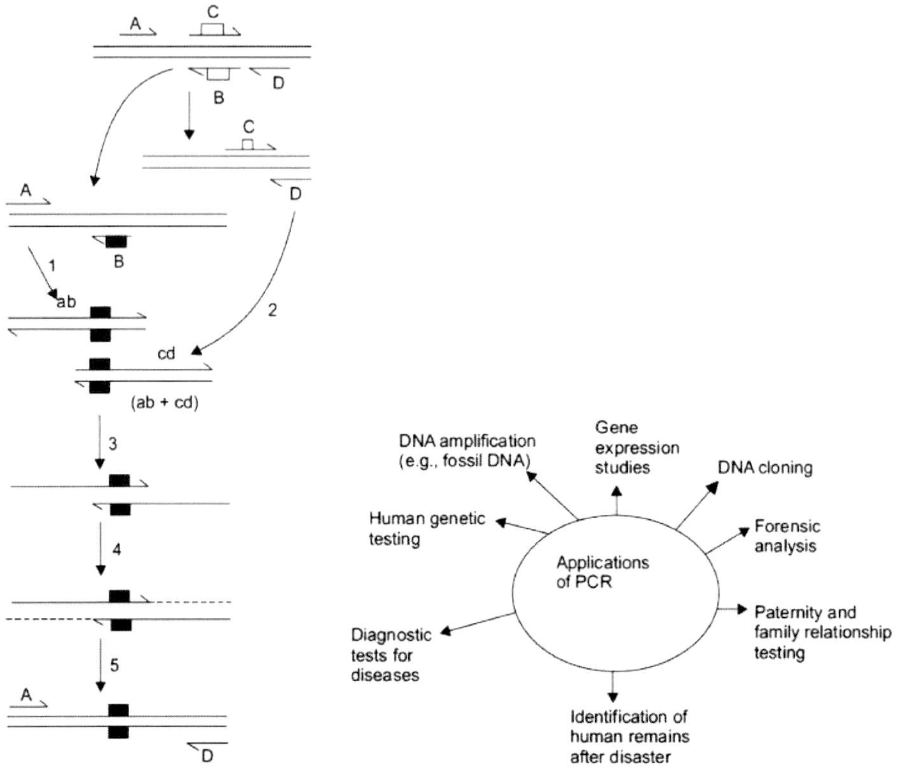

Fig. (21). On the left: Introduction of mutation at the internal site overlapping each other. On Right: Application of PCR.

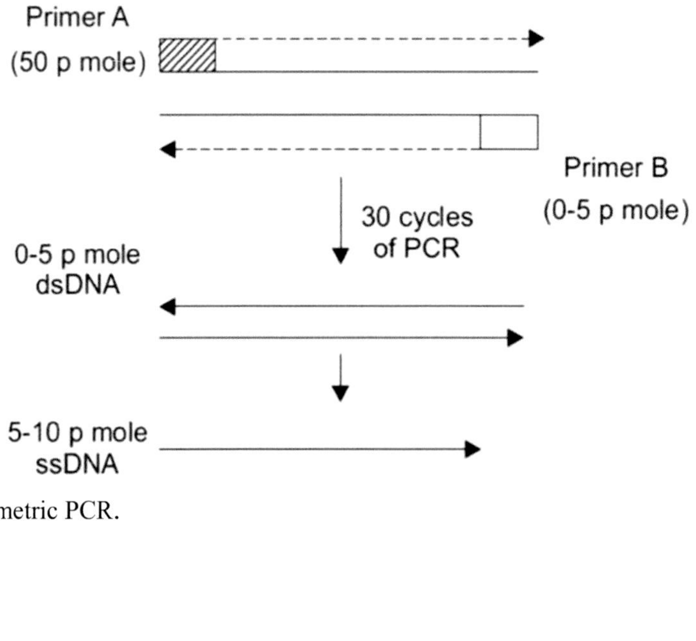

Fig. (22). Asymmetric PCR.

•To distinguish a gene for pseudogene.
•For genotypic SNPs.
•For determining haplotypes.

Using this technique, a single-stranded DNA can be produced by using two primers in 100: 1 ratio, and after 20–35 cycles of amplification. When one primer is exhausted, the single-stranded DNA is produced in the next 5–10 cycles.

It uses different concentrations of the two primers to generate more of one strand DNA than others.

•For sequencing purposes.
•For making single-stranded probes.
•For probe hybridization.

It allows amplification of DNA with unknown sequences that are present adjoining a known sequence within a DNA fragment.

It involves 3 steps:

1.Restriction enzymes to produce a large number of DNA fragments.
2.Ligation of adapters to restriction fragments.
3.PCR amplification using one adapter primer and other gene-specific primers.

RT is used to obtain cDNA for using it as a template for PCR reaction to examine mRNA transcripts.

Steps:

(i) Isolation, and purification of mRNA.
(ii) Reverse transcription of mRNA with reverse transcriptase enzyme to synthesize cDNA.
(iii) cDNA is used as a template for PCR using Taq polymerase and specific primers.

USE- Differences in two mRNA samples are identified by using these techniques.

BLOTTING TECHNIQUES

They include (Figs**. 24 and 25**):

1.Southern Blotting
2.Northern Blotting
3.Western Blotting

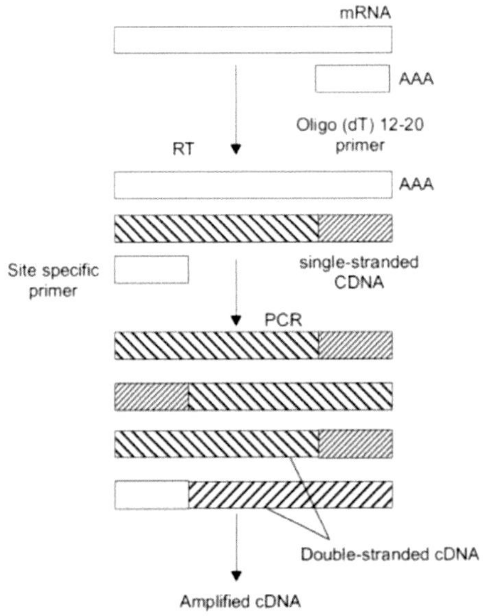

Fig. (23). RT- PCR.

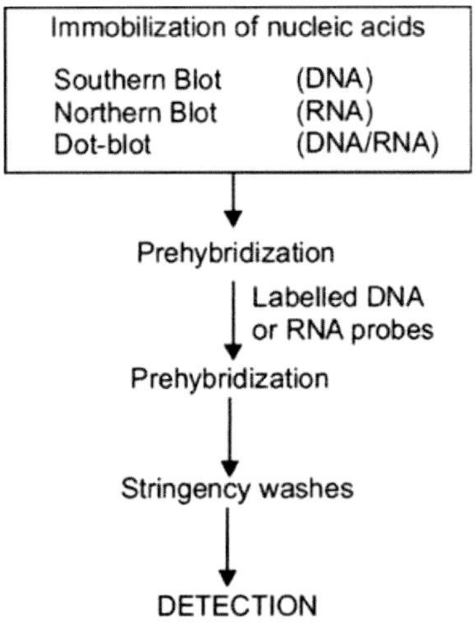

Fig. (24). Nucleic Acid Blotting Techniques – outline.

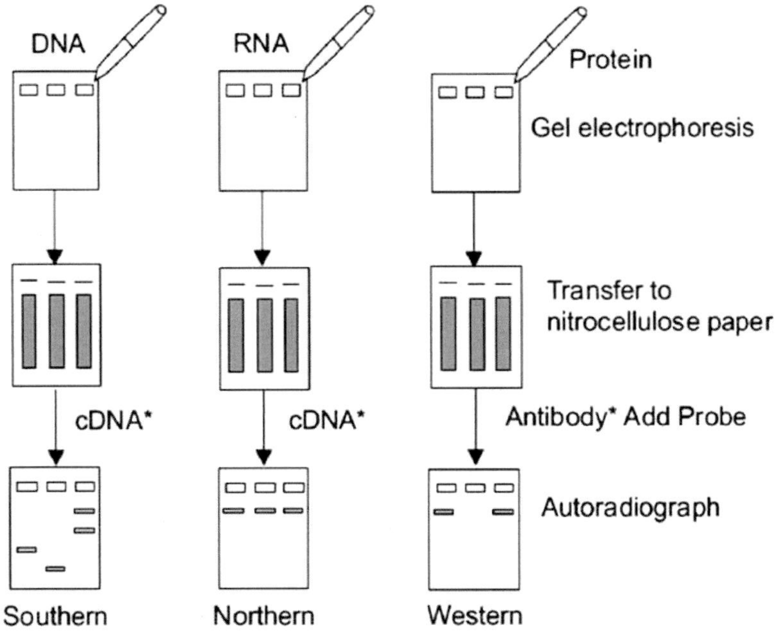

Fig. (25). Scheme: Blotting techniques.

Used to detect DNA.

Original sample DNA is digested by a restricted endonuclease, separated by agarose electrophoresis, and transferred by agarose electrophoresis to a solid support (Nylon or Nitrocellulose membrane) followed by selective visualization of the fragment using labelled hybridization probes.

•Reveals polymorphism in the DNA sequence based on RFLP
•Detect: Structural alteration

Deletion

Duplication

Insertion

Rearrangement

Uses RNA rather than DNA as the test nucleic acid.

RNA is transferred from the gel after electrophoresis onto a solid support followed by hybridization with a specific labelled probe.

Since RNA molecules are shorter than genomic DNA, no cleavage is required before electrophoresis.

Provides information about the size of mRNA transcript.

DNA SEQUENCING

DNA sequencing has now become a routine procedure. It determines:

•The actual nucleic acid sequence of a DNA fragment.
•Base changes resulting in an altered amino acid code, stop codon, deletions, or insertions.

Sequence alignment is used to get information from sequence data to discover information related to functions, structure, and evolution.

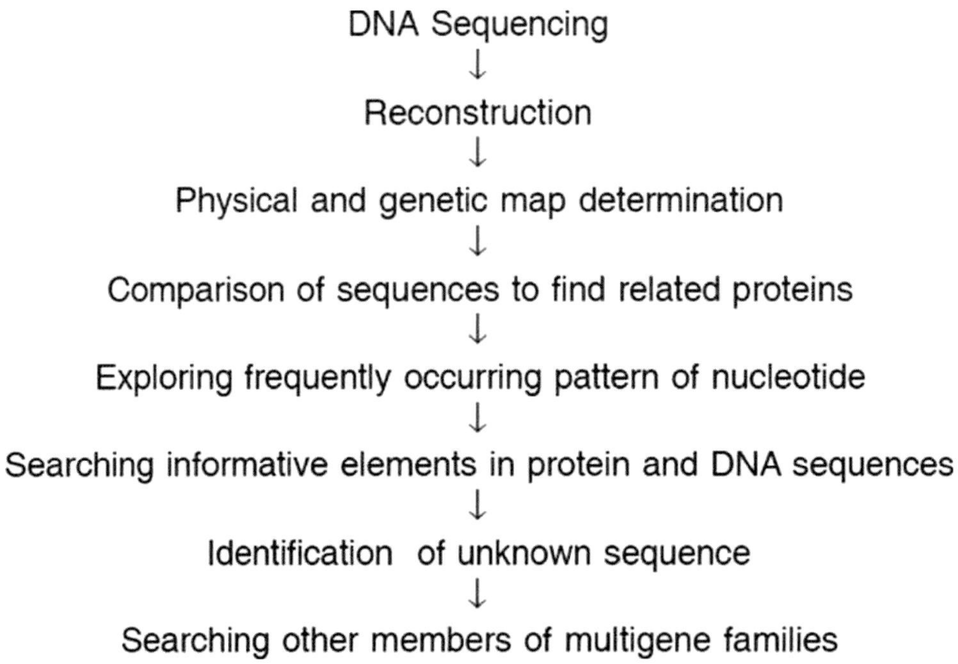

Fig. (26). Scheme of sequence analysis.

It is the process of determination of nucleotides or base sequence of a DNA molecule/fragment. DNA sequencing at present is possible only for 100–800 bp long DNA fragments.

In this technique, the DNA fragment to be sequenced is end-labelled by the addition of 32P-dATP either at the 5-ends (by the enzyme polynucleotide kinase) or at the 3-ends (by the enzyme deoxy nucleotidyl transferase) or its both strands.

This end-labelled fragment is digested with restriction endonuclease to generate two fragments of unequal lengths of which only one end would be labelled. These fragments are separated by gel electrophoresis and sequenced separately. Alternatively, end-labelled fragment is denatured and complementary strands are separated through gel electrophoresis and sequenced separately (Figs. **26**, **27** and **30**).

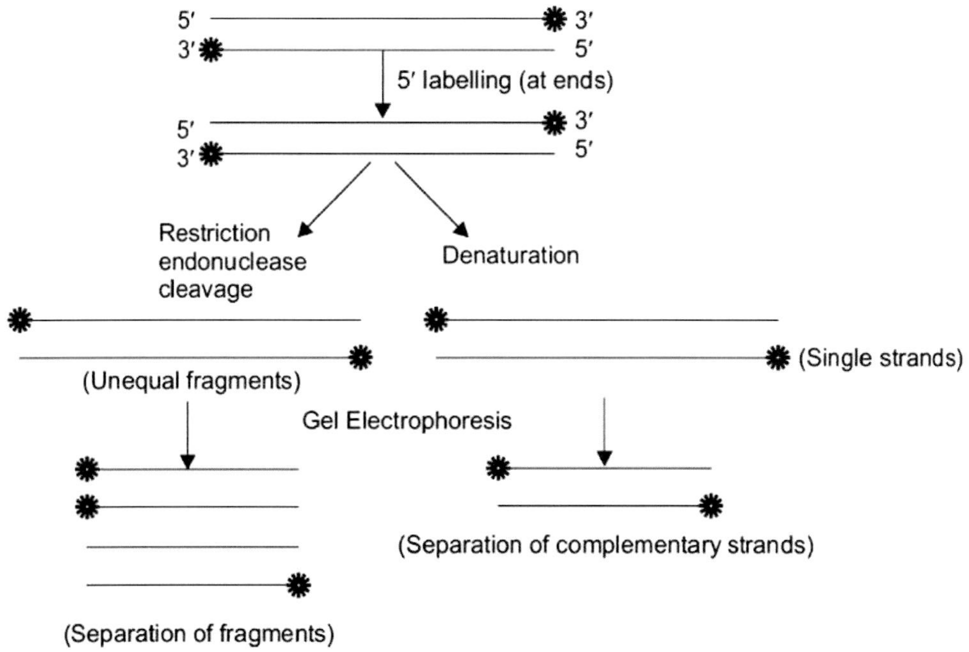

Fig. (27). Sequencing.

The single and labelled ds or ssDNA samples are subjected to base-specific chemical cleavage at four sites, namely, G, C, G + A/C + T. Then, in four separate reaction mixtures, the DNA samples are partially digested according to base specific sequences by the following steps:

(i) Modification of concerned bases.
(ii) Removal of a modified base from DNA strand.
(iii) Induction of strand break (break in the sugar-phosphate back-bone) in the position from which the modified base has been removed.

Such a cleavage generates a mixture of end-labelled DNA fragments of variable lengths. Digests of double-stranded DNA are denatured. Then, they are subjected to electrophoresis with separate lanes of the same gel to separate fragments according to their lengths by sequential reading of bands in the four lanes of the gel by autoradiography, in this way, the base sequence is determined.

This is also termed as an enzymatic procedure. The DNA fragment to be sequenced is denatured and the resulting complementary strands are separated by electrophoresis.

This technique generates fragments that are generated at various lengths by the incorporation of one 4 dideoxynucleotide base analysis during extension from the sequencing primer.

Dideoxynucleotides lack 3′ hydroxyl group and 2′ OH on pentose ring, and because DNA chain growth requires the addition of deoxynucleotides to 3′ OH group, the incorporation of this base analog terminates the chain growth.

Cycle sequencing is the most common method for generating these terminated fragments and involves repeating steps of annealing, chain extension and termination and denaturation by temperature cycling. The fragments generated are tagged with fluorescent dye, then separated by PAGE or capillary electrophoresis and detected by the fluorescent detector. Around 600 bases can be resolved in 2½ hour run.

DNA sequencing is most used in infectious disease testing:

•Genotyping of HIV for drug resistance
•Genotyping of HCV (Figs. **28** and **29**)

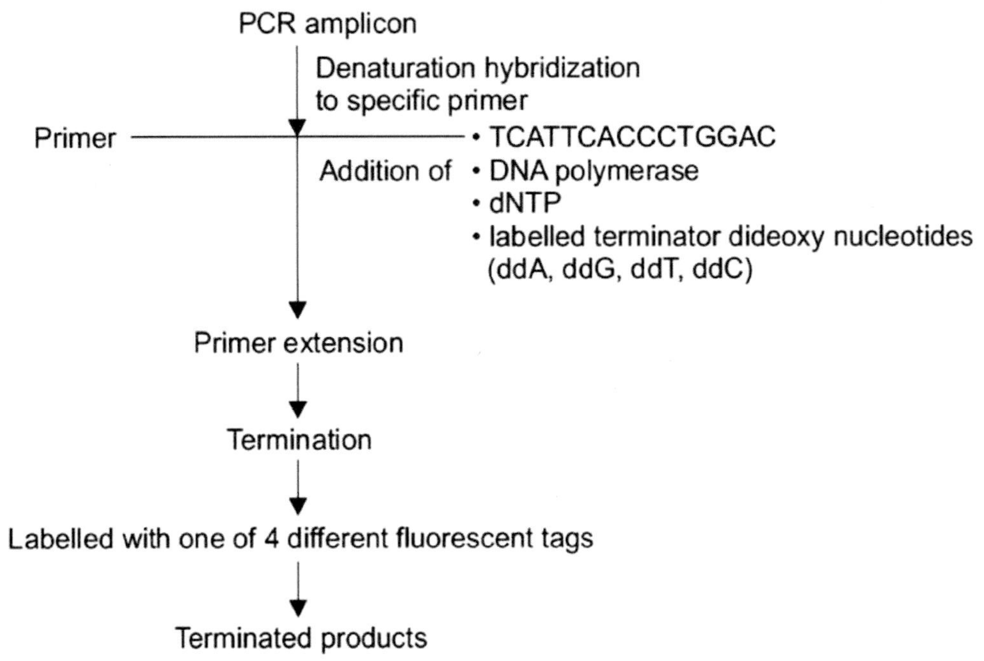

Fig. (28). Chain termination reaction (Sanger).

It is also based on Sanger- Coulson method with two differences:

(i)Labelling: fluorescent labelling is done instead of radioactive labelling used in the standard procedure.

(ii)Track system: A single-track system is used instead of the four-track system.

a.No use of radioactive labels, no radiation hazard

b.No need of autoradiography

c.Less time-consumption in data processing

d.Test can be repeated to recheck

e.Fast

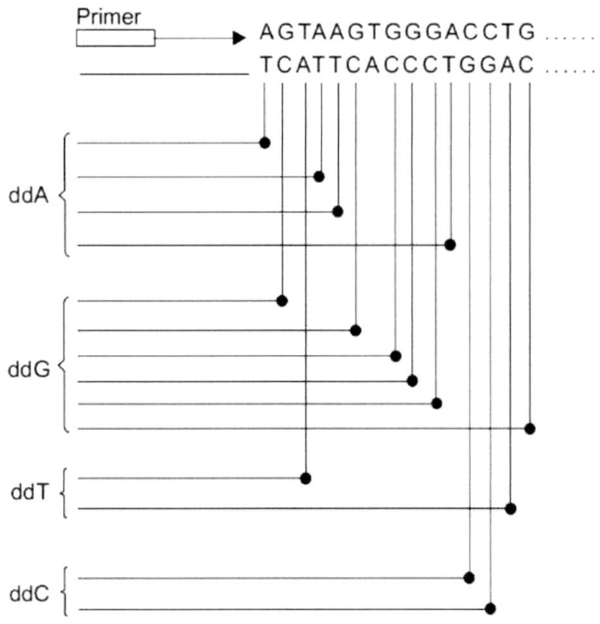

Fig. (29). Chain termination reaction (Sanger).

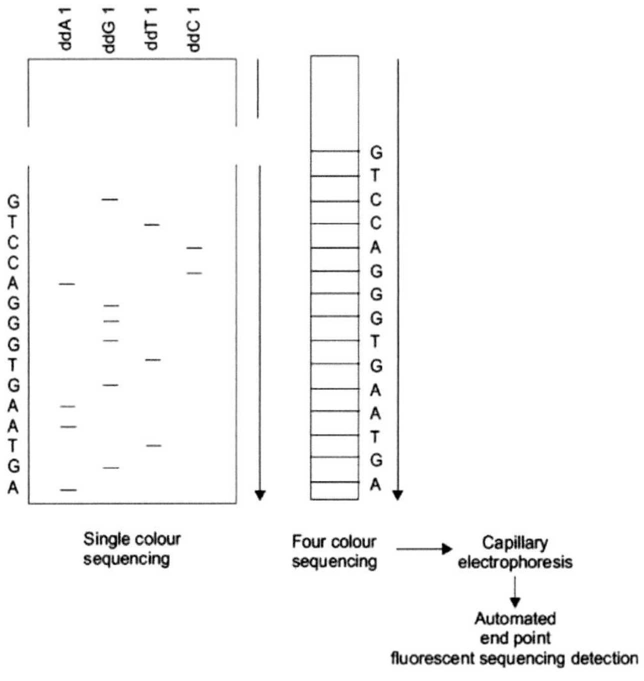

Fig. (30). DNA sequencing.

It offers automated specialised tools for working with the output from automated sequences and assists researchers with DNA sequencing using automated sequencers along with GCG. Mac vector and Gene work as a sequence entry and multiple sequences alignment editor to generate sequence data.

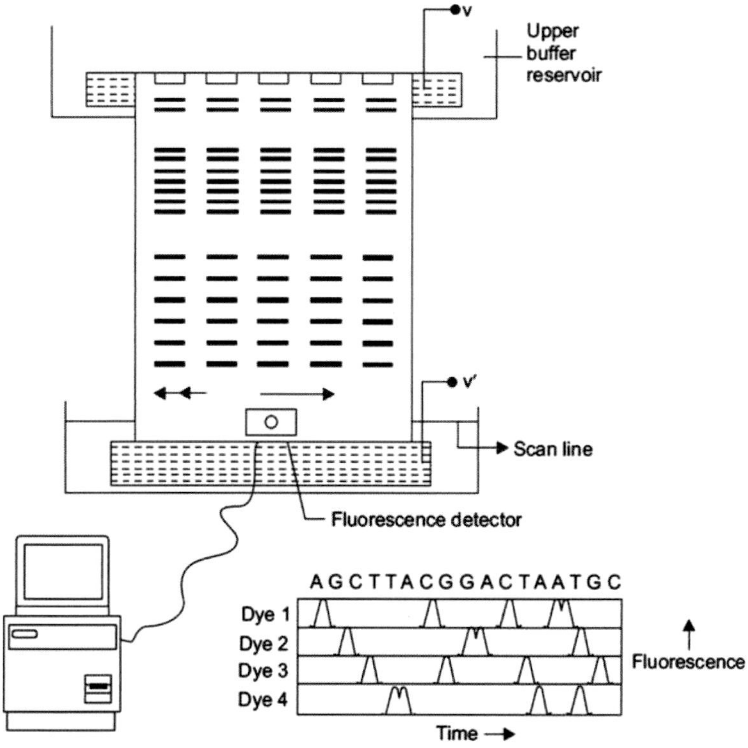

Fig. (31). Automated DNA sequencer.

Automated DNA sequencers are of the following types (Fig. **31**):

1.Slab-gel sequencing system
2.Capillary gel sequencing system
3.Direct DNA sequencing system using PCR
4.DNA sequencing through transcription
5.DNA sequencing by hybridization with micro arrays on DNA chips
6.DNA sequencing by DE-MALDI-TOF MS

Here, ultrathin (75 μm) slab gels and 96 lanes per gel runs are used. Automated sample loading into each plexiglass block well (filled with PCR dideoxy reaction mixture) is done with the help of capillary action followed by electrophoresis.

In this system, automated capillary gel electrophoresis is carried out in a 96 capillary tube filled with a polymerized gel system.

Commercial system available: Mega BASE 4000 (having 384 capillaries)

This is also called the ligation mediated PCR (LMPCR). This is a faster and more reliable method that can utilize either whole genomic DNA or cloned DNA fragments.

(i)Generation of ds or ss DNA sequencing templates by PCR
(ii)Sequencing of PCR product by:
a.Taq DNA polymerase (Thermostable)
b.Thermolabile DNA polymerase

Even asymmetric PRC can also be employed to sequence ds DNA

(iii)Termination of reaction by the addition of formamide stop solution.
(iv)Running the mixture on polyacrylamide sequencing gel, which can be read manually or by computer.

DNA sequencing through transcription is also called transcriptional sequencing. By using RNA polymerase enzyme, DNA sequencing is carried out using labelled 3′ dNTP. The labels used are fluorescent (rhodamine) labels.

This method is a superior method because it does not require a primer (making it faster) and it produces a large amount of product.

This method utilizes sequencing of oligonucleotides by hybridization with DNA microchips. This method can be applied to small fragments and SNPs only and longer fragments need to be fragmented for hybridization. But it cannot be applied to repeat DNAs such as microsatellites or minisatellites.

Matrix-assisted laser desorption/ionization mass spectrometry (MALDI-MS) can rapidly acquire DNA sequence information.

It can accurately determine the mass of each fragment arranged by the difference of single nucleotides. This method is applicable to short oligonucleotides and can be used in combination with Sanger's termination reactions.

It is quick, and requires only a few minutes for a sample with no gels, labelling.

GENE PROBE

A probe is a nucleic acid whose identity is known and is used to reveal the identity or abundance or a target or sample.

Probes can be unlabelled or labelled with one of a variety of reporter molecules (depending on the technique used.)

Probes can be:

•Cloned (recombinant)
•Generated by PCR or
•Synthesized (oligonucleotide)

They may be DNA, RNA, PNA and single stranded or double stranded.

Table 7. Nucleic acid probes

Probe	**Type**	**Label**
DNA	• Cell based DNA cloning (ds DNA) PCR	Random Primer
RNA	• RNA transcription from phage rectors (Single Stranded)	Run-off transcription

(Table 7) cont.....

Oligonucleotide	• Chemical synthesis (Single-stranded nucleotides)	End-labelling

Table 8. Labels used for probes.

DNA Probe	**Label used**
• End Labelling • Polymerase-based labelling • Nick-translation	^{32}P, ^{35}S ^{32}P, ^{35}S ^{32}P, ^{35}S
Labels used	Examples
Radioactive Non-radioactive	^{32}P, ^{35}S Biotin Streptavidin Digoxigenin

They consist of a known segment of DNA inserted into a plasmid vector that is propagated by growth in a bacterium.

P^{BR} 322 was one of the first in common use and now many different plasmid vectors are available.

Composition. They may consist of:

•Entire plasmid DNA (insert plus vector sequence).
•Or purified insert from vector sequences.
•RNA promoter regions adjacent to the inserted DNA sequence.

Since only one strand is copied, single-stranded RNA probes are generated that allow the production of transcripts in sense or anti-sense direction (Tables **7** and **8**).

They are simple to prepare and are labelled with nucleotides that are radioactive, or fluorescent or have attached affinity labels. Also, by using a biotin-labelled primer, single-stranded probes can be obtained (Fig. **32**).

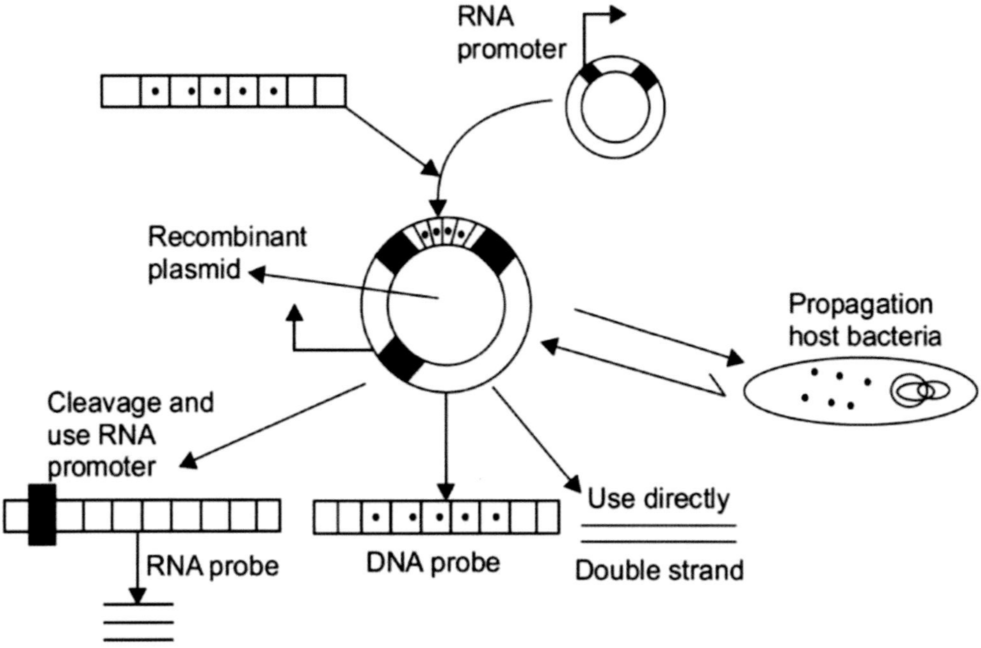

Fig. (32). Production of cloned probes.

Characteristic features of oligonucleotide probes:

•They are easier to obtain than PCR-generated ones.
•Contain 15–45 bases of single-stranded nucleic acids that are chemically synthesized to a specific base sequence.
•DNA oligonucleotide probes are commonly used, but RNA and PNA ones can also be used.
•Oligonucleotide probes are routinely available in a public database (*e.g.*, NIH genetic sequence database, public algorithms)

•Oligonucleotide probes are prcpared with covalent attachment of a reporter molecule (fluorescent dyes) or affinity labels that facilitate their attachment to solid supports.
•Real-time PCR uses fluorescently labelled oligonucleotides.

Nucleic acids are visualized or measured by ultraviolet absorbance and fluorescent dyes. However, they do not discriminate between different nucleic acid sequences *i.e.*, they are not sequence specific. Labelling of these probes solves the problem.

•Radioactive label
•Indirect probe detection
•Fluorescent label
•Electrochemical reporters (Figs. **32**-**37**).

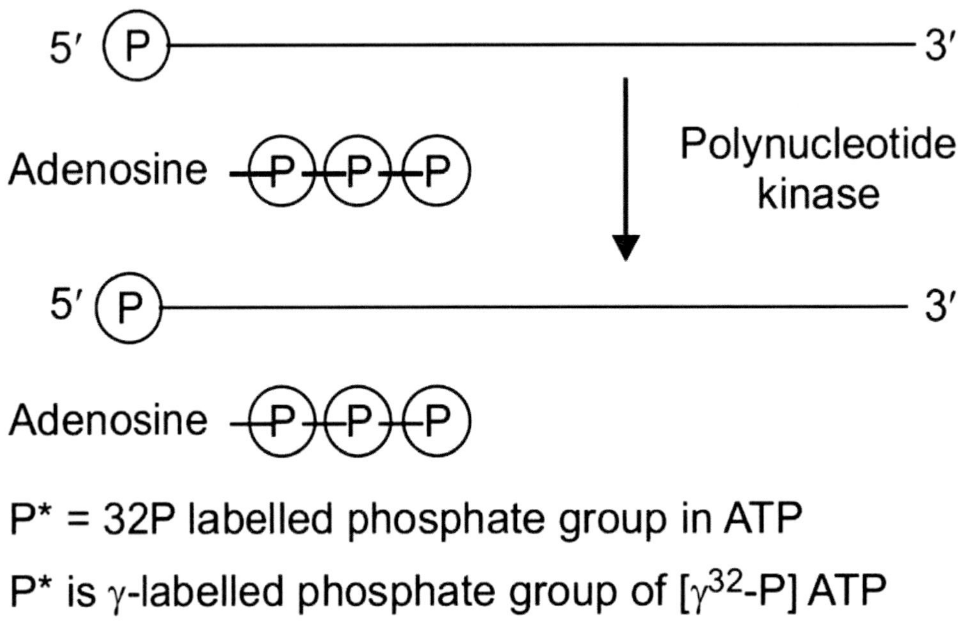

Fig. (33). End- labelling of DNA probe.

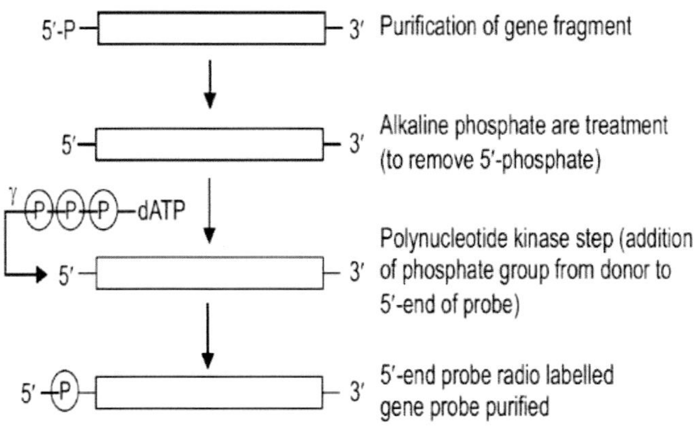

Fig. (34). End- labelling of DNA probe at 5' end.

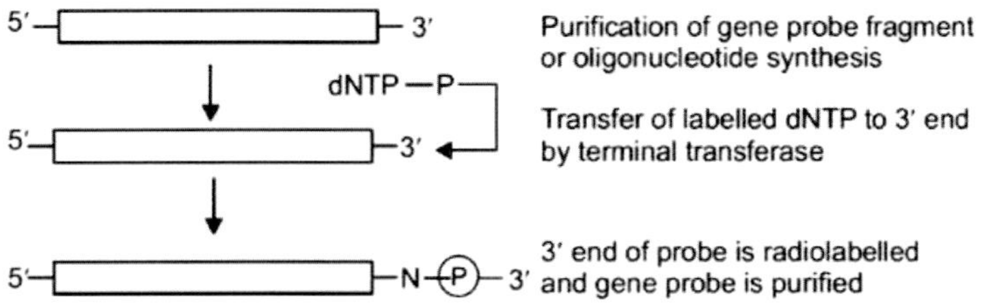

Fig. (35). End- labelling of DNA probe at 3' end.

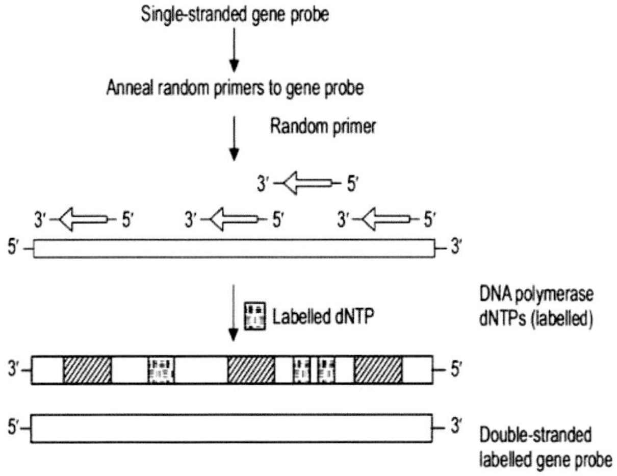

Fig. (36). Random primer gene probe labelling.

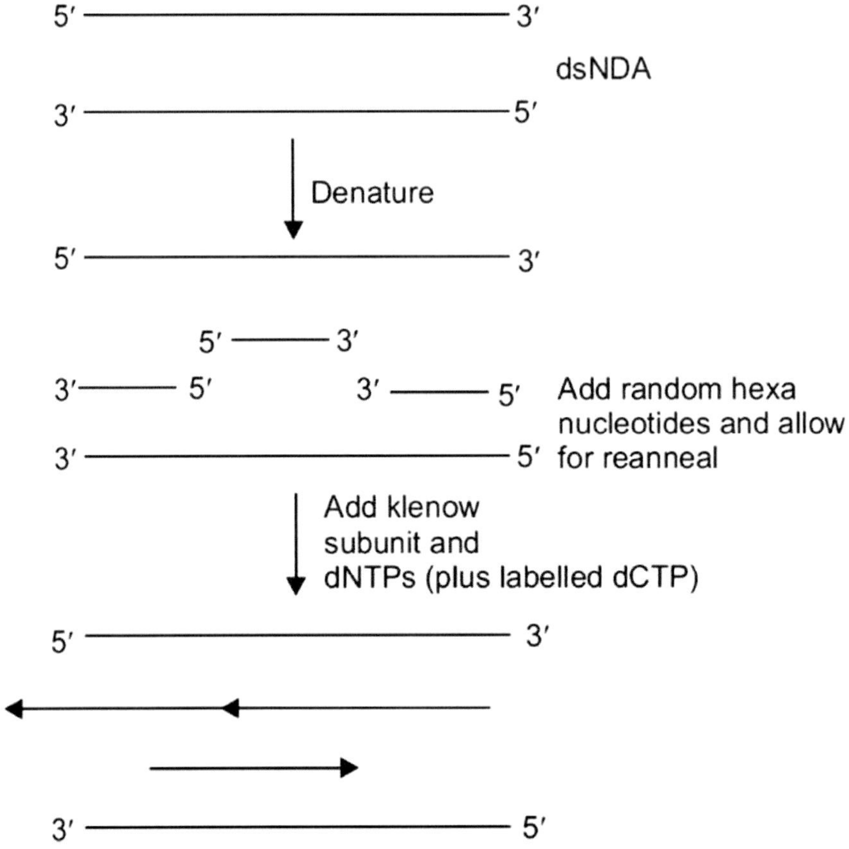

Fig. (37). Random primer blabelling of DNA probe.

These probes are:

•The first probe to be used in the detection of nucleic acid.
•Most frequently used isotopic labels are 32P and 33P.

(i)Nick translation: DNAse I introduces nick into each strand of DNA randomly and the resulting 3′ OH groups form priming sites for DNA polymerase.
(ii)Random priming: Nucleic acid is denatured and allowed to anneal with short hexamer oligonucleotides of random sequences. The 3′ end of annealed hexanes forms the initiation site for DNA polymerase.
(iii)By PCR: Labelled nucleic acids can also be synthesized by PCR.

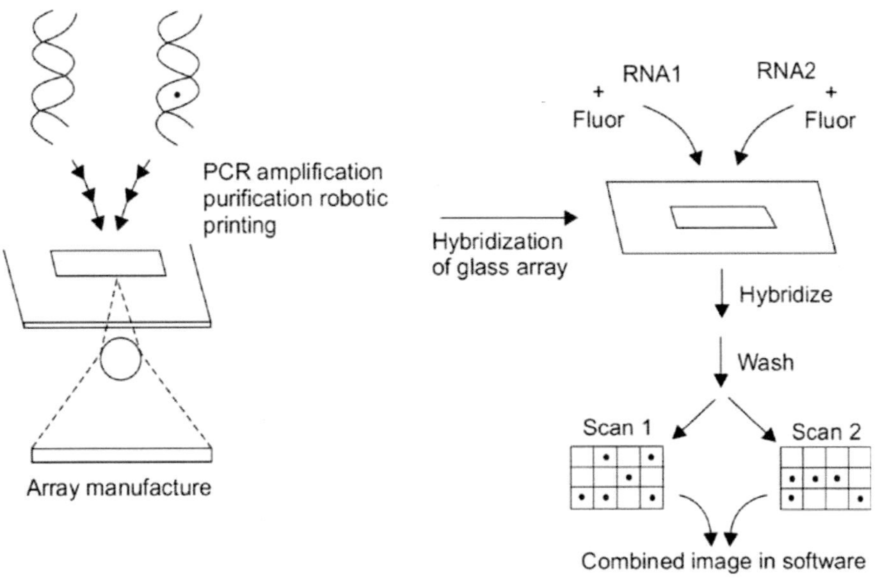

Fig. (38). Microarrays.

•They are sensitive
•They have high specificity
•Short half-life
•Inherent instability
•Problem of radio isotope safety and disposal.

It involves non-isotopic probe labelling by using:

•Biotin-labelled analog of dUTP
•Digoxigenin labelled analog of dUTP

These affinity labels (biotin, digoxigenin) do not generate detectable signals on their own. They can initiate signal amplification mediated by high-affinity binding with antibodies linked to enzymes (horse-radish peroxidase or alkaline phosphatase) or avidin or streptavidin.

Enzyme activity is monitored according to the enzyme-substrate used (Chemiluminescent, Colorimetric or Fluorescent).

(i)Biotinylated label: Biotin is an affinity label. Biotinylated probes can be affixed to a streptavidin-coated surface. Following incubation with the target nucleic acid, a second probe is added to amplify the signal.
(ii)Chemiluminescence: Nucleic acid can be linked to organic indicator molecules that emit light when exposed to certain chemicals, *e.g.*, acridinium esters when exposed to H_2O_2 at high pH produce light emission.
(iii)Bioluminescence: Biomolecules produce light through the catalysis of certain substrates, *e.g.*, alkaline phosphatase and peroxidase act on luminescent substrates to emit light. Luciferase is also a bioluminescent molecule used as an indicator of ATP generation in pyrosequencing.
(iv)Electrochemiluminescence: It is initiated at an electrode surface in the presence of certain chelates of ruthenium.

Fluorescent labelled probes are a preferred reporter for nucleic acid analysis.

•DNA Sequencing
•Fragment Length Analysis
•DNA Arrays
•Real-time PCR
•Fluorescence polarization
•Fluorescence resonance energy transfer
•Fluorescence quenching

They detect hybridization-induced changes in electrochemical parameters, such as conductivity or capacitance.

Different designs available are:

(i)Attachment of oligonucleotide to the electrode surface: Its binding to a complementary target and to an electroactive reporter labelled with ferrocenyl derivative can be detected by voltammetry.
(ii)Tethered oligonucleotide: A reporter probe is attached to a metal nanoparticle that changes conductivity between electrodes.
(iii)Unlabelled probes anchored to the field-effect sensor: They are used to detect the increase in change following hybridization of the target.

DNA probes have an advantage of detecting the presence of a gene rather than its product. DNA probe signals need to be amplified with the help of the following steps.

1)Developing rRNA probes because rRNA genes are present in thousands, thus amplifying the target.
2)Using PCR technology to generate millions of copies of target DNA sequences to be identified by standard methods.
3)Increasing the signal generating capacity of probe by the following ways:
(i)Concentrating more label at the site of target molecule (by attaching multiple enzyme molecules to each of its DNA probe)
(ii)Use of multiple probes.
(iii)Attaching multiple enzymes to each of these multiple probes, *i.e.*, multiple secondary probes.
(iv)Amplifier technology uses multiple secondary probes to hybridize secondary probes that hybridize multiple target specific primary probes.

Table 9. Properties of different types of DNA array for expression analysis.

Property	**Spotted Microarray**		**Affinities**
	Nylon	**Glass**	**Gene chips**
Target size	Typical 100–300 bp	–	• Typical 20–25 ntd
Target source	Maintained Clone sets	–	• Sequence derived from public and/or Private databases • Chemically synthesized
Target composition	ds DNA fragments	– –	Single-stranded oligonucleotides
Probe labelling	Radioactive or enzymatic	Dual Fluorescent	Fluorescent
Detection	Autoradiography	Confocal scanning	Confocal scanning
Cost	Low	Moderate	High

Microarrays represent high-density miniaturized arrays of molecular samples. The technology involves a series of probes immobilized on a glass slide as microdots, which are then hybridized with a mixture of test DNA sequences labelled with a fluorochrome (Fig. **38** and Table **9**).

Prepared either by the synthesis of oligonucleotides on a DNA chip, or by deposition of available DNA sequences on a DNA chip.

A microarray, also known as gene chip iOS, is created by using a small glass microscope slide and single-stranded DNAs are attached or spotted on it.

1.DNA Microarray: Contains cloned gene sequences, cDNA, ESTs
2.Antibody Microarray: Contains sports of different antibodies.

EXERCISE

1. How can you isolate and separate nucleic acids?
2. What are the tools of molecular biology?
3. Short notes: (i) Restriction enzymes. (ii) RFLP. (iii) Cleavage pattern of restriction enzymes.
4. What is temperature cycling in PCR?
5. Enumerate different amplification methods for target amplification.
6. What are the different schemes of PCR?
7. Discuss different schemes of PCR.
8. Describe nucleic acid blotting techniques.
9. Describe Sanger's reaction.
10. Discuss Maxim Gilbert's procedure of sequencing.
11. Give an account of automated sequencing.
12. Discuss automated DNA sequencers.
13. What is ligated mediated PCR?
14. What is transcriptional sequencing?
15. Describe different methods for sequencing a DNA segment. Discuss its advantages and disadvantages.
16. Discuss microarrays.
17. What is a gene probe?
18. How probes are labelled?
19. What are electrochemical reporters?
20. Describe the amplification of the DNA probe signal.
21. Draw a scheme for restriction mapping of a DNA fragment.

22. What are the cleavage patterns of various restriction enzymes?
23. Give a comparative account of different schemes of PCR.
24. Give a comparative account of different gene probes.
25. Prepare a list of applications of microarrays.
26. Calculate a comparative account of probes.
27. Prepare a flow chart outlining the process of isolation of DNA.
28. Outline the steps of isolation of RNA.
29. Tabulate tools of molecular biology with their functions.
30. Figure out how restriction enzyme recognizes sequences.
31. What are RFLPs?
32. Prepare a list of molecular markers used for genetic mapping apart from RFLPs.
33. Give an outline of the PCR cycle.
34. How contamination control for PCR is enforced?
35. Outline steps and uses of Southern blot.
36. Outline steps and uses of Northern blot.
37. Give an outline of nucleotide sequencing of DNA.
38. What is automated DNA sequencing?

CONCLUSION

In this chapter, various techniques and tools in biotechnology are discussed right from the isolation of nucleic acid, its handling, and precautions in DNA mapping to automated DNA sequencing. With the advancement in various molecular techniques, biotechnology has varied applications namely, the production of genetically modified (GM) crops, newer drugs, vaccines, enzymes, chemicals (for industrial use), diagnostics, for increasing the crop yield and waste management.

PCR is a revolutionary procedure with innumerable uses, and it allows *in vitro* amplification of discrete segments DNA to a million-fold. DNA sequencing has become a routine procedure nowadays. It is necessary to know the complete sequence of a cloned gene and dideoxynucleotide method of Sanger is often used for this process. There are four approaches for isolating a human gene: positional cloning, candidate gene cloning, restriction mapping *e.g.*, RFLPs, position candidate gene cloning or cytogenetic mapping.

The DNA fragments can be identified by gene (DNA) probes or microarrays. Microarray or chip technology holds great promise to biotechnologists in future.

BIBLOGRAPHY

[1] Rapley R. Molecular biology, bioinformatics and basic techniques.Principles and Techniques of Biochemistry and Molecular Biology. Cambridge: Cambridge University Press 2010; pp. 138-94. [http://dx.doi.org/10.1017/CBO9780511841477.006]

[2] Karp G. Cell and molecular biology: concepts and experiments. John Wiley & Sons; 2008 Oct 19.
[3] Daniel L. Hartl, Elizabe Genetics: Principles and analysis. 854.
[4] Sambrook J, Russell DW. (David William), 1957 and Cold Spring Harbor Laboratory Molecular cloning: A laboratory manual / Joseph Sambrook, David W. N.Y.: Russell Cold Spring Harbor Laboratory Cold Spring Harbor 2001.

CHAPTER 2

Recombinant DNA Techniques

LEARNING OBJECTIVES

This chapter gives an overview of the basic tools of cloning, gene cloning, gene expression and its analysis, DNA-finger printing, setting up a new lab, quality management in the lab, and lab safety.

Abstract: Following the success of the human genome project with 99.99% sequence accuracy, with no gaps, biotechnology has been revolutionized. Recombinant DNA technology comprises a battery of experimental procedures to isolate (clone) pieces of DNA containing specific genes. The usage of restriction enzymes for manipulating DNA and producing recombinant DNA along with advances in gene editing technology has paved way for diagnosing the candidate disease genes and treating human genetic disorders by restoring functional genes through the modification of the mutant gene or by introduction of a functional gene by Gene therapy. Array technology helps in the validation of recognized sequences, proteins, other biomolecules, drugs, *etc.* on a miniaturized platform. Quality management in the lab along with lab safety plans for biomedical labs requires adherence to various governmental regulations for protecting health and safety of lab employees and for the maintenance of safe working environment.

Genome analysis is carried out by genome mapping. Genetic maps can be linkage, cytogenetic or physical maps. Gene expression can be analyzed by genomics and proteomics Microarrays are emerging as useful closed systems for genomic (DNA microarray) and proteome (protein chip) analysis.

Keywords: Biohazard, DNA Libraries, Knockout mice, Lipofection, Palindromic, Transgenic mice, Transcriptome, Transduction, Vectors.

THE HUMAN GENOMIC PROJECT

The Human Genomic project deciphered 3 billion base pairs that make up the genetic code. In 1988, US National Research Council's special committee formulated a 15-year human genome project, costing some $200 million a year. In September 1994, a genetic map with 1cm resolution was accomplished and a physical map involving 52000 sequence-tagged sites (STSs) was completed in October 1998.

The International Human Genome Sequencing Consortium consisting of investigators from 20 centres located in six countries—UK, US, Japan, France, Germany, and China announced completion of a draft sequence in July 2000. The

Simmi Kharb, Akshat Singh, Abhyuday Singh & Deepa Kharb (Eds.)

final sequence was accomplished in April 2003, with 99.99% sequence accuracy, with no gaps.

HUMAN GENOME

Of the total 3.2 Gb DNA of human genome, 2.9 Gb consists of weakly, staining gene-rich euchromatic proteins and only 1.1–1.4% sequence encodes proteins. The estimated number of genes in the human genome is between 26,000 and 31,000.

With the decoding of the basic sequence, even more difficult task is the elucidation of biological function of these str*etc*hes of DNA.

From the data generated from the Human Genome Project, new disease-associated genes are being discovered every week. Also, it has allowed us to develop a test for molecular diagnosis and development of new targets for the pharmaceutical industries.

Hap Map Project

International Hap Map Project has been launched to study the patterns of linkage disequilibrium and haplotype across the human genome and to characterize SNPs (Single nucleotide polymorphisms).

Encode (Encyclopedia of DNA Elements)

This project aims to identify all the functional elements in the human genome.

Human Epigenome Project

This project aims to elucidate all the methylation sites in 30,000 human genes.

RECOMBINANT DNA TECHNOLOGY

Definition

Recombinant DNA Molecule

It is a vector into which the desired DNA fragment has been inserted to enable its cloning in an appropriate enzyme.

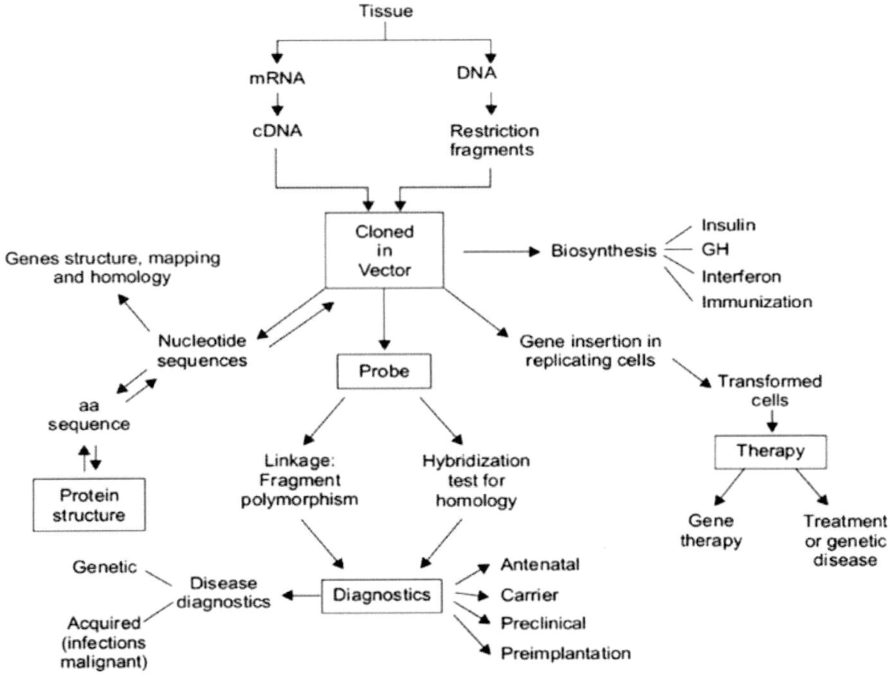

Fig. (1). Applications of DNA technology.

By using restriction enzymes, DNA is cut into suitable fragments and then ligated with appropriate fragments to produce a recombinant DNA.

Objective of Producing Recombinant DNA Molecule

1. To obtain a large number of copies of specific DNA (Fig. **1**).
2. To recover large quantity of protein produced by a gene of concern.
3. To integrate the gene of interest into the chromosome of the target organism.

From Protein to Gene	From Gene to Protein
Isolation of protein (on basis of its molecular function)	Isolation of genomic clone
↓	↓
Determination of partial amino acid sequence of protein	Isolation of cDNA
	↓

(Fig. 2) contd.....

↓

Synthesis of oligonucleotides

↓

Selection of cDNA or genomic clone

by oligonucleotide probe

↓

Isolation of gene

Sequence cDNA to deduce

amino acid sequence

↓

Comparison of this deduced

amino acid sequence with that of known proteins

↓

Production of encoded protein

Fig. (2). DNA Technology.

DNA Technology

Identification of restriction endonuclease, development of the DNA cloning vectors, introduction of southern blot technique and Sanger sequencing and more recent development of Polymerase Chain Reaction (PCR) are important development in the field of molecular biology (Fig. **2**).

DNA technology has two main areas:

• DNA cloning or gene cloning

• Methods of DNA analysis

DNA Cloning or Recombinant DNA Technology

It is selective amplification of a specific DNA fragment (or sequence) to produce relatively large amounts of the DNA fragment.

It is of two types:

1. *In vivo* cell-based mechanisms of DNA replication

2. *In vitro* polymerase chain reaction

1. *In vivo* cell-based cloning: It includes generation of DNA fragments by restriction enzymes and recombination of DNA fragments to form a recombinant DNA molecule.

2. Cell-free DNA cloning or *In vitro* Polymerase Chain Reaction (PCR): It can be used to produce vast quantities of a target DNA fragment of known sequence (This has been already discussed in Unit I).

BASIC TOOLS FOR DNA CLONING

Restriction Enzymes

They cut DNA at specific locations. Endonuclease enzymes that cut DNA at specific DNA sequences within the molecule are called Restriction Enzymes. They are key tools in recombinant DNA research. They are named so because their presence in the bacterium restricts the growth of certain bacterial viruses called bacteriophages.

Restriction enzymes recognize a palindromic nucleotide sequence of DNA between 4 and 8 nucleotides in length. Well over 300 different restriction enzymes have been isolated from various bacteria.

Restriction enzymes cut the DNA of any source into short pieces in a sequence-specific manner. They are named after the bacterium from which they are isolated, *e.g.*, Eco RI is from E. coli, Bom HI is from Bacillus amyloliquefaciens (Table **1**).

Nomenclature

The 1st 3 letters in the restriction enzyme name consist of 3 letters of the genes (E) and the 1st two letters of the species (co). These may be followed by a strain designation (R) and a roman numeral (I) to indicate the order of discovery (*e.g.*, Eco RI, EcoRII).

Recognition

Each enzyme recognizes and cleaves a specific double-stranded DNA sequence that is 4–7 bp long.

These DNA cuts result in:

(i) Blunt ends, *e.g.*, Hpa I

(i) Sticky (overlapping) ends, *e.g.*, Bam HI: useful in constructing hybrid or chimeric DNA molecules.

Recognition Sequence

The recognition sequence for type II endonucleases form palindrome with rotational symmetry (Table **1**), (Fig. **3**).

Table 1. Selected Restriction Endonuclease.

Endonuclease	Sequence specificity	Source (bacteria)
Taq I	↓ TCGA AGCT ↑	Thermus aquaeticus YTI
ST I	↓ CTGCAG GACGTC ↑	Providencia stuartii 164
Eco RI	↓ GAATTC CTTAAG ↑	*E. coli* RY 13
Eco RII	↓ CCTGG CGACC	*E. coli* R 245

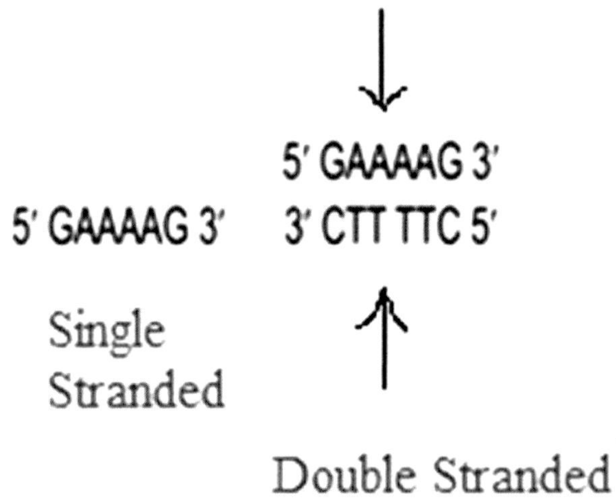

Fig. (3). Palindromic sequence (Arrow represent axis of symmetry).

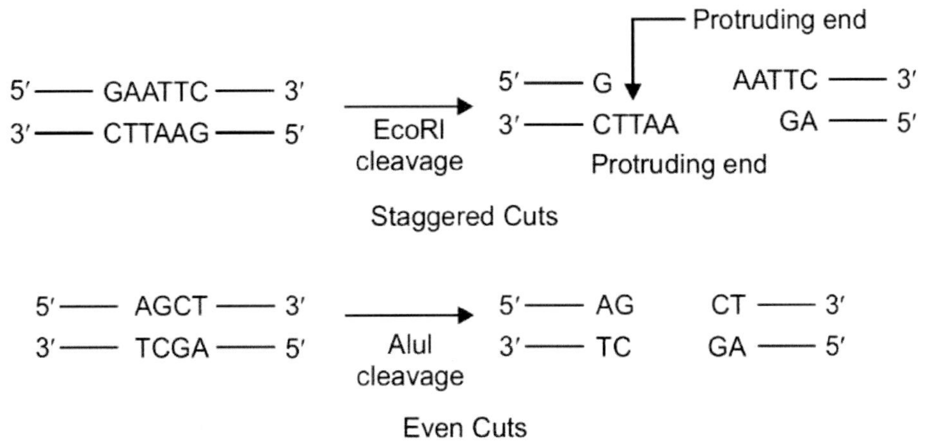

Fig. (4). Isolation of Desired Gene.

Cleavage Patterns

The DNA fragments used for cloning are generally obtained in the following ways:

(i) Genomic DNA fragments from DNA library

(ii) cDNA from cDNA Library

Recombination of DNA Fragments

When DNA has been cleaved by a restriction enzyme that produces staggered termini, these are referred to as being sticky or cohesive; since they will unite under appropriate conditions with complementary sequences produced by the same restriction enzyme on DNA from any source by enzyme (Figs. **4** and **5**).

Purify specific protein

↓

Raise Ab against it and precipitate polysomes

↓

Isolate mRNA

↓

Reverse transcriptase

↓

cDNA synthesis

↓

Cloning of cDNA

(Fig. 5) contd.....

↓

Confirm identity of cDNA

↓

Colony Hybridization

↓

Select clone

↓

Isolation of gene

Fig. (5). Isolation of a gene for a specific protein.

DNA Ligase

The union of two DNA fragments from different sources produces a recombinant DNA molecule.

Vectors

They are carrier DNA-molecules used in the cloning process by its own independent replication within a host organism to produce multiple copies itself (Table **2**).

5 main types of commonly used vectors:

Plasmid, Bacteriophage, cosmid, bacterial (BAC) and yeast artificial chromosomes (YAC).

Plasmid and bacteriophage have a limitation of size of DNA that could be inserted.

Cosmid can take up upto 50 kb in size. BACs and YACs allow cloning DNA fragments between 300 kb-1000 kb in size.

Table 2. Properties of vector.

Properties of Good Vector
• Replicates autonomously
• Size less than 10 kb.
• Easy to isolate and purify
• Easy to transform host
• Suitable marker gene for selection
• Ability to integrate into the host genome
• Unique target sites for restriction enzymes.

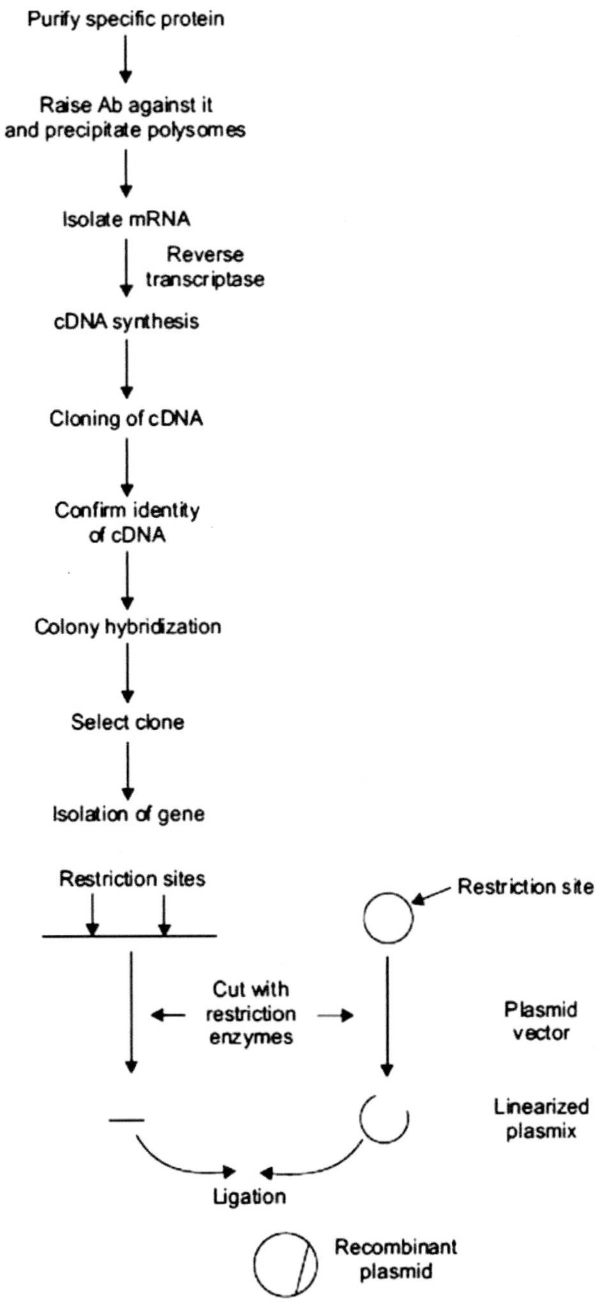

Fig. (6). Cutting and joining of DNA.

Cloning Vector

Vector used for propagation of DNA insert in a suitable host is called cloning vector Fig. (**6**).

Expression Vector

Vector designed for expression of DNA insert, *e.g.*, for production of protein specified by the insert is termed as expression vector. Expression vector and constructed by translational and transcriptional fusion.

GENE CLONING

Recombinant DNA is product of breakage of a DNA molecule at two desired places to isolate a specific DNA segment and its insertion in another DNA molecule at a desired position Figs. (**7** and **8**). The technique of obtaining recombinant DNA is genetic engineering.

With the help of this technique, a single copy of gene can be isolated and cloned into an indefinite number of identical copies. This technique is termed as gene cloning and the vector are called cloning vectors (Fig. **9**), (Tables **3** and **4**).

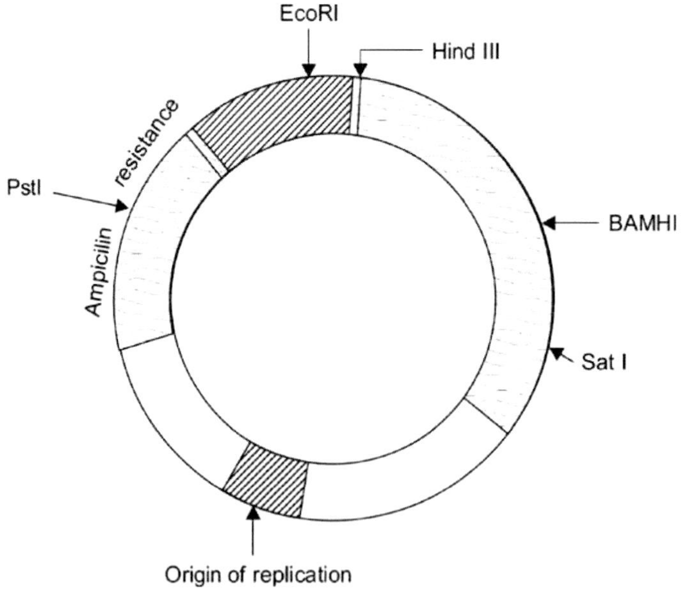

Fig. (7). Genetic map of plasmid cloning vector pBR322.

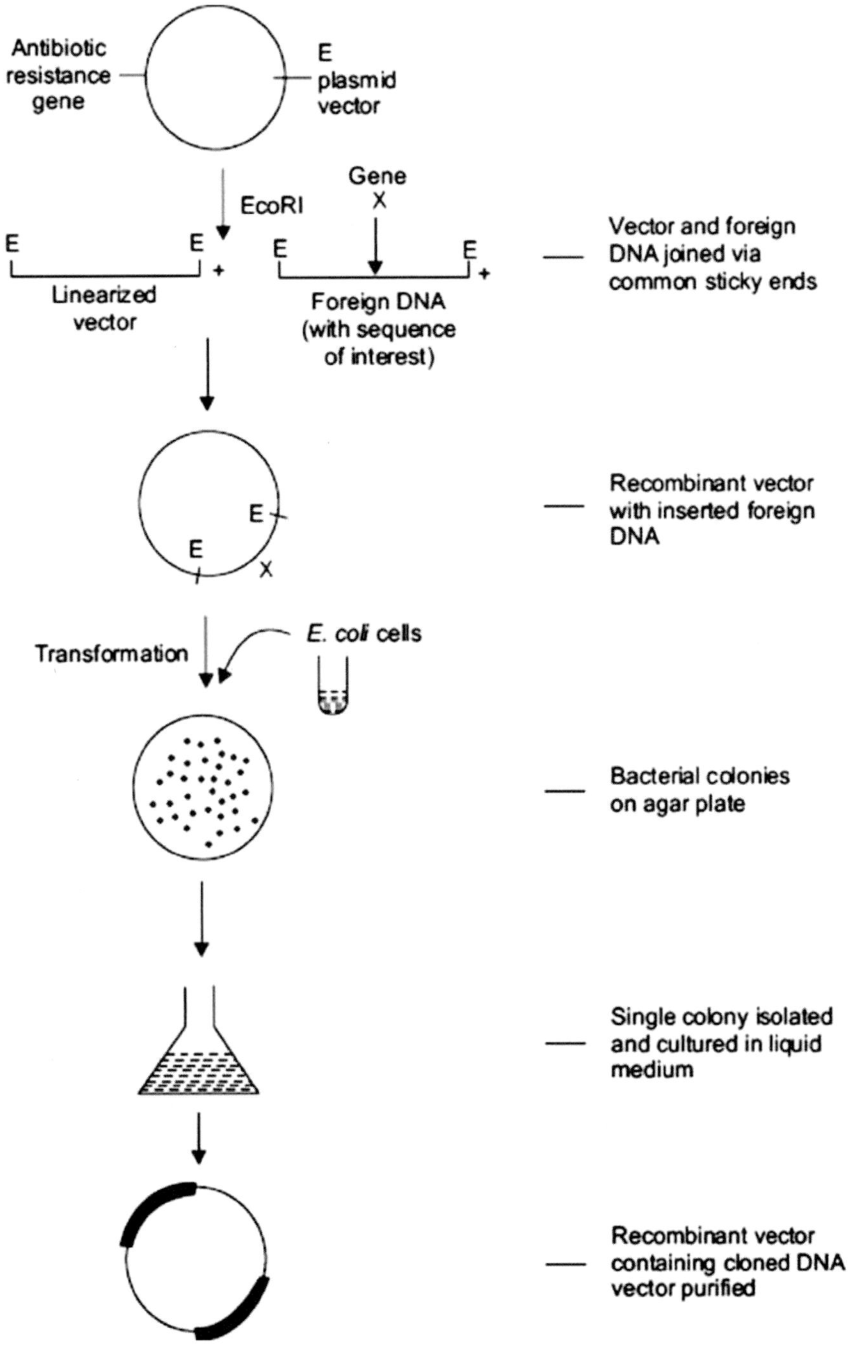

Fig. (8). Cloning with plamsids.

Table 3. Cloning Vectors.

Cloning Vectors	Foreign insert size kb
Phage I	5–25
Cosmid	35–45
Plasmid Artificial Chromosome (PAC)	100–300
Bacterial Artificial Chromosome (BAC)	100–300
Yeast Chromosome	200–2000

White colonies

Contain insert

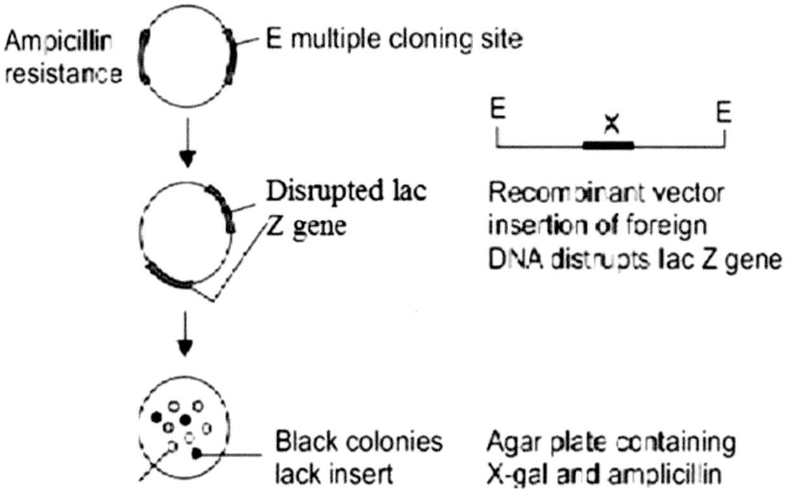

Fig. (9). Insertion of foreign DNA molecule inactivates lac Z gene and recombinant colonies appear while on agar plate containing X- gal.

Choice of Vector

The maximum size of insert that the different vectors will accommodate is shown in Fig. (**10**) the following Tables **4** and **5**:

Table 4. Maximum DNA insert possible with different cloning vectors.

Vector	Host	Insert size
λ phage	*E. coli*	5–25 kb
λ cosmid	*E. coli*	35–45 kb
P1 phage	*E. coli*	70–100 kb
PACs	*E. coli*	100–300 kb
BACs	*E. coli*	< 300 kb
YACs	*S. cerevisiae*	200–2000 kb

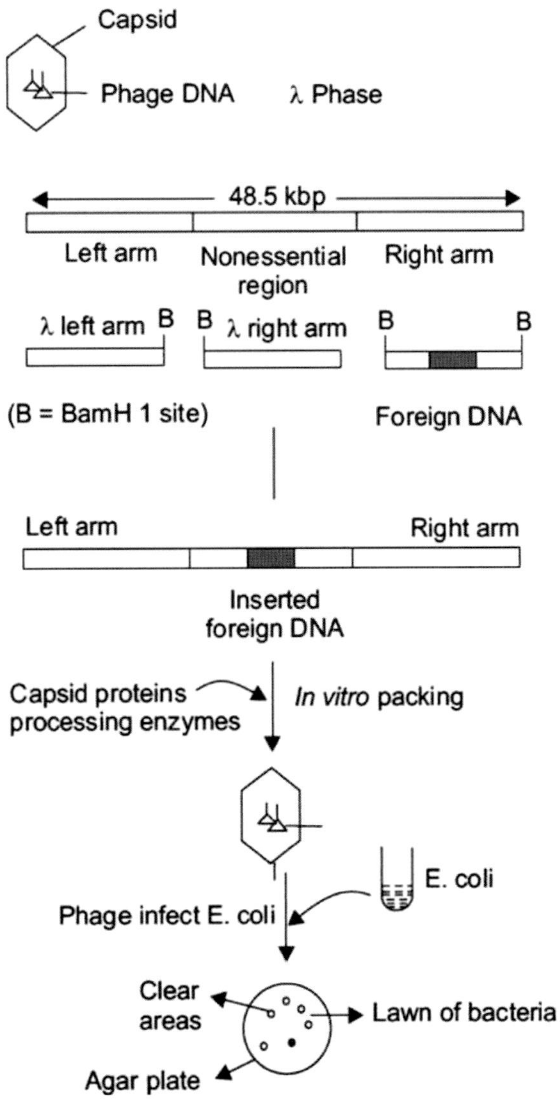

Fig. (10). Lambda phage as cloning vector.

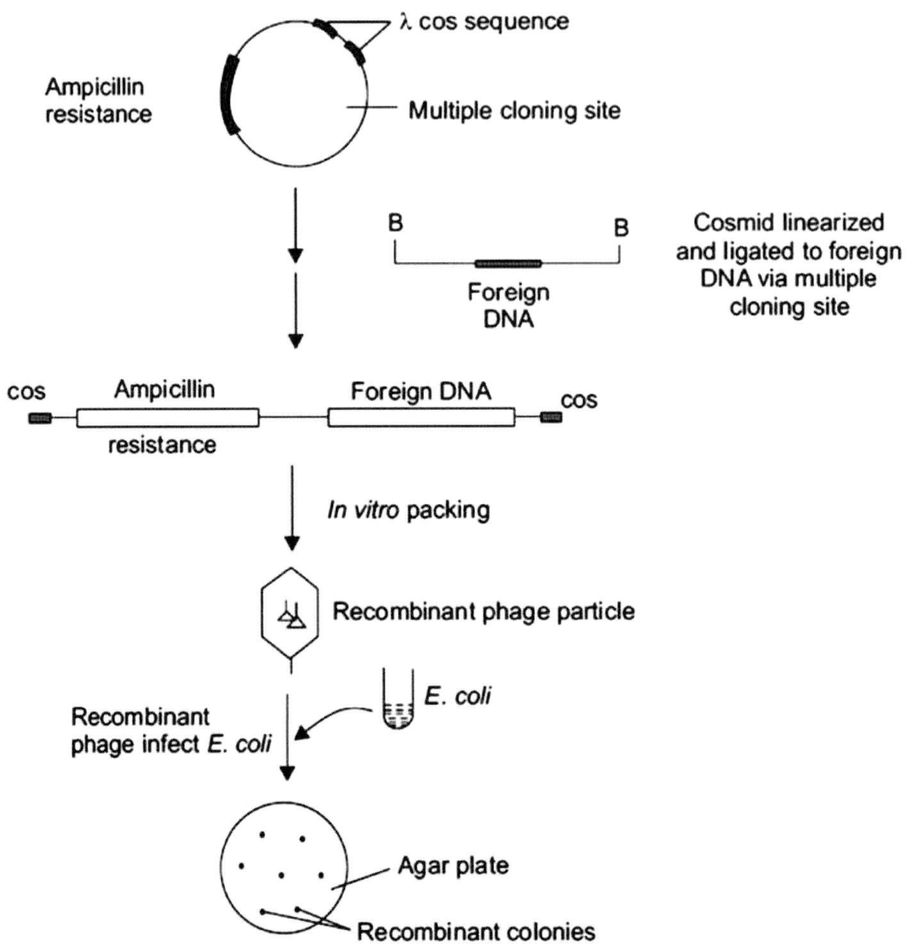

Fig. (11). Cloning.

Table 5. Different cloning vectors.

Organism	**Haploid genome size**	**Cosmid (40 kb)**	**P1 (85 kb)**	**PAC/PAC (250 kb)**	**YAC (1000 kb)**
E. coli	4.70×10^6 bp	118	55	19	5
S. cerevisiae	1.35×10^7 bp	338	159	54	14
D. melanogaster	1.80×10^8 bp	4500	2118	720	180
H. sapiens	2.80×10^9 bp	70000	32941	11200	2800

Transformation of Host Organism

Following introduction of foreign DNA fragment into vector, the recombinant vector is introduced into modified bacterial or yeast host cell, which multiply and produce large quantities of identical copies of original single target DNA or CLONES.

Recombination Vectors Screening

The recombinant vectors can be screened by various detection system, *e.g.*, loss of antibiotic resistance, immunological or activity assay of protein; products encoded by cloned gene; DNA hybridization with a probe (Figs. **11** - **14**).

Clone Selection

Several techniques are available for detecting presence of clones within specific DNA sequence inserts and nucleic acid hybridization is most widely used method.

DNA Libraries

A library is a collection of recombinant clones.

Types of Libraries

Genomic Library

Prepared from total DNA of a cell line or tissue.

cDNA Library

Comprises of complementary DNA copies of mRNAs.

Genomic Library

It is prepared by partial digestion of total DNA with help of restriction enzymes to generate large fragments so that most genes remain infected. BAC, YAC, and Pl vectors are preferred as they can accept very large fragments of DNA (Figs. **15** and **16**).

cDNA Library

It is a population of bacterial transformants or phage lysates in which mRNA isolated from an organism is represented as its cDNA insertion in a plasmid or a phage vector.

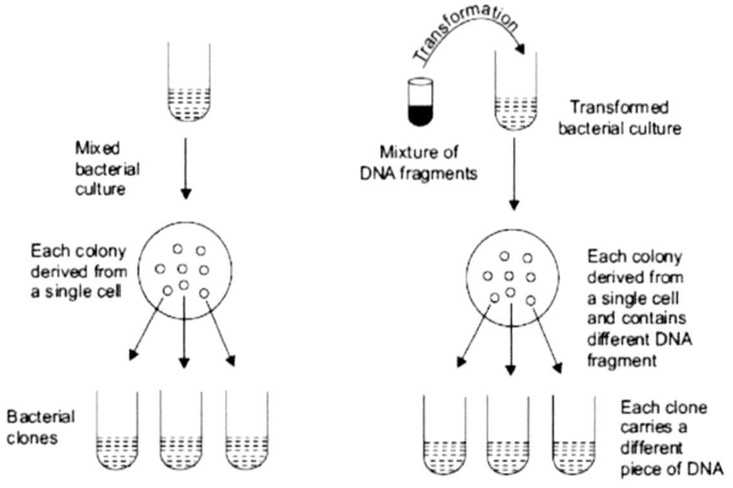

Fig. (12). Bacterial cloning and gene cloning.

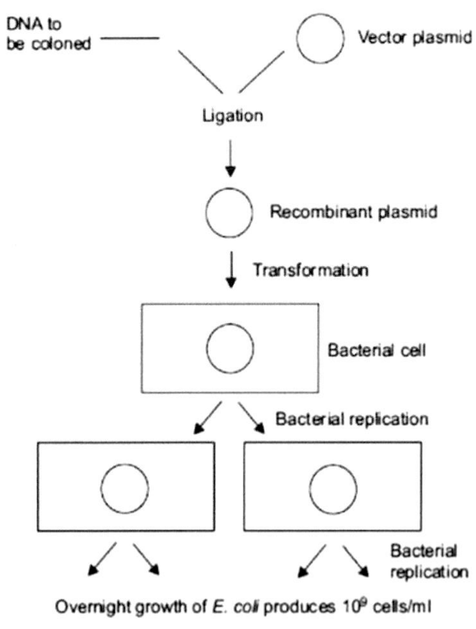

Fig. (13). Gene cloning.

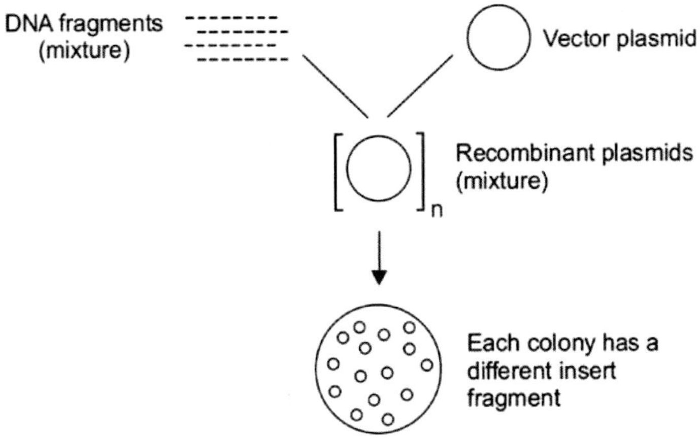

Fig. (14). Preparation of genomic library.

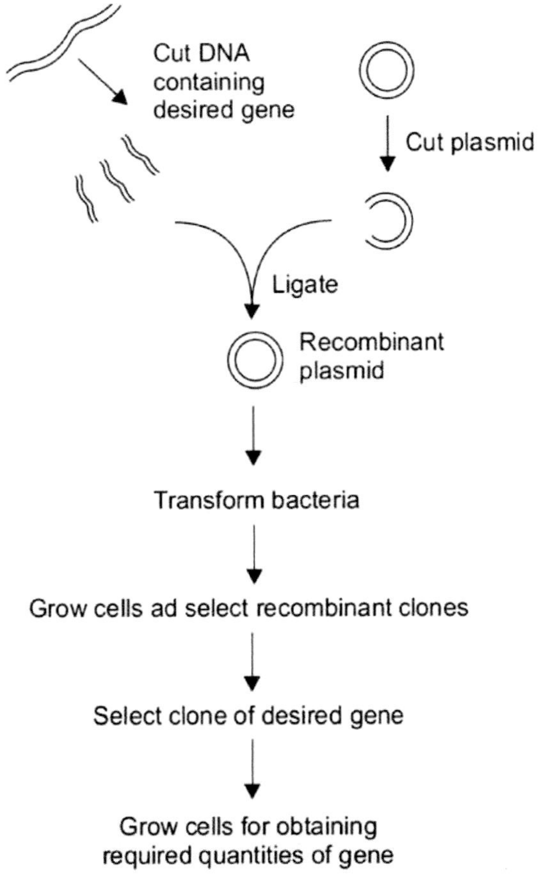

Fig. (15). Gene cloning outline.

Colony Hybridization for Screening of Libraries

Once a genomic library or cDNA library is available, gene sequence can be isolated by colony hybridization technique. In this technique, bacteria carrying chimeric vectors are grown into colonies, which are lysed on nitrocellulose filters. Their DNA is denatured in situ and fixed on the filter, which is hybridized with radioactively labelled probe carrying a sequence related to the gene to be isolated, usually cloned cDNA for screening of a genomic library. The colonies carrying these sequences are identified by autoradiograph as dark spots Fig. (**17**).

cDNA Library	Genome Library
Extract mRNA	Extract chromosomal DNA
↓	↓
Product cDNA	Digestion with restriction endonuclease
↓	↓
Insert cDNA into vector	Insert DNA fragment into vector
↓	↓
Recombinant DNA	Recombinant DNA
↓	↓
Transform bacteria	Transform bacteria
↓	↓
Clone each recombinant	Clone each recombinant

Fig. (16). Comparison of genomic and cDNA libraries.

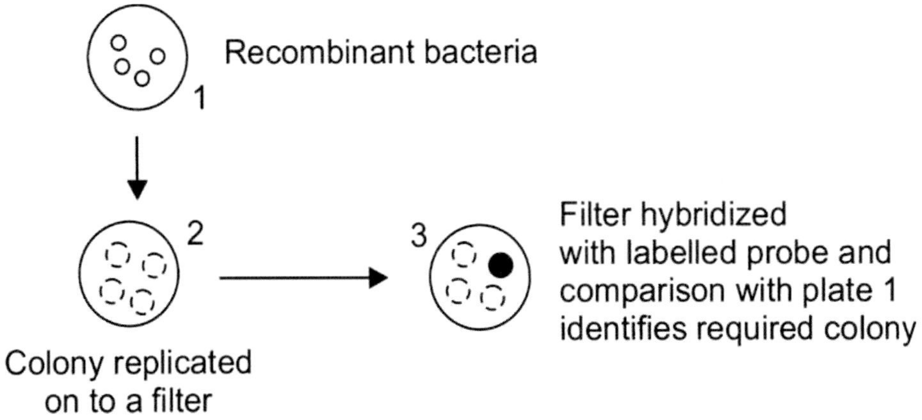

Fig. (17). Colony hybridization.

If chimeric page particles are taken as vectors, the plaques develop overnight. These plaques can be treated like colonies and the technique is then described as plaque hybridization.

Searching Specific Genes or cDNA Molecules in Libraries

Probes are used to search for a specific genes or cDNA molecule or to quantitate and define DNA or RNA separated by gel electrophoresis.

Applications of DNA Technology

Gene mapping, Study of gene structure Table **6** and function:

Table 6. Gene structure and functions.

Genetic	➢ Population genetics ➢ Clinical genetics • Preimplantation genetic • diagnosis Prenatal genetic • Diagnosis Carrier detection
Molecular	➢ In diagnosis and pathogenesis of diseases:
Diagnostics	➢ Genetic ➢ Acquired: • Infective • malignant

(Table 6) cont.....

Synthesis of biologicals	➢ Synthesis of hormones: • Insulin • GH ➢ Products of immunity • Interferon • Vaccines
Treatment of genetic disease	➢ Gene therapy • Cloning

FOREIGN GENES: EXPRESSION

DNA Transfer into Eukaryotic Cells and Mammalian Embryos

Manipulating the sequence of a gene in a test tube is not sufficient for discovering its function. It remains to study the functioning of the gene in a living cell, and this requires persuading a cell to take up the gene. Cells do not take up DNA easily and geneticists devised methods to bypass natural barriers to gene transfer (Fig. **18**).

One of the most widely used strategies to introduce genes into eukaryotic cells, where they are generally transcribed and translated.

Transduction

Viral-mediated gene transfer where DNA is incorporated into genome of a non-replicating virus and then virus infects the cell. Bacteriophage, monkey tumor virus SV40, severe commonly used for gene transfer earlier. Now, many viruses, lytic viruses and nonlytic viruses (retro-, adeno- and adeno associated viruses) have been modified to transfer genes to animal cells.

Transfection

Naked DNA is introduced into cultured cells by treating them with calcium phosphate or DEAE dextran and gets incorporated into chromosome. Also, electroporation and lipofection can transfect cells.

Electroporation

Cells are incubated with DNA in special vials that contain electrodes which deliver a brief electric pulse that cause plasma membrane to become transiently permeable to DNA molecules. These DNA molecules may find way into the nucleus and get incorporated into chromosomes.

Lipofection

Cells are treated with DNA found attached to cationic liposomes (Positively charged lipids) that fuse with lipid bilayer of cell membrane and deliver DNA to cytoplasm.

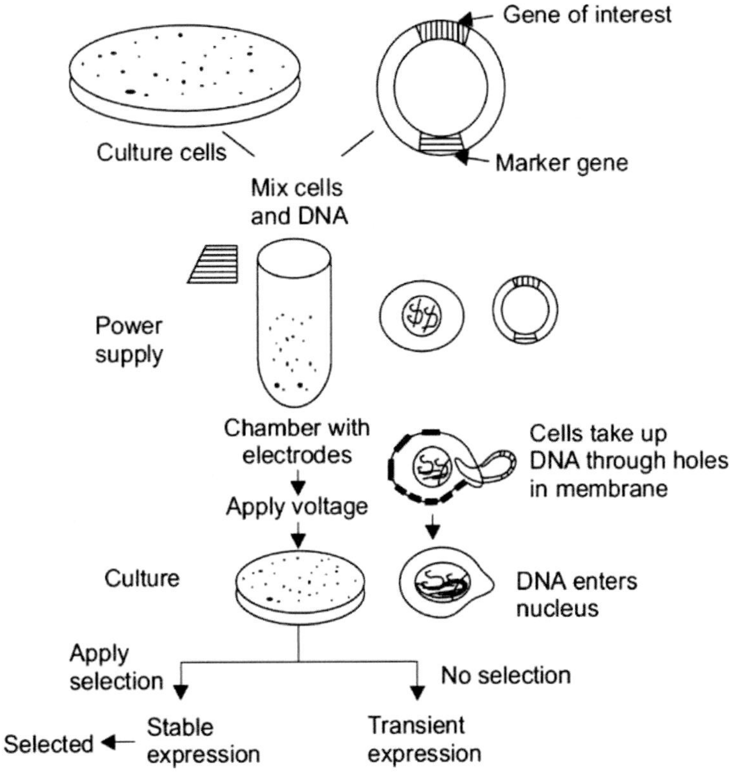

Fig. (18). Mapping methods.

Introduction of Foreign Genes into Cells

By microinjection of DNA directly into the cell's nucleus, foreign genes are introduced into cells. This approach is best suited for nuclei of oocytes and eggs, *e.g.*, Xenopus oocytes are used for studying expression of foreign genes. The oocyte nucleus contains machinery necessary for RNA synthesis and when foreign DNA is injected into nucleus, it is readily transcribed, and RNA is transported to cytoplasm to be translated into proteins.

Another target for injected DNA is nucleus of a mouse embryo to have foreign DNA getting integrated into egg's chromosomes to passed onto all the cells of the embryo and subsequent adult. Such animals that have been genetically engineered so that their chromosomes contain foreign gene are called Transgenic Animals. Transgenic animals provide a means to monitor when and where in the embryo particular genes are expressed. Also, they help to determine the impact of extra copies of genes on the development and life of the animal.

Table 7. Foreign proteins.

Proteins made in plants
Human serum albumin
α-interferon
α1-antitrypsin
collagen
Recombinant antibodies
Subunit vaccines

Many organisms can be used for making "foreign" proteins. Many proteins can be successfully expressed and purified from the bacteria, usually E. coli and in yeast cells. The major drawback of protein expression in bacteria and yeast is that they cannot modify proteins the way they do in animal cells. Also, proteins from higher organisms have different post translation modifications. Insect virus called baculovirus, plant systems have been developed for protein expression (details are given under "protein expression systems") (Table 7).

TRANSGENIC ANIMALS CAN BE MADE BY INJECTING DNA DIRECTLY INTO EMBRYOS

Genes can be directly injected into fruit flies, worms, zebrafish, and mice to create animals carrying integrated genes.

Transgenic Mice

Most effective technique is microinjection of cloned genes into fertilized eggs that contains two pronuclei (one from sperm and other from egg) and ultimately form one-celled embryo. About 2 picolitres of solution (containing few hundred copies of foreign DNA) are microinjected into one of the two pronuclei and injected embryo are transferred to oviduct of foster mother for implantation in uterus where many develop to term (10–30%). Introduced DNA appears to integrate randomly without preference for a particular chromosomal location. Mice that carry foreign gene are referred to as Transgenic and foreign DNA is Transgene.

Mice derived analysis injected with cloned human interferon DNA or rabbit β-globin DNA transmit transgenes to offspring as Mendelian Trait and every member of a line of mice has some transgene at identical position in its genomes (Fig. **19**).

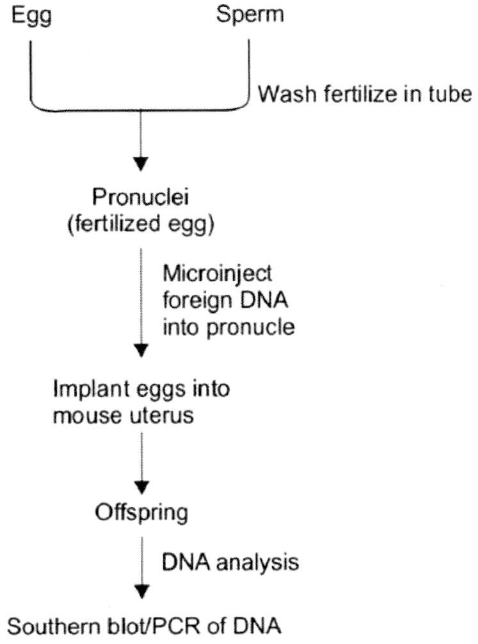

Fig. (19). Genomic maps: types.

TRANSGENE EXPRESSION CAN BE TARGETED TO SPECIFIC TISSUES

A transgene integrates in a chromosome different from that of its endogenous counterpart and is often expressed in a pattern that mimics expression of endogenous gene.

Various tissues can be analyzed for presence of RNA or proteins products encoded by transgenes. *e.g.*, Transgenic mice harbouring human insulin. RNA was found in pancreas and showed that transcription of this transgene can be induced by same signals that induced endogenous mouse insulin gene. Thus, a foreign transgene can be expressed in the correct tissue and may be subjected to the same regulatory signals as endogenous genes.

Similar results have been obtained using many genes introduced into transgenic mice by embryonic stem cell (ESC) transfer.

If tissue-specific regulatory sequences are known, expression of a protein can be targeted to a tissue in which it is not normally expressed, *e.g.*, Promoter-enhanced control region of rat insulin gene (RIP) can target expression of SV 40 large T antigen (Tag), a viral oncogene, to β cells of islets. Mice with RIP-Tag transgene died at 9–12 weeks of age and pathological analysis showed hyperplasia and tumor of islets of Langerhans. All other tissues of transgenic mice containing the transgene were normal showing that tissue-specific expression was occurring in the islets.

MICE WITH ALTERED GENOMES CAN BE CREATED BY INJECTING ESC INTO EMBRYOS

Direct transfer of DNA into embryonic stem cells (ESC) and then injected transfecting cells into embryo is an efficient method of manipulating and controlling DNA integration. ES cells are obtained from inner cell mass (ICM) of mouse blastocysts and are grown in tissue culture with feeder layer (Fig. **20**) of fibroblasts or leukaemia inhibitory factor (LIF) to prevent differentiation.

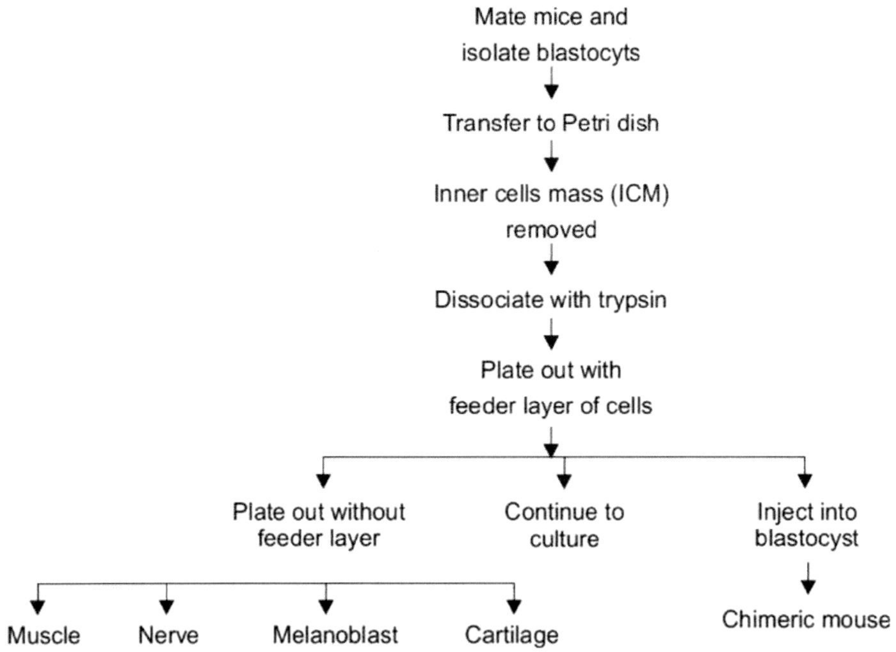

Fig. (20). ESC produced from mouse blastocyst.

These ES cells are injected into mouse blastocyst and can participate in the formation of all tissues including germ cells.

Advantage of ES cells for gene transfer in mice is that it allows manipulation of transgene *In vitro* before injecting cells into embryo. DNA can be introduced into ES by transfection, retroviral infection, or electroporation. Also, cells carrying properly expressed transgenes can be selected to be injected into blastocyst. Recombination techniques along with ESC can be used to produce transgenic mice with mutation in specific gene, replace mutant gene with normal one, gene of interest at a specific location into the genome.

HOMOLOGOUS RECOMBINATIONS TO KNOCK OUT GENES IN MICE

Following gene transfer foreign DNA taken up by cells is lost from 90% or more of the cells that originally take it up. Only rarely, it gets stably integrated into lost cell genome. Thus, wide fluctuations in transferred gene expression and its regulation occurs. If foreign gene gets integrated near highly expressed cellular gene, high levels of foreign gene expression occur, and expression is suppressed if foreign gene gets inserted into quiet areas of genome.

Gene can recombine in two ways:

Homologous: Recombines precisely into identical sequence.

Heterologous: Recombines into unrelated sequence

Homologous recombination is a powerful tool to study gene function, gene targeting (placing foreign DNA into precise locus). Gene targeting is used to inactivate mammalian genes by homologous recombination of disputed transgene into target gene of interest and is termed as Gene Knockout. Gene knockout can be used to introduce new sequences in a defined location of genome using targeting vectors along with selectable marker gene by homologous recombination

Knockout Mice can provide insight into genetic basis of a human disease and mechanism for studying cellular activities for producing product from a particular gene.

Double Knockout is compensation by one gene for another by producing mice that lack both genes in question.

Conditional Knockouts where a particular gene is knockout only in one or more desired tissues and is expressed in rest of the tissues and animals survive to adulthood allowing researchers to study role of gene on development or function of affected tissue.

In vitro Mutagenesis is another way of determining eukaryotic gene/function by gene elimination. Site directed mutagenesis (SDM) makes small specific changes in a DNA sequence (substitution of base or deletion or insertion) in form of oligonucleotide which hybridizes to a single-stranded preparation of normal DNA and polymerizes and cloned to determine gene expression and effect of changes in regulatory region on gene expression.

GENE THERAPY MAY PERMIT MANIPULATION OF GENE EXPRESSION IN HUMANS

Treating human genetic disorders by restoring functional gene through modification of mutant gene or by introduction of a function gene by Gene therapy using viral vectors is an alternative strategy. However, it continues to pose many challenges. Cloning, sequencing, modifying genes and introducing modified genes into cells and animals has transformed biology and these tools continue to reveal unsuspected facets of life.

Analysing Genes

The isolation of a specific gene from an entire genome that will discriminate one part in a million and recombinant DNA technology can accomplish this.

Terminology

Genome: Genome represents the total genetic information present in them.

Genome analysis: It refers to analysis of structural and functional organization of complete genome and it is commonly termed as genomics. This initial phase of genomics is development of genome maps.

Genome map: It is a detailed schematic description of the structural and functional organization of the complete genome of an organism.

AIMS OF GENOMICS

To obtain DNA sequence of the complete genome which can provide complete nucleotide sequence of genome.

Gene Mapping

Localizing specific genes to distinct chromosomes is termed as gene mapping.

Three approaches: Physical mapping, cytogenetic mapping, linkage analysis.

Physical mapping—determined by physical distances between genes. It is of the two types:

- Low resolution (1-several mega base)
- High resolution (Hundreds of kB to a Single Nucleotide)

Low resolution physical mapping techniques include:

- Somatic cell hybridization
- Chromosome specific libraries
- Fluorescence in situ Hybridization (FISH)

High resolution physical mapping techniques include:

- Pulses field gel electrophoresis
- High resolution FISHDNA sequencing
- DNA sequencing

FISH

Fluorescently labelled DNA probe is hybridized to metaphase chromosomes and examined using fluorescent microscopy. It is a very sensitive technique.

Genetic Map

They depict relative chromosomal locations of DNA markers (genes and other identifiable DNA sequences) by their pattern of inheritance. Three different strategies have been used to construct genetic maps (Fig. **21**), (Table **8**).

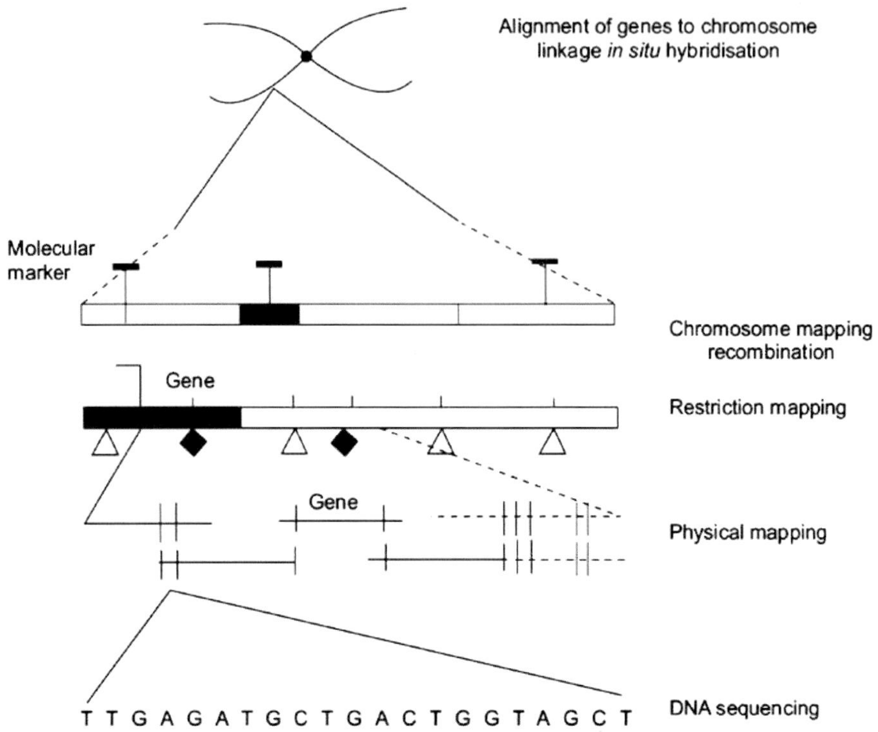

Fig. (21). Mapping.

Types of Genetic Maps

- Linkage maps
- Cytogenetic or cytological maps
- Physical maps

Linkage Map

It depicts order of genetic markers and relative distances between them.

Cytogenetic Map

It depicts location of various genes in a chromosome relative to specific microscopically visible landmarks in the chromosome.

Physical Map

Here, genes are depicted in the same order as they occur in chromosome (Fig. **22**).

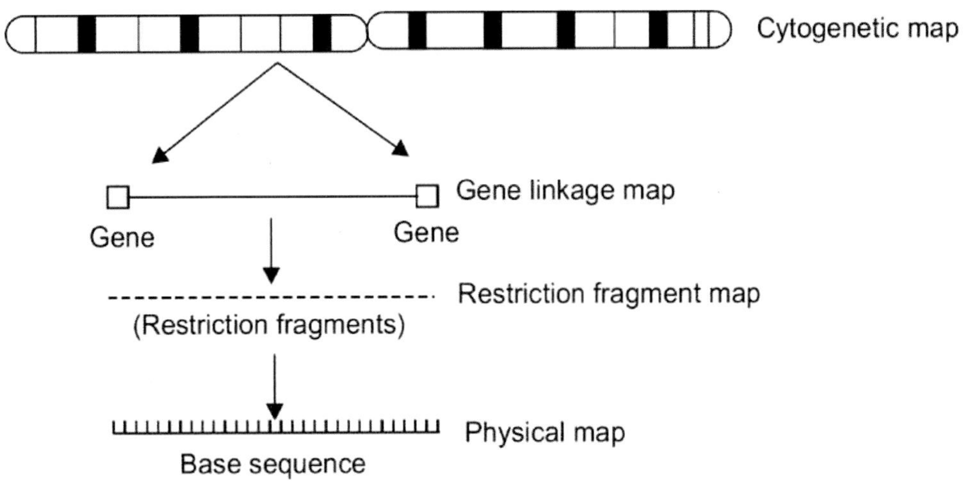

Fig. (22). Physical Map.

Table 8. Methods for genome mapping.

Method	Application
DNA sequencing	Identifies physical map of DNA
Probe	Identify RFLPs, STS, SNPs
Radiation hybrid mapping	To fragment genome into large piece and locate markers and genes.
STS mapping (sequence tagged site)	DNA sequencing
EST mapping (expressed sequence tag)	Mapping of expressed genes
PCR	To amplify gene fragments
Cloning (Plasmid, Phage, cosmid, YAC, BAC)	Isolation of DNA fragments
Chromosomal walking	To clone overlapping (fragments upto 200 kB in size)
Chromosomal jumping	Circularization of large DNA fragments to be used in chromosomal walking
Cloning of detective gene	Diagnostics

IDENTIFICATION OF GENES IN CLONED DNA

Several techniques are used to identify coding sequences or genes with DNA fragments of clones. These include:

1. HTF CpG Islands

2. Zoo blotting

3. Exon trapping

4. Expressed sequence tags (ESTs)

1. HTF/CpG Islands

Some infrequently cutting restriction enzymes such as Hpa II contain one or more CpG dinucleotide (cytosine-guanine dinucleotide with intervening phosphate molecule) in its nucleotide recognition sequence. This dinucleotide pair following methylation of cytosine residue prevents cleavage of DNA by these restriction enzymes.

CpG dinucleotides occur with one-quarter of the frequency in genome and are non-randomly distributed in genome. Clusters of methylation free Hpa II tiny fragments: HTF or CpG islands are found near transcription initiation sites at 5′ end of genes.

About half of genes are associated with HTF/CpG island and 40% of genes show tissue-specific expression of HTF/CpG islands and 40% of genes show tissue-specific expression of HTF/CpG islands.

2. Zoo Blots

The structure and relative positions of many genes have been highly conserved during evolution and in closely related species are termed as Homologs and usually they are sequences of an important functional gene. Southern Blots of DNA from several different species is termed a Zoo Blot.

3. Exon Trapping

By using expression cloning vectors, a suitably modified eukaryotic cells line is transfected to transcribe inserted target DNA into RNA that gets spliced subsequently. Production of abnormal splice product indicates presence of an exon in cloned DNA fragment.

4. Expressed Sequence TAGs (ESTs)

Sequence specific primers from cDNA can be designed to identify sequences of expressed genes (ESTs). ESTs can be assigned to a particular chromosomal location by the following methods:

i. Chromosomal hybrids
ii. Radiation hybrids
iii. FISH
iv. PCR analysis of gridded arrays

ESTs provide a rich source of partial sequences of many positional genes responsible for inherited diseases in humans.

ANALYSIS OF HUMAN GENOME DATABASE

Genomic DNA sequence databases of sequence homology to known genes as well as DNA sequences specific to all genes are available.

About 1500 human disease genes have been identified using positional cloning (based on its chromosomal location of a gene).

POSITIONAL CLONING

Positional cloning can be done by Linkage analysis:

e.g., Cystic Fibrosis (CF) has been linked to chromosome 7 and gene was mapped to a region of 500 kb between markers MET and DTS 8 at chromosome band 7q 31–32.

Also, positional cloning is associated with:

i. Chromosomal abnormalities *e.g.*,
a. Duchenne muscular dystrophy (DMD)
b. Retinitis pigmentosa
c. Chronic granulomatous disease
d. All these are X-linked
ii. Homology to genes in model organisms

Genetic disease	→	Map to a chromosome site	→	Retrieve genomic clones from the mapped site	→	Identify and analyze exons
↓		↓		↓		↓
Implement mutation detection assays	→	Characterize in the genomic clone	→	Select a genomic clone	→	Isolate a cDNA clone

CANDIDATE GENES

Those genes which are likely to be involved in the pathogenesis of the inherited disorder are known as candidate genes.

Mutations in candidate genes can be screened for by a variety of methods of DNA sequencing. It has been observed that candidate gene is expressed in the appropriate tissues and at the relevant stages of development (Figs. **23** and **24**).

Genetic disease
↓
Analyse symptoms
↓
Predict possible proteins
↓
Pick a candidate gene
↓
Implement mutation detection assays

Fig. (23). Candidate gene cloning.

ANALYSIS OF GENE EXPRESSION

Gene Expression

Two main phases of gene expression are:

- Transcription
- Translation

Terminology

Genome: Genome is complete set of genetic information. The complete collection of mRNA transcripts in a cell, tissue or organism at a particular time is referred to as Transcriptome and comparative study of mRNA transcripts in Transcriptomics.

Protein with a known function
↓
Determination of amino acid sequence
↓
Deduce the nucleotide sequence
↓
Synthesis of oligonucleotide probe
↓
Isolation of cDNA clone
↓
Selection of genomic clone
↓
Characterization of genomic clone
↓
Implementation of mutation detection arrays

Fig. (24). Functional gene cloning: Isolation and identification of gene where sequence if gene product is known.

Proteome: Proteome is a complete set of translated proteins and study of translated proteins is Proteomics.

The first methods that were developed allowed investigators to study the expression of a specific RNA or a specific protein. Gradually, methods to compare complex mixtures of gene products have been evolved over time and recent advances have created new terms: transcriptomics, proteomics, metabolomics, epigenomics *etc*

Analysis of gene expression will be discussed in this section under the assumption that polypeptide chain is the product of gene expression (Fig. **25**).

Initially study of products of single genes will be discussed followed by study of complex samples.

ANALYSIS OF TRANSCRIPTION

Techniques for analysis of transcription are:

a. Analysis of products of single gene:

Northern blot

RNase protection assay

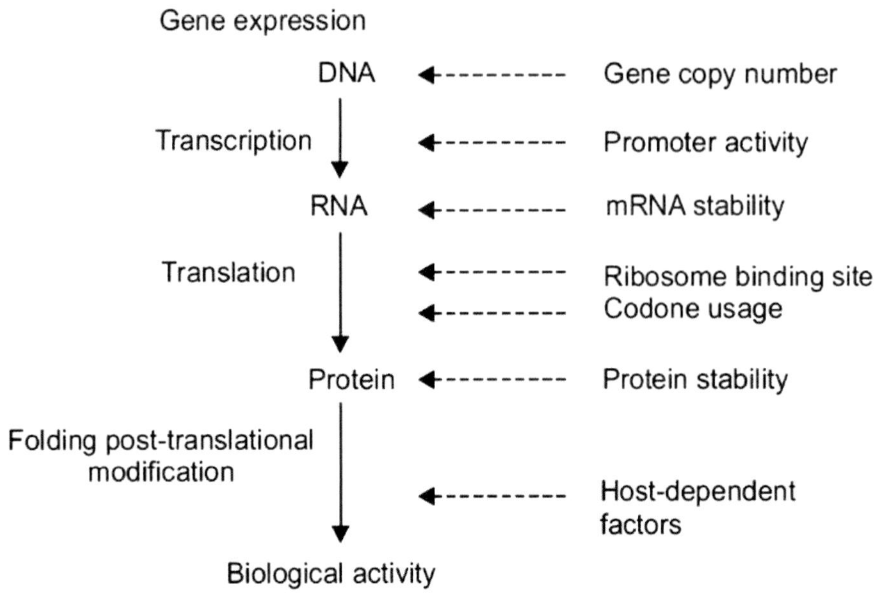

Fig. (25). Gene expression.

Reverse transcription PCR

Real-time—RT PCR

In situ—hybridization

Primer extension assay

b. Study of complex samples:

(Comparing transcriptomes)

Differential screening

Subtractive hybridization

Differential display

Array-based methods

EST arrays

PCR based arrays

Two Important Points Concerning Measurement of mRNA are

1. Amount of a specific mRNA in a cell at a point of time is influenced both by level of transcriptional activity and stability of that message.
2. Amount of mRNA present does not necessarily correlate with the amount of protein produced.

Analysis of Whole Genome

Each human cell contains two copies of a 3.2 million sequence code of nucleic acids on 46 chromosomes.

Intergenic DNA

Three quarters of human DNA is intergenic or between genes 60% of which consists of parasitic DNA regions of transposable elements (*i.e.*, 3.2 million in each copy of genome). These elements are responsible for genetic recombination and chromosome structure.

SSRs

Simple sequence repeats, present in the form of micro-satellites or short tandem repeats (STRs) (1–13 base repeat unit) and mini-satellites or Variable Number of Tandem Repeats (VNTRs) (14–500 base repeat unit) are present in intergenic DNA. One STR on average occurs every 2000 bases.

USES of STRs

STRs serve as markers in:

- Genetic linkage studies
- Forensic medicine
- Medical identity testing

Evolution of STRs

They are formed by slippage during replication, *e.g.*, ACACAC, ATAT are most common dinucleotide repeats.

There are 30,000 genes in human genome and each gene covers 27,000 bases of which only 1300 code for amino acid sequence. These coding regions are exons, and 9 exons are present per genc (5%). The intervening noncoding regions are introns (95%).

Sequence Variation

Approximately 99.9% of sequence is identical between randomly selected copies of genome (*i.e.*, 1 difference on every 1250 bases).

Most common sequence variations are single base changes termed as SNPs (Single Nucleotide Polymorphisms pronounced snips). Majority of SNPs (97%) occurs in non-coding regions and only 3% are associated with exons.

Of the sequence alternations (mutations) that are known to cause disease, about 70% are SNIPs, of which most are missense mutations (49%), fewer are nonsense mutations (11%), 9% are splicing and less than 1% are in regulatory regions.

TECHNIQUES FOR STUDYING ANALYSIS OF PRODUCTS OF A SINGLE GENE

Northern Blot

It detects specific mRNA by hybridization to specific labelled probes. A northern blot involves electrophoretic separation of a purified extract of RNA from the cell, followed by immobilization onto a membrane and hybridization with a specific probe (Fig. **26**).

Advantage

1. Risk of artefact is much smaller than the PCR-based methods.
2. It is the only method for determining size of a specific transcript and for detecting presence of different transcripts for a particular gene.

Disadvantage

1. Technique is not very sensitive.
2. It sequences fairly large amounts of RNA (1–10 mg of total RNA). Sometimes it may not be possible to get enough specimen *e.g.*, in case of gene expression of pathogenic bacterium at mRNA level in material obtained by biopsy.

Still this technique is very important tool for detecting products of gene.

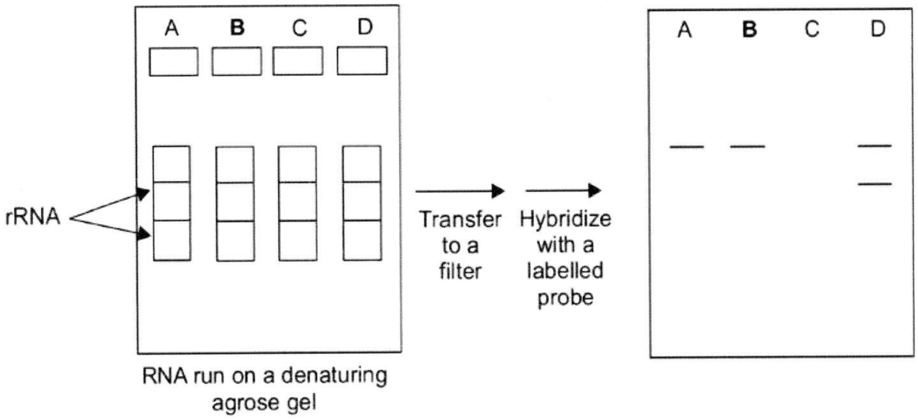

Fig. (26). Northern Blot.

RNase Protection Assay

When labelled antisense RNA is added to mRNA preparation, it will anneal to the specific RNA to be measured, forming double-stranded RNA, while non-specific RNA molecules remain single-stranded (Fig. **27**).

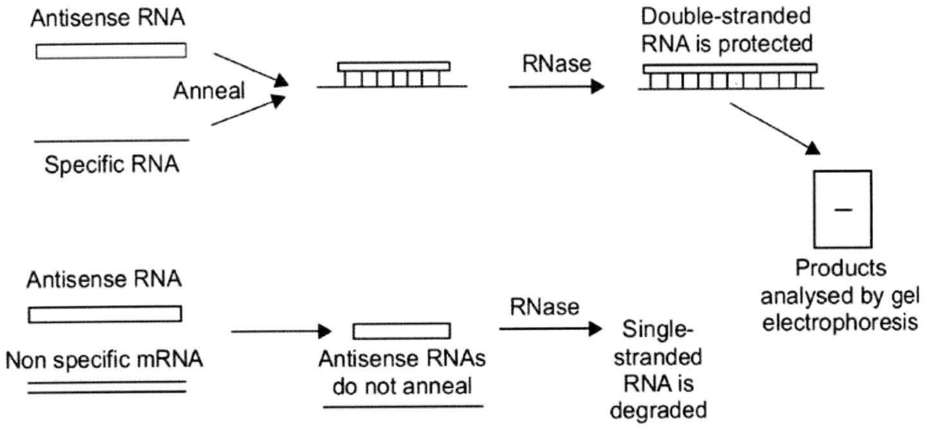

Fig. (27). RNase Protection Assay.

When RNase (ribonuclease) is added, it will degrade all the single stranded RNA and double stranded hybrids formed by annealing the antisense RNA probe to specific mRNA are protected. After RNase digestion, the hybridization mixture is separated by PAGE and radiographed.

Advantage

It is more sensitive, quantitative, and more tolerant of partial degradation of RNA than northern blotting.

Disadvantage

1. It does not allow determination of size of transcript.
2. It demands more work than northern blotting.

Reverse Transcription PCR (RT-PCR)

RT-PCR is a much more sensitive way of detecting specific mRNA by copying mRNA into cDNA by reverse transcriptase enzyme. It is very sensitive to detect a specific mRNA in a single cell. It has now been superceded by more accurate and simple method of real-time PCR. Since there is no reliable relationship between amount of template (Fig. **28**) added and ultimate amount of product detected after a fixed number of cycles.

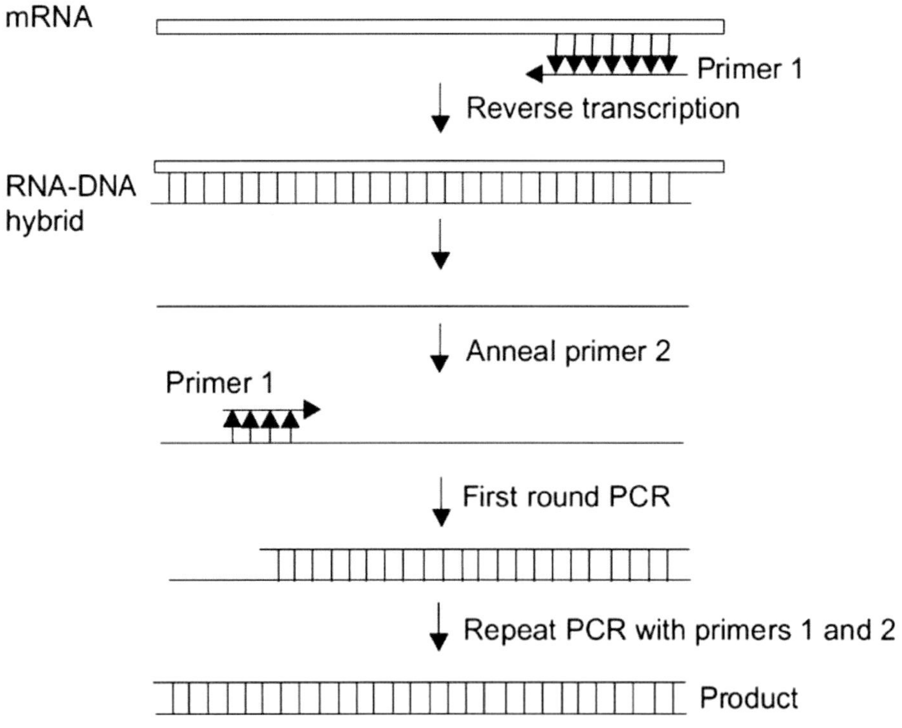

Fig. (28). RT-PCR.

Real-time RT-PCR

In real-time PCR, there is more reliable relationship between the amount of template and the number of cycles of amplification needed to produce a detectable product. This is achieved by using combination of dyes to label probes (that will bind to specific product). As amplification proceeds, double-stranded product is formed and resulting fluorescence is detected by the machine. The level of fluorescence will increase over several cycles and by extrapolation of resulting curve back to zero, one can determine number of cycles needed for formation of detectable amount of product. This value is known as CT value and is related to the initial amount of template "higher the value of initial template initially, will result in lower CT values". *e.g.*, if a sample A produced a detectable single after 20 cycles, it has a CT value of 20 (Fig. **29**).

- Real-time PCR is also an important technique for:
- Quantitative detection of specific DNA sequences
- Identification of specific alterations in DNA sequence
- Medical diagnostic applications

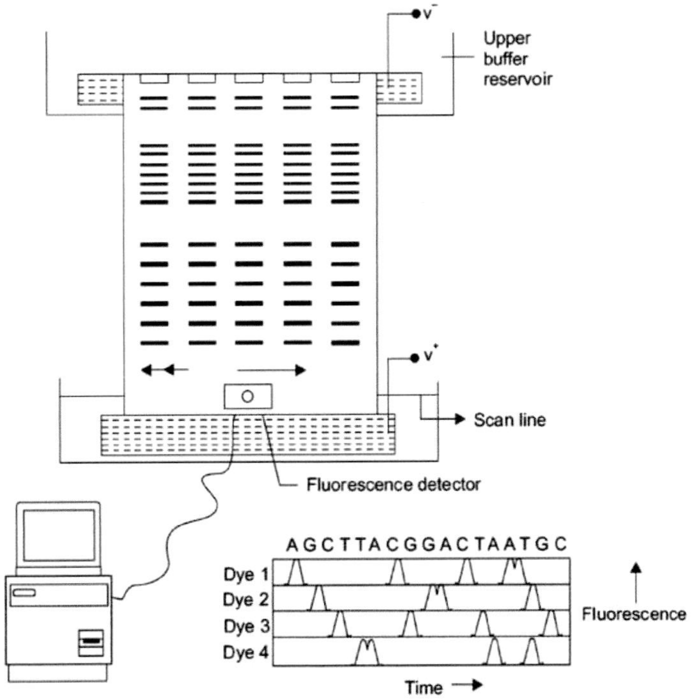

Fig. (29). Representation of correspondence between fluorescence in a single electrophoresis gene and nucleotide sequence.

In situ Hybridization

In this method, the target is found immobilized within a cell on a microscopic slide and labelled probe is hybridized to cell with metaphase chromosome and following counter staining gene is localized. DNA target is used for gross chromosomal mapping of genes.

Uses:

1. Identification/localization of gene
2. Detection of viruses

Primer Extension Assay

While studying gene expression, it is important to know how much mRNA is made and where does it start and stop. Studying the 3′ end of a eukaryotic mRNA species is rarely a problem. While construction of cDNA library, 5′ end is not always incorporated into cDNA.

The primer extension assay is used for exact mapping of 5′ terminus of mRNA. Firstly poly-A RNA is purified from a tissue or cell and mixed with radio-labelled oligonucleotide primer, complementary to region close to 5′ end of the sequence. Addition of reverse transcriptase extends primer to the very 5′ end of mRNA where polymerization automatically terminates. Then this new radioactive cDNA strand is run in gel for optimum resolution along with sequencing reaction of the same gene with same primer to identify transcription site down to the first base. In automated sequencers, fluorescent labels can be used to perform this assay.

TECHNIQUES FOR STUDY OF COMPLEX SAMPLES (COMPARING TRANSCRIPTOMES)

Norther blotting is suitable for comparing expression of a small number of genes and identification of disease genes when a limited number of strong candidate genes are known. Newer techniques have been developed for comparing mRNA species expressed in different samples. They include hybridization, array-based methods, *etc* (Figs. **30** and **31**).

Differential Screening

It is the most primitive method for identifying cloned genes in a gene library. Two identical filters containing DNA imprints of gene library are produced. Two complex mRNA mixtures (A and B) are used to prepare a probe by reverse transcription in the presence of radio-labelled nucleotides.

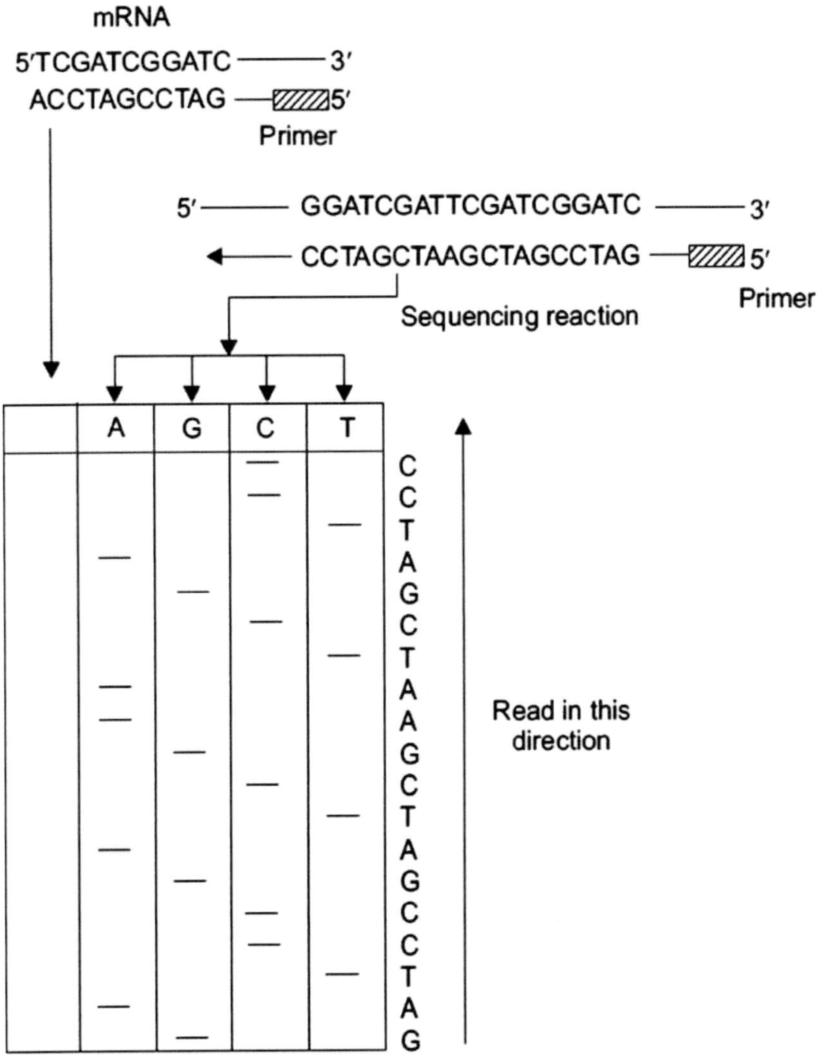

Fig. (30). Primer extension: determination of 5' end of mRNA.

Then, these pools of radioactive cDNA hybridize with duplicate filters separately. Clones that show a positive signal with one probe (say, in B) but not the other, are the candidate clones of expressed genes.

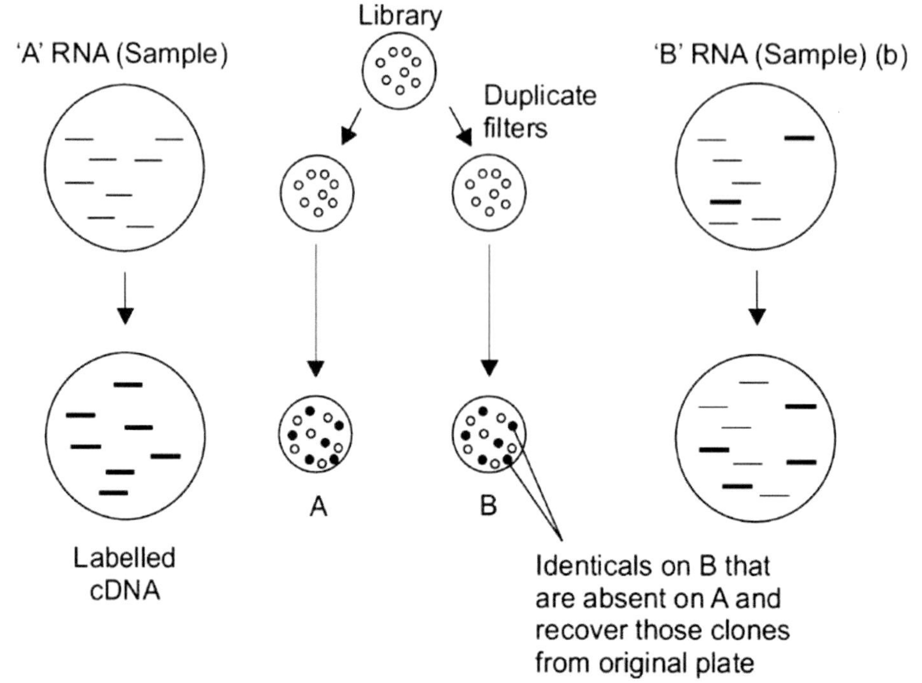

Fig. (31). Differential Screening of a gene library.

Subtractive Hybridization

It is an alternative procedure to remove common sequences from the probe and leaving only those which are present in test material (Fig. **32**).

Use

Subtractive tester transcript can be used as a probe for screening a gene library.

Disadvantage

It requires large amounts of mRNA, so, PCR combined with principle of above method is preferred. (Known as representational differential analysis, RDA).

Differential Display

It is a PCR-based method for comparing two cDNA populations. Two primers are used: one binds to poly—A tail and the other to random sequence.

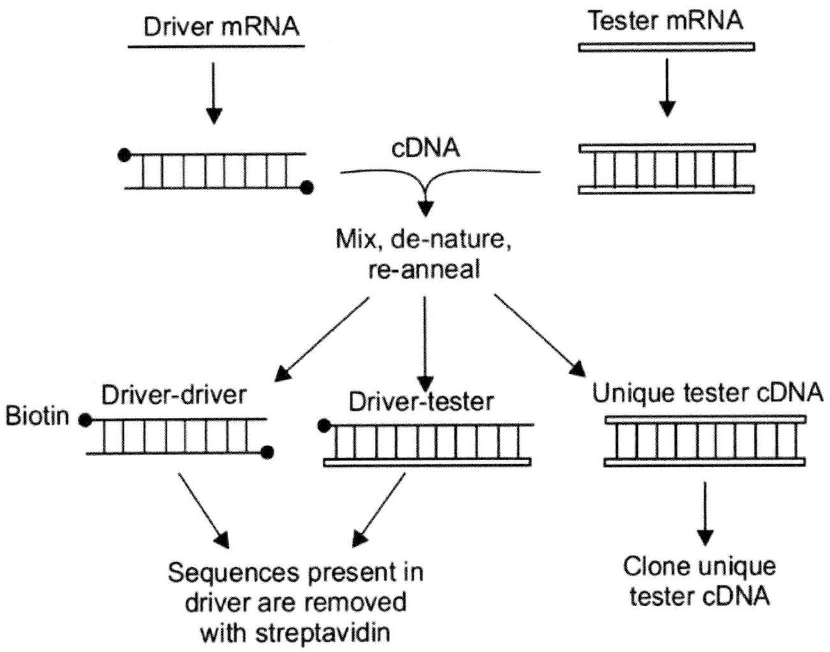

Fig. (32). Subtractive Hybridization.

Following PCR at very low annealing temperature the resulting subpopulation is small enough to be resolved in PAGE and sequenced. This procedure must be supplanted by more sophisticated techniques such as array technology, RDA.

Array-Based Method

Array—Array is a recent approach to analyze human genome. It involves production of a series of PCR products (oligonucleotides) which correspond to all predicted genes from a specified organism.

To analyse small genome, one can use sequences spaced at regular universals over the whole genome. A robot is used to produce tiny spots of each fragment in a precisely defined pattern on a treated glass slide. This is the Microarray.

Once the fragments are made, the machine is set up that can produce many identical copies of the same microarray. The sequence in the microarray represented in target organism result in a positive signal, while deletions will show up as absence of a signal.

Thus, microarrays are a very effective method of detecting insertions and deletions. Also, microarray of oligonucleotide sequences of known mutations or polymorphisms in a gene allow quick screening.

Also, presence of wide range of cDNA molecules derived from different environment can be tested.

WHOLE GENOME ARRAYS AVAILABLE

1. EST arrays
2. PCR based arrays

1. EST Arrays

ESTs are cDNA cloned where a lab is equipped with a robot to pick every clone from a library.

Also, transcriptome fingerprint for cDNA clones from different tissues can be treated. Systematic computer comparison has made it possible to identify which cDNA clones are unique. Also, cDNA arrays with non-redundant clones can be produced. By spotting these clones onto a membrane (macroarrays) or glass slide (microarrays), simultaneous study of majority of genes in humans, mouse and rat genome have been possible.

These microarrays used both 33P-label and fluorescent labels and data are collected by phosphoimager and microarray readers respectively.

2. PCR Based Arrays

In PCR, at least one clone representing each gene is obtained. However, this objective was not quite achieved in case of human genome.

ESTs are helpful in identifying genes with open reading frames. Mammalian genomes are much larger and complete array of PCR amplified products covering all genes in the entire human genome is possible.

TRANSLATIONAL ANALYSIS

The methods for studying protein expression are developed earlier than DNA cloning methods.

Western Blot

With SDS-PAGE, protein produced by cell can be analyzed and much higher resolution can be obtained by 2D-SDS-PAGE.

To detect a specific protein and for analysis of its expression, specific antibodies are used in combination with SDS-PAGE. These antibodies can be either labelled themselves or more commonly detected by second labelled antibody.

The analogy with a Southern blot led to this technique being termed Western Blotting. It identifies both presence or absence of a protein that reacts with the antigen as well as its size and estimation of relative levels of expression Fig. (**33**).

Immunochemistry and Immunohistochemistry

They help in intracellular localization of protein and thus give important clues to its function. Incorrect transport of a protein gives important information about a disease phenotype.

2-D-Electrophoresis

It involves isoelectric focussing in one direction and SDS-PAGE in the other.

Isoelectric Focussing

All proteins have a characteristic isoelectric point (pI) *i.e.*, the pH at which they are electrically neutral until they reach a pH equal to their pI at which they are no longer charged. The result is that each protein will focus at a characteristic point on the pH gradient (Table **9**), (Figs. **34**, **35** and **36**).

The second dimension separates the protein according to the size. Thus, a pattern of spots is finally obtained that can be compared with other patterns to identify proteins.

Table 9. Characteristics of isoelectric focussing.

pH	Charge on protein	Movement
At		
pH values below pI	Protein is positively charged	Move towards cathode (–ve)
pH values above pI	Protein is negatively charged	Move towards anode (+ve)

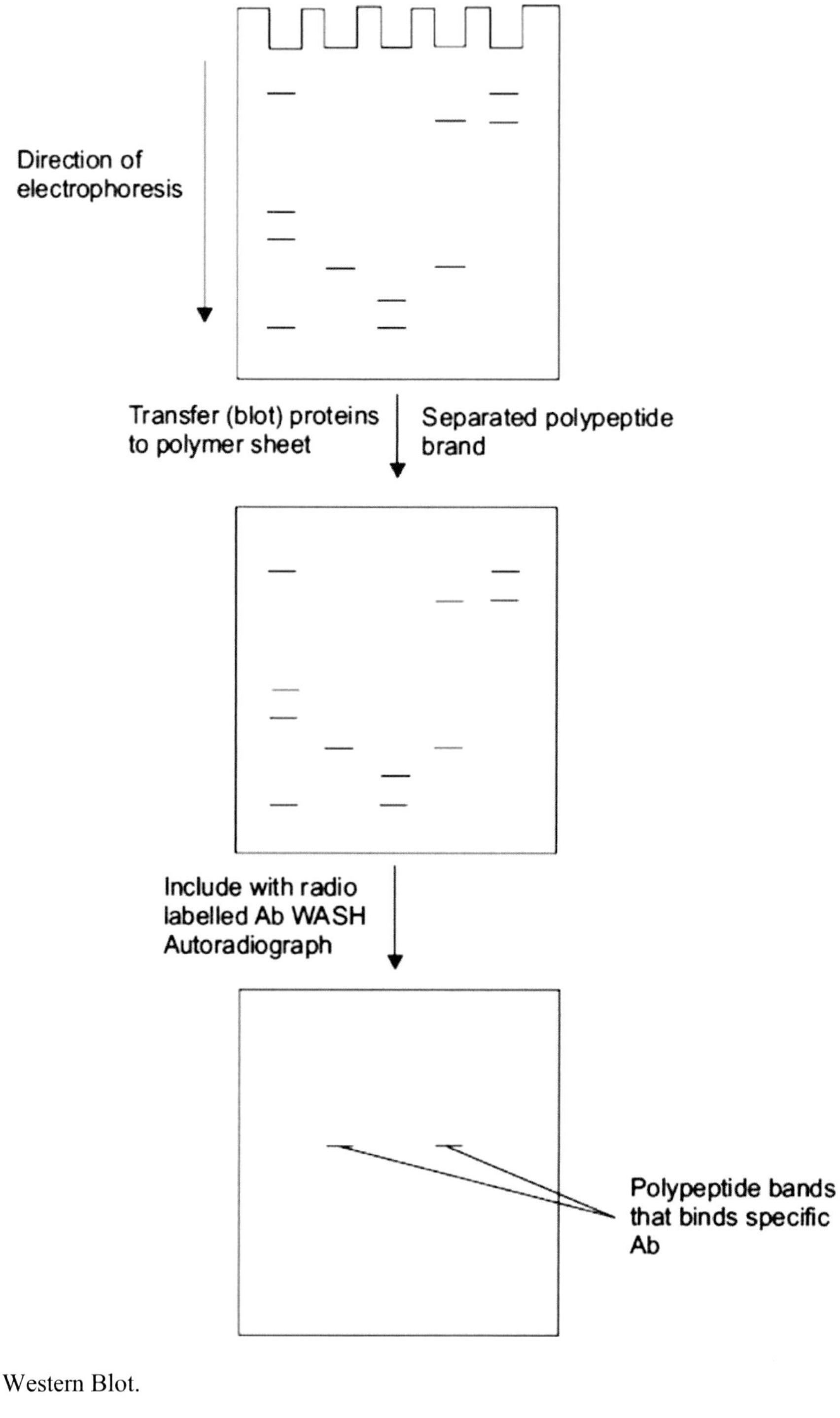

Fig. (33). Western Blot.

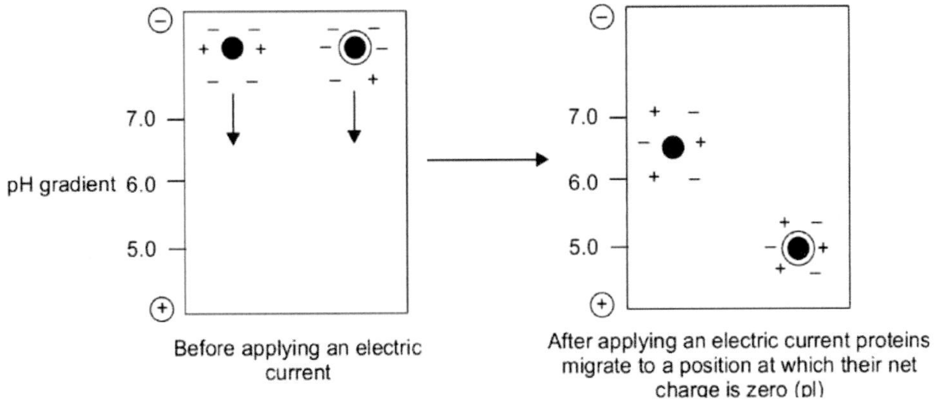

Fig. (34). Isoelectric Focussing.

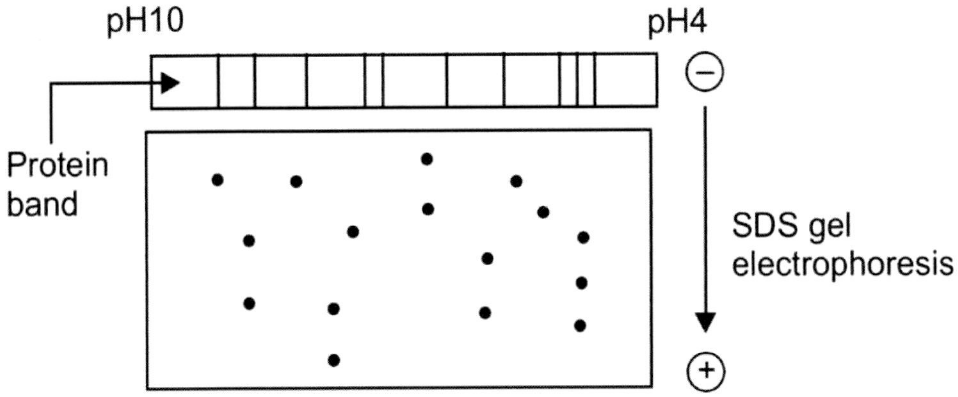

Fig. (35). 2-D-gel Electrophoresis.

ALTERNATIVES TO 2 DE

2DE is the workhouse of proteomics and recently this technique has been combined with Reverse Phase Microcapillary Liquid Chromatography (RPMLC) for enhancing the protein separation. Also, a procedure involving cation-exchange liquid chromatography followed by RPMLC has been combined with MS recently.

MASS SPECTROMETRY (MS)

It involves ionization of target molecules in a vacuum and accurate measurement of mass of resulting ions Fig. (**37**).

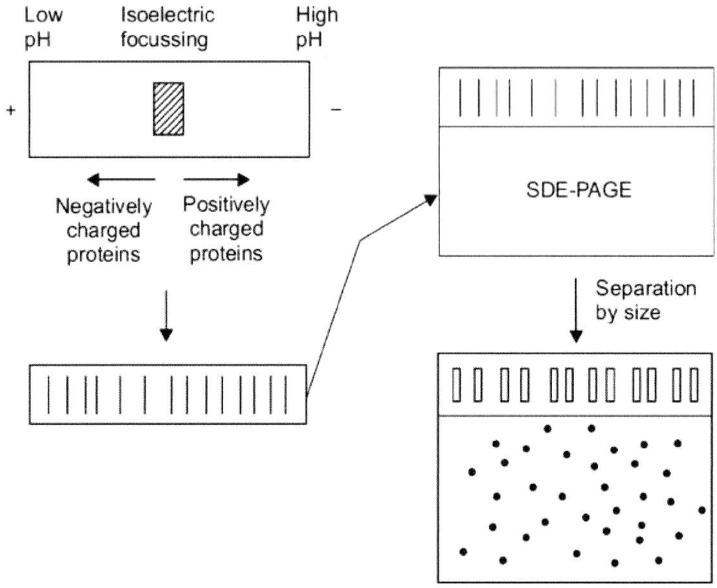

Fig. (36). 2-D-protein Electrophoresis.

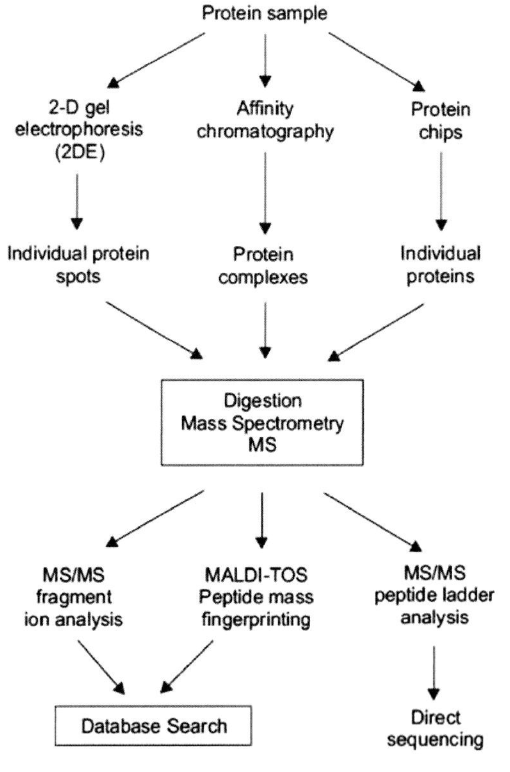

Fig. (37). Proteomics.

Two Strategies to Annotate Proteins

1. Peptide mass fingerprinting

It is carried by using MALDI-TOF analyses (matrix assisted laser desorption source coupled with a time-of-flight analyser) (Fig. **38**).

2. Fragment Ion searching.

It is carried out by using tandem MS and the database is searched for peptide mass and mass of its fragment ions.

Three Components of MS

1. Ionizer: It converts analyte into gas phase ions.
2. Mass analyzer: This separates ion according to mass: charge ratio.
3. Ion detectors.

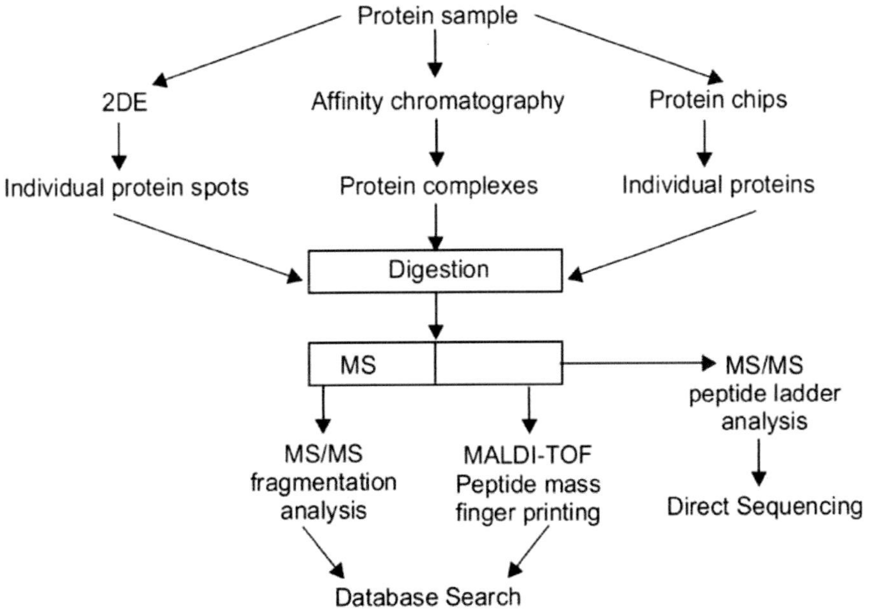

Fig. (38). Peptide mass fingerprinting.

PROTEIN ARRAYS AND PROTEIN CHIPS

2DE is an open system for proteomic analysis in which all proteins can be detected. For their characterization, it relies on MS.

Protein Arrays are emerging as useful closed system for proteome analysis. These are miniature devices in which proteins or molecules that recognize proteins are arrayed on a surface. In concept they are no different to DNA array, but they suffer from many practical limitations:

1. No amplification procedure exists for DNA.
2. Recognition parameters vary widely so the same reaction conditions could never be used for all proteins.
3. Labelling of proteins is variable since it could interfere with protein folding, binding.

General Protein Array

The device that can contain any type of proteins and is used to array protein-protein interactions with other molecules. And defection strategies include labelling, surface plasmon resonance Table **10**.

Different protein-arrays system:

1. UPA—Universal protein array with 96-well microtitre plates
2. Glass microarray—Protein array on glass slides.

Types of protein microarray available:

1. Antibody arrays (micro immuno-assays)
2. Antigen arrays (reverse immuno-assays)
3. General protein arrays
4. Arrays of specific capture agents, *e.g.*, aptamers, biochips, SS nucleotides

Table 10. Comparison of DNA and protein array.

	DNA array	**Protein array**
Amplification	Nucleic acid sequence can be amplified	No amplification procedure exists for protein
Sequences	Made up of 4 nucleotides	No such sequences
Principle of molecular Recognization	Hybridization between complementary base Paris	Recognition parameters vary widely
Number of probes	Single complex probe used	Same probe cannot be used
Labelling	Labels are incorporated evenly, does not interfere with hybridization	Labels are much more variable. Labelling of protein interfere with protein binding

MOLECULAR IMPRINTS OR PROTEIN CHIPS

They contain artificial recognition sites for proteins.

Molecularly Imprinted Polymers (MIPs)

MIPs depend on ability to emboss a polymeric substrate with recognition molecules. It is yet to be applied to proteome-wide expression analysis on mass-scale.

Broad-Capture Agent Biochips

These devices use broad specificity capture agents. They are commercially available. (Cipherigen Biosystems inc.) Protein chips bind different classes of proteins and they can be integrated with MS. Also, surface plasmon resonance-based protein chip integrated with MS are available.

SOLUTION ARRAYS

Next generation of miniature protein array platforms would be based on microfluidics.

DNA FINGER PRINTING AND FORENSIC ANALYSIS

Introduction

In 1985, after the emergence of PCR, this new forensic tool was used by investigators to look at a new kind of "fingerprint", the unique signature present in each person's genetic makeup.

DNA FINGERPRINT

Since every human being carries a unique set of genes novel assemblage of 3 billion base pairs formed into 23 pairs of chromosomes gives unique genetic identity to all individuals.

The uniform nature of DNA in a single individual and genetics availability between individuals make DNA fingerprinting possible. Also, each cell in a body shares the same DNA. This, cells collected in buccal swab (from check of a person) will perfectly match with those found in WBCs, skin cells or other tissues.

DNA TYPING

How is DNA Typing Performed?

Only 1/10th of 1% of DNA (~ 3 billion bp) differs from each person and unique DNA profile of an individual is observed using blood, bone, hair, body fluids.

Two Main Types of Forensic DNA Testing

- RFLP
- PCR

RFLP requires testing of large amount of DNA and DNA must not be degraded. PCR based testing is less time-consuming requires less DNA than RFLP and is effective in partially degraded samples.

But PCR-based tests are sensitive to contaminated DNA at crime scene and in lab.

VNTRs (variable number tandem repeats). VNTRs are of particular interest in determining genetic identity. They are inert portions containing repeated sequences of 1–100 bp. Each person has VNTRs inherited from his parents and no person has VNTRs identical to that of either parent (this could only occur in case of cloning). This uniqueness of an individual, VNTRs provides scientific marker of identity known as a DNA Fingerprint.

DNA fingerprints are restricted to detection of presence of microsatellites that are 1–6 nucleotide repeats dispersed throughout the chromosomes. The probes used to identify the DNA regions that surround specific microsatellites. Microsatellite short repeat segments are also termed Short Tandem Repeat or STR. Combined DNA Index System (CODIS) of FBI has 13 unique STRs for testing the DNA profiles.

PREPARING A DNA FINGERPRINT

Specimen Collection

Routinely investigators search for sources of DNA at the crime scene such as piece of cloth, licked envelope, cigarette but used cup or glass or anything else that might be a source of human cells. Tiny blood stains, smear of dried semen or trace of saliva often helps in cracking of a case.

Precautions at Crime Scene

- Wear disposable gloves and change them frequently
- Use disposable instruments, if not available, instruments should be thoroughly cleaned before and after handling each sample.
- To prevent contamination with microdroplets of saliva, avoid speaking, sneezing, and coughing
- While handling evidence, avoid touching any item that might contain DNA. Pack them in specifically designed evidence bags. Before packaging, air-dry the evidence. Mould/fungus can contaminate a sample

Enemies of Evidence

- Sunlight and high temperature can degrade the DNA.
- Bacteria can contaminate a sample before or during collection
- Mould/fungus due to moisture

Ideal Sample

1 ml or more of fresh whole blood treated with EDTA (ethylene diamine tetra acetic acid, anticoagulant): This quantity of whole blood contains an adequate number of WBCs with nuclear DNA (normal complement of human chromosomes).

Sources of Contamination of DNA Evidence

- Human error—major cause
- Sneeze, improper storage, failure to label every single sample
- Damage during analysis: DNA from technician or from other sources.

Agencies That Provide Accreditation to Forensic Labs

- American Society of Crime Lab Directors (ASCLD)
- National Forensic Science Technology Center (NSFTC)
- College of American Pathologists (CAP)
- FBI: has its own standard operating procedure.

Extraction and Purification of DNA is carried out in lab and unique signatures of DNA are transformed into visible evidence.

RFLP Analysis

RFLP: restriction fragment length polymorphism to isolate VNTRs, DNA is treated with restriction endonuclease that cuts DNA helix at specific sequences. Then, the DNA fragments are separated by gel electrophoresis (based on size of genetic fragment) and DNA is denatured chemically or by heat. DNA fragments are transferred from gel to nitrocellulose membrane by Southern Blot Technique and radioactive or fluorescent short strand probe are added.

Using single-stranded probes, unique DNA sequences are separated. Probes can be single locus or multilocus probes. (Usually 17 or more of bases). X-ray film is placed on the nitrocellulose and autoradiograph is generated which looks like a bar code. The bands produced are matched.

RFLP is not used as much as it once was in human analysis because it requires relatively large amounts of DNA.

PCR and DNA Amplification

Several thousand cells are required to do an RFLP analysis. Whereas PCR can be used to 'grow' or amplify sample into an amount that can be analyzed. In about three hours, the DNA segment can be increased by millions or billions. This rapid growth is very sensitive to contamination and a small error in laboratory procedure can result in duplication of a useless DNA sample a million times.

Dot Blot Analysis

DNA produced by PCR is identical to the original sample and DNA is applied to blot strips with dots containing a different DNA probe from human DNA. The DNA probe present in "dots" on the nitrocellulose strip are attached to an enzyme complex that converts a colourless substrate into a coloured are following binding (Figs. **39** and **40**).

STR (Short tandem repeats) Analysis

The specific regions (loci) with in nuclear DNA are evaluated by STR technology. Variability in STR regions can be used to distinguish a particular DNA profile from another. FBI uses 13 specific regions for CODIS and chances of two individuals having same 13 loci-DNA profile are more than one in a billion.

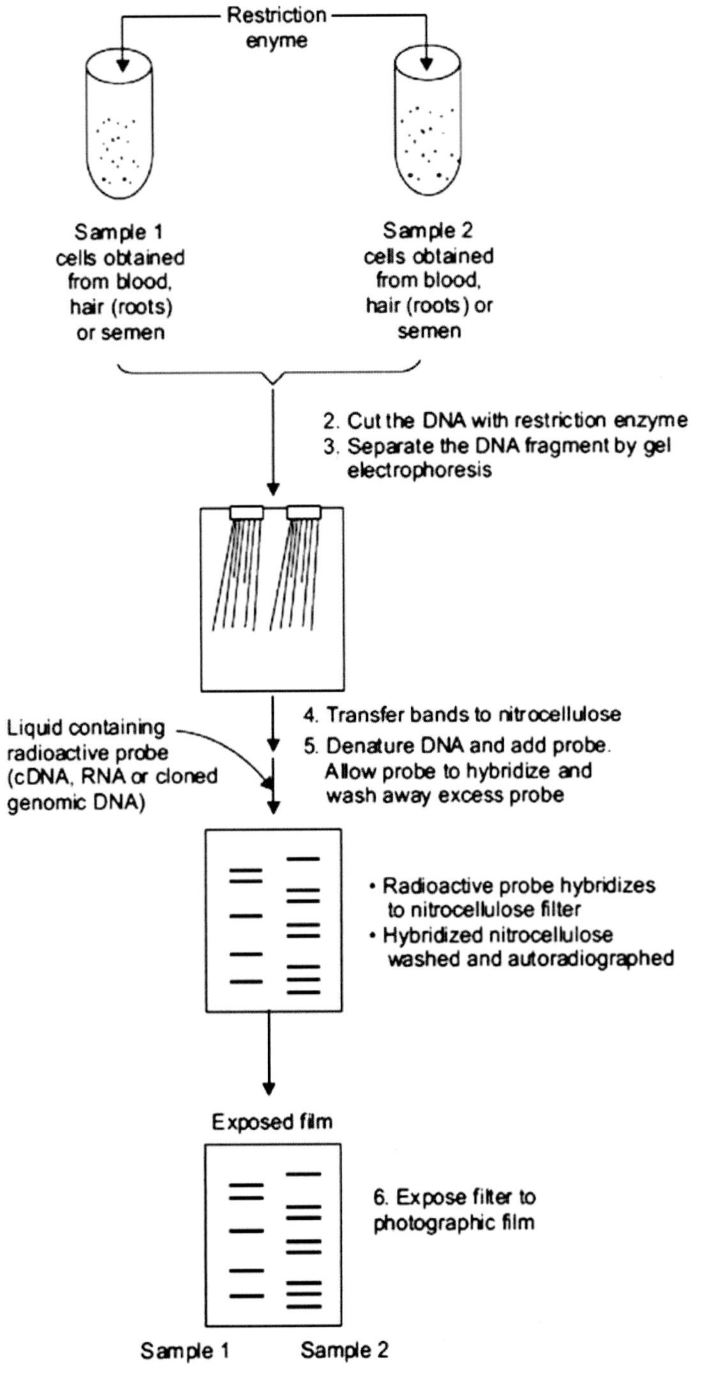

Fig. (39). Blot Analysis.

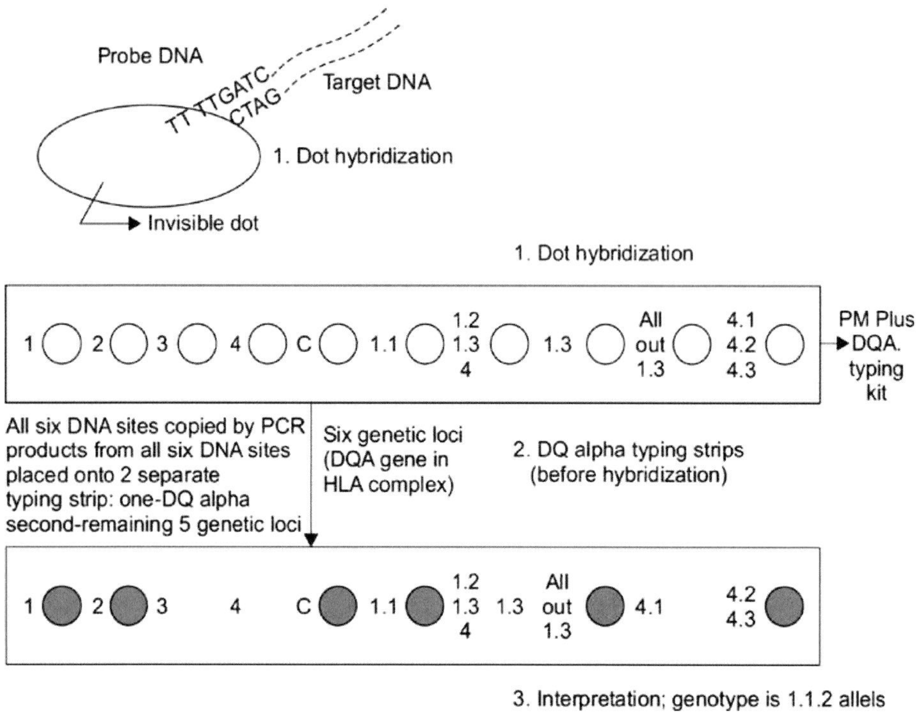

Fig. (40). Dot blot process: Example PMDQA 1 typing kit.

Mass Fatality Identification System (M-FI Sys)

In response to major acts of terrorism, namely, 9/11 tragedy and, natural disasters namely, South Asian Tsunami (2004), several companies developed new software programs to help match samples Isolate Chromosomal DNA from a sample of cells submitted four family members to DNA profiles obtained from victims. Myriad Genetics, Inc., gene code Forensics, DNA-View, Celera Genomics Bode Technology Group, Orchid Gene screen were several companies that assisted identification of victims of 9/11. Thailand Tsunami Victim Identification effort along with M-FI Sys software (by gene codes) were customized to analyze male-specific variations in Y chromosome (termed Y-STRs) in addition to mitochondrial DNA to aid identification of 2004 Tsunami victims.

Also, Gene Codes has established DNA Shoah Project to establish a genetic database of Naziera Holocaust survivors to reunite an estimated 10,000 post war orphans around the world.

DNA Profiling and Familial Relationships

Apart from crime solving, DNA shared by members of the same family, their relationships can be conclusively determined by comparing samples between two individuals.

Another use of DNA fingerprinting is paternity testing to resolve child support or custody disputes. New reproductive technologies such as *In vitro* fertilization artificial insemination with donor sperm, and surrogacy has raised issues of custody and paternity. Also, sperm mix-ups in fertility clinics can be resolved by DNA profiling. With amniocentesis it is possible to verify a child's parentage even before birth.

Debate

DNA Finger-printing a crime-fighting tool or invasion of privacy?

DNA-profiling databases, CODIS (Combined DNA Index system) run by FBI contains profiles of both convicted offenders and unidentified DNA profiles from crime scenes. Also, DNA profiles from illegal immigrants and detainee captives in war on terrorism will also be added to CODIS.

Some people are advocating that DNA profiles should be taken from all individuals at the time of birth to create database. Also, mass testing of individuals is advocated.

Opponents believe that even routine guest for DNA evidence during a criminal investigation continues to undermine fundamental right of privacy. Also, they believe that technique may be abused. They point out that taking a blood sample is a more invasive process than taking a set of fingerprints also, there is a possibility that DNA information could be some day used to discriminate against job seekers or those applying for health insurance. Hence, some people demand that all samples be destroyed after investigation of a specific case is completed.

People in favour of DNA collection pain out that trained professionals collect the blood sample DNA databases are regulated and secure future will prove whether it is a reasonable tool in effort against crime or an unwarranted invasion of privacy?

Mitochondrial DNA (mt DNA) Analysis

mt DNA can also be used to examine such DNA from samples that cannot be analyzed by RFLP or STR. RFLP, STR and PCR require nuclear DNA. Whereas mt DNA analysis uses DNA extracted from cellular organelle: mitochondrion. Older biological samples lack nucleated cellular material (*e.g.*, hair, bone, and teeth) and cannot be analyzed by STR and RFLP. They can be analyzed with mt DNA.

Mitochondrial DNA has maternal inheritance, *i.e.*, mitochondria of each new embryo come from mother's egg and father's sperm contributes only nuclear DNA, and no mitochondria mt DNA remains virtually the same from generation to generation and changes only about 1% every million years due to random mutations. Thus, DNA can be traced through maternal line with fingerprinting of mt DNA (Fig. **41**).

Y- Chromosome Analysis

Y-chromosome is passed directly from father to son, and this makes analysis of genetic markers on Y-chromosomes for tracing relationship among males. Y-chromosome can be analyzed by nuclear DNA (Mainly PCR) methods.

Other Advances in DNA Profiling

In addition to crime solving, DNA profiles from animals have been used in biological research and to preserve the 'pure' herds of domestic livestock.

mt DNA analysis has proven to be on good tool in evolutionary biology.

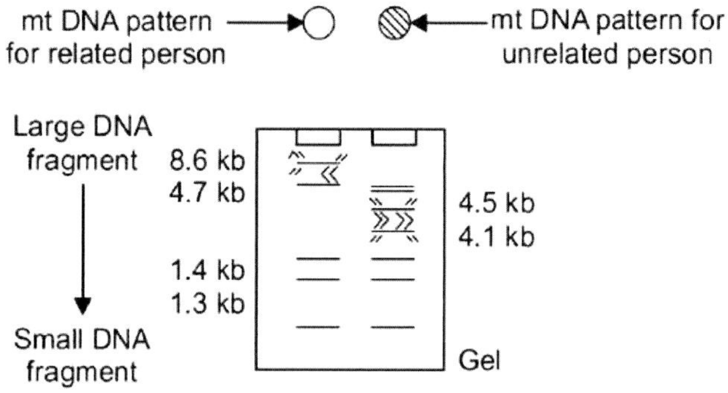

Fig. (41). Mitochondrial DNA pattern of inheritance. (Some gene show variation due to mutations).

Mitochondrial clock: Since mitochondria mutate 2%–4% per million years, gene frequency changes through time can be traced by the scientists. This help to differentiate between similar animal species and examine the role of base substitution during evolution. "Eve" hypothesis that used mt DNA evidence to trace majority of people now living an earth to a single female ancestor from ancient Africa, is based on mt DNA analysis. Also, royal blood lineage has been traced using mt DNA.

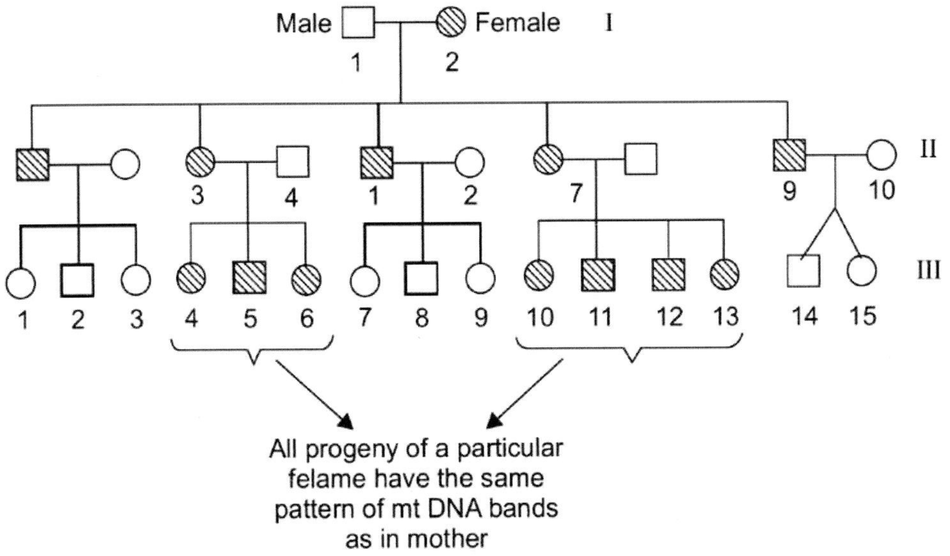

Fig. (42). Inheritance of mt DNA from mother.

Analysis of Non-human DNA

DNA evidence has been used to generate genetic profile of animals and plants. DNA profiling is regularly conducted by wildlife management authorities.

SETTING UP A NEW LAB

Introduction to Biotechnology Lab Notes and Labels

It is the duty of researcher and student to keep an orderly laboratory notebook to save and report their activities while preparing, executing, and analyzing all their experimentations including those that 'did not work'. Also, takes organisms, media and reagents must be adequately labelled to avoid confusion.

Chemical Handling and Storage

Clear protocol for handling and storage of chemicals should be established.

Maintenance of Equipment

Specific personnel/technician should be assigned the maintenance of specific instruments, apparatus, or bench spaces to have functional equipment.

Preparation and Storage of Buffers, Reagents

It is important to have proper stock of buffers and reagents to run a lab since biological materials require buffered solutions, expiry and storage of buffers and other reagents are fundamentally important.

Culture: Care and Maintenance

Maintenance of microorganism required for research is very important and bacteria and yeast are easily cultured by streak planting (once or twice a week). While criminal cell culture and subculture is performed by dissociating cells from culture flask with trypsin and diluting with a serum based medium and transferring them to new flasks.

Aseptic technique is required to prevent contamination that include filtration, autoclaving or irradiation of solutions, use of disposable or sterile culture ware; wearing the gloves and mask; cleaning and sterilization of work surfaces.

Handling and storing microbial strains correctly are most important in molecular biology.

Culture Preservation

Most cultures are preserved frozen in liquid nitrogen or in –80°C freezer, to prevent cell lysis by freezing and ice crystal formation intercellularly, 10%, (v/v) glycerol is added.

Cryogenic vials are used for preserving E. coli and yeast containing 1/3 full of 2 mm glass bead and 250 μL of 20% glycerol).

To reactivate a culture, remove from freezer, break away several glass beads, pour fixed beads onto agar plate and incubate.

Protein Handling: Precautions

Being extremely sensitive to denaturation and consequent loss of biological activity under typical lab condition require proper handling.

Precautions- Reasons

Wear gloves: protease from skin can degrade or contaminate

Mix and dissolve mildly: vigorous stirring can degrade integrity of protein molecule, they can foam.

- Maintain high concentration of protein solution (> 1 mg/ml): more stable.
- Wash or since glass ware or plastic ware with deionized water: washes away metal ions, prevent protein adsorption to glass.
- Store proteins at low temperature 4°C, frozen, lyophilized.
- Buffer condition of protein solution should be maintained (pH, salt concentration *etc.*)
- 50% (v/v) glycerol addition is useful for long term storage.
- Antimicrobial agents, *e.g.*, sodium oxide is appropriate to limit microbial growth during storage.
- Avoid repeat freezing and thawing

Nucleic Acid Storage

DNA being very stable and can be stored for years in dry or frozen form. Addition of EDTA preserves sample since it chelates Mg+2 required for nuclease activity. Autoclaving also helps to destroy most nucleases.

RNA isolation and storage is more difficult since RNases tend to be more thermostable and difficult to destroy. Ribonuclease free water and reagents are used.

LAB SAFETY

Safety in lab is very important and personnel should be assigned responsibility of ensuring lab safety, for researchers and students.

OSHA (Occupational Safety and Health Act) safety plan directs that each operation that uses potentially hazardous chemicals shall have a safety plan including equipments in labs such as pumps, hoods, electrical components, *etc.*

Lab Safety Plans

1. Material Safety Data Sheets (MSDS): Safety plan containing set of specifications for hazardous materials used.
2. Emergency exit routes: Map of building identifies the lab in terms of floor and rooms of interest.
3. Chemical waste disposal: Keep solid, liquid, and mixed wastes separately.
4. Biological waste: Includes vector, bacteria, enzyme, and autoclaving.
5. Radioactive waste: Should be carefully monitored.

Rules of Lab

- No smoking, drinking, eating (even storing food) in the lab.
- Wear lab coat, gloves, safety glass and masks (wherever applicable) and proper shoes. Tie back long hair and loose clothing.
- Remove gloves after handling hazardous substances and wash outsides of the glove.
- Dispose of microorganisms include tubes for their growth in Orange Bags marked "Biohazard" for autoclaving.
- Dispose of glass in designated marked boxes. Do not put glass or sharp objected in orange bags.
- Wear ear protection while working with sonicator.
- While working transilluminator, wear UV protective googles and face shield.
- Clean up spills immediately.
- Report all accidents to concerned person.
- Wash your hands before leaving lab.
- Know location of fire extinguisher, eye, wash station, emergency shower.

If there is trouble with a power supply or leads to a gel, report it to concerned person.

Good Lab Practice (GLP)

Good laboratory practice has become a major criterion in all biotechnology research (Fig. **43**).

Test Facilities

Test facilities include persons, premises, and operational unit necessary for conducting a study.

Study

Study is an experiment or set of experiments where a test substance is examined to obtain data in terms of its properties and/or safety with respect to human health and environment.

Study Plan is a document that defines scope of the study.

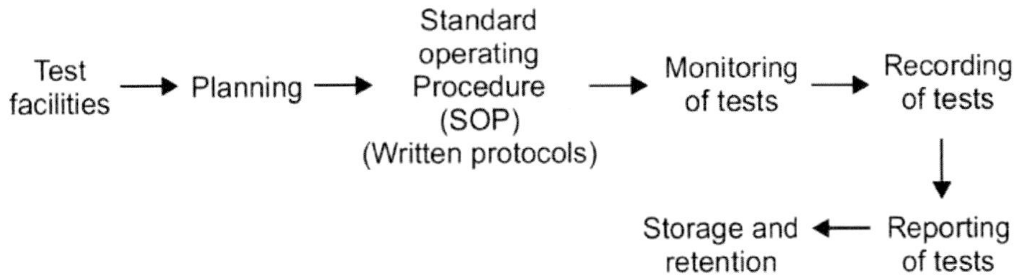

Fig. (43). Good lab practice.

Test Guidelines

They mean a set of test guidelines recommended for use.

Test System

Test system can be any animals plant, microbes, cellular, subcellular, chemical, or physical system or a combination.

Raw Data

Raw data is all original records and documentation that are result of original observations and activities in a study.

Specimen

Specimen can be any material derived from a test system for examination, analysis, or storage.

Test Substance

Test substance is a chemical substance or a mixture that is under investigation.

Reference Substance

Reference or control substance is any well-defined chemical substance or mixture other than the test substance to provide basis for comparison with the test substance.

Sample

Sample is any quantity of test or reference substance.

Batch

Batch is a specific lot of tests produced/done during a defined cycle of manufacture/procedure.

Vehicle

Vehicle or carrier is any agent which serves as a carrier to mix, disperse the test to facilitate its administration to the test system.

Organization of Test Facilities

It is the responsibility of person/organization to manage the test facilities according to principles of good lab practice.

Prerequisite:

1. Qualified personnel's, study director.
2. Availability of equipment, materials, and appropriate facilities.
3. Periodic training of professionals and technical staff.
4. Health and safety precautions are ensured according to regulations.
5. Quality assurance programme.
6. Maintenance of records: Study plan, standard operating procedures, and study results.

Quality Assurance (QA)

Quality assurance programme should be adopted and implemented by the test facility to ensure that principles of good lab practice are adhered to QA program is carried by an individual designated by the management and both external and internal quality assurance programmes are adopted.

Facilities

Test facility should be of suitable size, construction, and location to meet the requirements of the study and minimize interferences.

Also, design of test facility should provide an adequate degree of separation of different activities to assure proper conduct of each study.

Infrastructure

Test facility should have enough rooms or areas to isolate test systems and individual projects; storage areas for supplies and equipment; pre sample analysis area and cleaning and washing rooms. Also, separate area for receipt (sample receiving); Storage of substances (preferably cold room); record keeping. Also handling and disposal of wastes should be carried out according to regulatory requirements.

Test Systems

Test systems include physical/chemical systems (apparatus, chemicals reference substances) biological system (microbial, plant, animal, human, other cellular and subcellular systems).

Standard Operating Procedures

Each lab unit should have standard operating procedures/mammals to ensure quality and integrity of the data generated from the study.

Components of Test System

- Room preparation
- Receipt, transfer, proper placement, identification, and care of test system
- Test system preparation, observation
- Collection, identification, and handling of specimens
- Quality assurance procedures
- Health and safety precautions
- Reporting system
- Storage and retention of records and material

Quality management in lab

There is a growing interest in accreditation of medical laboratories throughout the world to implement quality and competence in medical laboratories.

ISO (International Organization of Standards)

ISO 9000:2000 defines quality as "the degree to which a set of inherent characteristics fulfils requirements".

QUALITY MANAGEMENT

Quality management in lab involves specifying the requirements passed by different clinical situations and ensuring that inherent characteristics of laboratory parameter fulfils the specified requirement. This means that lab parameter is fit for its intended purpose.

Quality Management System (QMS)

Quality management system is a mechanism for quality management, and it ensures quality. QMS has been described as "Integration of organizational structures, processes, procedures and resources needed to fulfil a quality policy and thus meet needs and requirements of users"

Accreditation

Accreditation system include four elements:

1. Accreditation body
2. Standards
3. Assessors
4. Laboratory

Accreditation body

It oversees the assessments and grants accreditation.

Standards

A laboratory must comply certain standards to gain accreditation.

Assessors

Assessor is a person who establishes compliance with the standards by conducting an assessment.

Laboratory

Laboratory is required to or voluntarily seeks to comply with the standards.

International Standards

To reflect quest for quality and harmonization of practice from laboratory to laboratory, from country to country, ISO has published international standards (www.iso.org)

ISO 900:2000	Quality management systems requirements: For certification of QMS
ISO/IEC 17025:2005	Central requirements for the competence of testing and calibration laboratory: For accreditation of quality and competence of testing and calibration lab.
ISO 15189:2007	Medical lab: requirements for quality and competence; For accreditation of quality and competence of medical lab.

Accreditation Bodies and Standards

General Assembly of International Laboratory Accreditation Corporation (www.ilac.org) has published guidelines for laboratory accreditation.

Unsatisfactory Aspect: ISO

17035:2005:	Does not address issues related to medical lab.
9001–2000:	Does not include competence requirement
1589:2007:	QMS (management) and (competence) technical requirements.

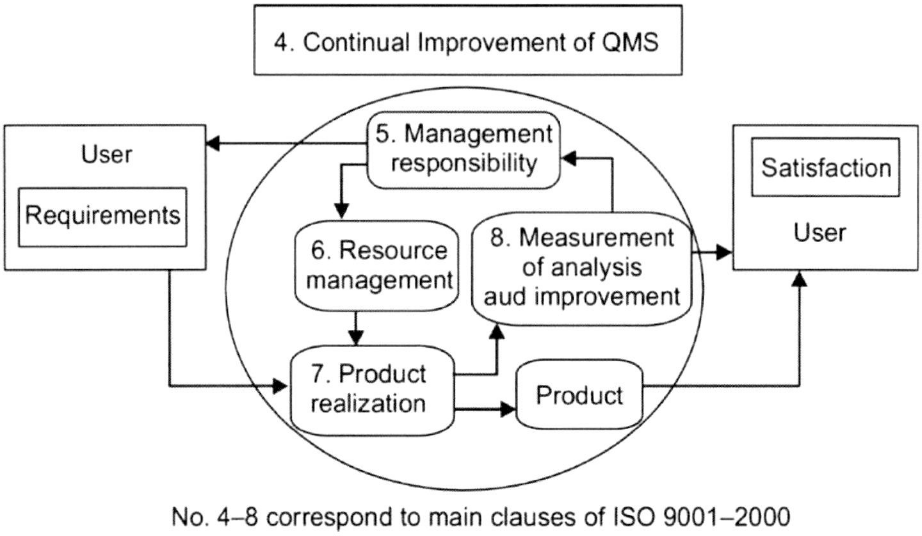

Fig. (44). ISO 9001-2000 model for QMS.

Actions in Quality Management

There is a sequence of action in quality management: Ist step is creation of policies that can be defined as overall intentions and directions of an organizations. 2nd step is objectives and plans involve making of plans and setting objectives to enable fulfilment of intentions expressed in policies. Third step involves definition of activities needed to carryout intentions. Fourth step procedures are practical way in which intentions are translated into action. Fifth step: records, provide evidence, on a day-to-day basis, that procedures have been carried out correctively and intentions have been fulfilled (Fig. **44**).

Documentation

The primary requirement for evidence is to enable the lab to reconstruct its examination and processes because of questions asked by the users of lab concerning performance.

Documentation

Quality manual should not be more than 25 pages in length and should contain quality policy, processes that take place in the lab.

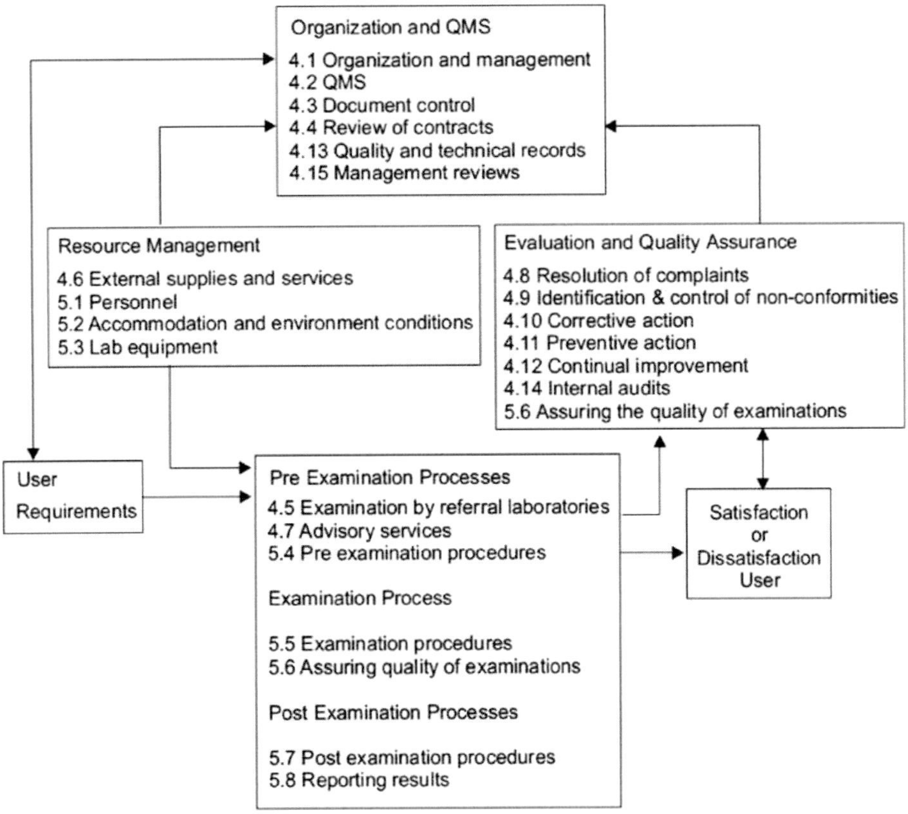

Fig. (45). ISO 15189-2003.

To pursue and maintain a particular time of action, objectives must be set, and plans executed.

There should be reference to procedures. SOP (standard operating procedures) are procedures where policies have been translated into actions. Procedures should contain references to (working) instructions. This level of documentation involves practical day-to-day work instructions that are needed near the work situations for easy reference (Fig. **45**).

Forms are final level in hierarchy of documentation. Forms are the evidence that a procedure and/or related instructions have been carried out.

Document Control

Control of documents requires their approval for adequacy, review and update as required prior to their release. It should be decided at an early stage in which form document register should be prepared. Nowadays, off-the-shelf commercial products are available, namely, Q-pulse by Gael Quality (free 30-days trial version is available at www.gaelquality.com)

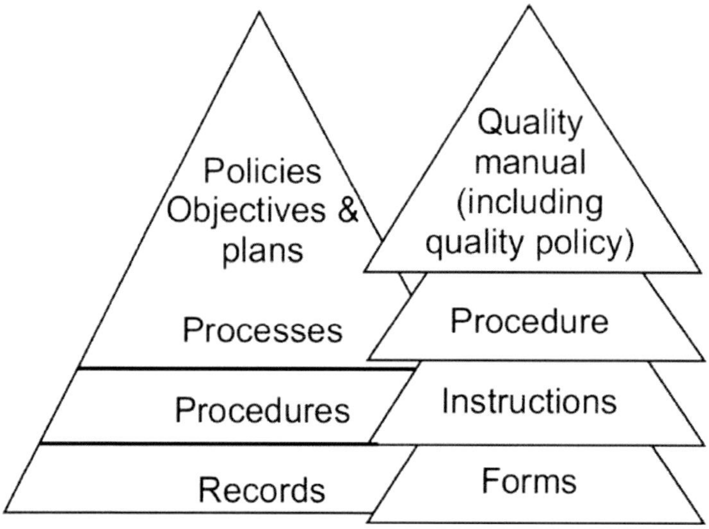

Fig. (46). Quality Management.

Control of Records and Clinical Material

ISO 9001 says "records shall be established and maintained to provide evidence of conformity to requirements and of effective running of QMS ISO 9001, being a quality standard, refers to retention and storage of quality records.

ISO 17025 and ISO 15189 being lab focused standards, refer to retention and control of quality and process record and in case of ISO 15189, clinical material as well.

Review and Improvement

Any lab should be evaluating its activities constantly and seek to continually maintain and improve quality terms as "quality assurance".

Internal Audit

Audit (ISO) is systematic independent and documented process after obtaining evidence and evaluating it objectively to determine the extent to which audit criteria are fulfilled.

Internal audit is conducted by the lab itself (or occasionally on behalf of a lab by an outside auditor) on some aspect of lab activity.

External Audit

As termed assessment is conducted by some persons or bodies interested in the organization or regulatory authority.

Cooperative Audit

It is conducted between the lab and another party for mutual benefit.

Non-conformities (Corrective or Preventive Action). It can be identified as

i. Reactive audit in response to a problem occurring in the conduct of an established process and leading to need for remedial and/or corrective action or continual improvement.
ii. Proactive audit that can identify potential non-conformities that require preventive action, that removes root cause of potential non-conformity.

Both corrective and preventive action are at the core of continual improvement. Management review is a crucial part of a quality management system of a lab. It sets overall objectives for the following year and within the lab they are translated into objectives for the staff and training needs of staff (Fig. **46**).

Inputs to a Management Review

- Assessment of user satisfaction and complaints
- Internal audit of QMS
- Internal audit of examination process
- External quality assessment reports
- Reports of Assessment by outside bodies
- Status of preventive, corrective, and improvement actions
- Major changes in organization and management, resource, or process.

Safety in Biomedical Research Laboratories

The safety operations of a lab that focuses on biomedical research is difficult. There are numerous aids available for developing safety plans for biomedical lab. There are extensive governmental regulations focussed on protecting health and safety of lab employees and many governmental and non-governmental organizations provide guidance concerning safety regulations and maintenance of safe working environment.

Internet Resources on Lab Safety

www.osha.gov	Occupational Safety and Health Administration, USA
www.cap.org	College of American Pathologists
www.cdc.gov	Centers for Disease control and Prevention
www.fda.gov/cber	Food and Drug Administration, Center for Biologic Evaluation and Research
www.absa.org	American Biological safety Association
www.epa.gov	Environment Protection Agency
www.cdc.gov/niosh/database.html	National Institute for Occupational safety and Health
www.lbl.gov/ehs/pub 3000/ch08-html	Lawrence Berkeley National Lab Health and Safety

Training in Safety

Training in each area of safety (*e.g.*, biohazards and chemical hazards) follows the same general approaches and has the same general requirements. Training in each area of safety that is important to a specific employee should be provided by trainers before he begins work in the lab.

Biological Safety

All human tissues and animals are inherently dangerous and should be handled with universal precautions. Also, all employees of the organizations handling human and animal tissues should be educated in the potential hazards/dangers of human tissues. They should be educated regarding what to do to avoid exposures *via* cuts, sticks, splashes, oral, and respiratory transmissions, and actions to take if exposure occurs. Also, they should be familiar with applicable governmental regulations related to exposure to human tissues.

Biohazards in Lab

- Infections
- Prions (CJ disease mad cow disease scrapie)
- Anthrax (in animal tissues)
- HIV, hepatitis
- Transfecting cells with specific genetic products: self-replicating viral vectors.
- Reagents and research products derived from human or animals: CJ disease, mad cow disease
- Spread of newly identified infections, *e.g.*, SARS access the countries
- When a "new" disease is notices which may be studied or diagnosed or to which employee may be exposed, planning should be done to deal with such situations.
- Bioterrorism agents: Anthrax, smallpox
- Lab equipment, ventilation, cooling system, drains, sinks, inoculators cell culture, culture media, refrigerators, leftover food may develop colonization.

Chemical Safety

Written chemical hygiene plan should be planned that can protect employees from hazardous chemicals in the lab and keeping chemical exposures below the action level.

Also, formaldehyde standard should be incorporated into safety plan of lab involved with fixation of tissue specimens.

Regulations related to Chemical Safety

- 29 CFR 1910, 1450 (Occupational exposure to hazardous chemicals in lab)
- 29 CFR 1910–1200 (Hazard communication standard)

- 29 CFR 1910, 1048 (Formaldehyde standard)

MSDS: Material Safety Data Sheet

- MSDS are prepared by manufacturers and are available from manufacturer of the chemical.
- MSDS lists various hazards of specific chemicals, namely, toxicity, explosive potential, and categories of danger (strong oxidizers).
- Also, procedures to minimize toxic exposures and contact information for additional information about chemical can be obtained.
- Combinations of chemicals that may be serious hazards may not be specified in MSDS.
- Also, for biomedical research lab MSDS do not address specific uses or conditions to which a chemical must be exposed.

Chemical Hazards

Toxic, carcinogenic, teratogenic.

Explosive

Opening of old ether, picric acid bottle.

Accidental

Unaware combinations of chemicals.

Electrical Safety

By ensuring that all electrical equipment is grounded and tested before first purchase and yearly inspection, electrical injuries can be avoided. Care should be taken with electrical appliances around water sources.

Fire Safety

Local fire department inspections, yearly fire drills, and posting of emergency exit pathways should be carried out. Also, emergency exists should never be blocked, obstructed, or locked and hallways must not be obstructed or clutter. Similarly, access to fire blankets, showers and fire equipment must not be impeded.

Store flammable agents appropriately and only in a fire cabinet which should be placed away from exit of room/areas. Regulate smoking and furniture, rug and equipment should be constructed of non-flammable material.

Physical Safety

Physical safety ranges from preventing falls to ensuring employees are not physically injured or intimidated by others.

Sources of Physical Injury in Lab

- Tears in rugs
- Broken steps
- Water, soap, paraffin, and other slippery substances on floors
- Inappropriate use of ladders, chairs
- Unrestrained gas cylinder
- Unbalanced fire cabinets
- Inadequately secured shelves
- Temperature burns: cold (liquid nitrogen) and hot
- Unauthorized personnel in lab.

Radiological Safety

Radioactive material should be stored according to radiological safety plan. Extensive training should be imparted to personnel who utilize or encounter radioactive material. Periodic survey of lab area to detect contamination by strong β and γ-emitters. Personnel should be shielded from exposure to radiation by using shielding, appropriate lab clothing and safety equipment. Avoid contamination by containing all radioactive spills and contamination and cleaning up all spills.

Thus, lab safety can be maintained by careful evaluation of all safety incidents and safety plan.

Biological Hazards of DNA Technology

Recombinant DNA technology is used to improve animal and plant stocks for food production, and recombinant microbial strains are being used to deal with environmental waste products. With the introduction of use of these techniques, serious potential consequences can follow, *e.g.*, if engineered microbe strains are released into the environment can cause more problems than they solve!

Danger of producing transgenic organisms that could contain genes for antibiotic resistance or cancer susceptibility. GMAG (Genetic Manipulation Advisory Group, UK) and NIH (National Institute of Health, USA) have laid down careful guidelines for use of recombinant DNA techniques.

Ways to Minimize Biohazards Physical Containment Methods

Effort should be made to contain potentially dangerous microorganisms in specially designed lab having special ventilator systems. Grading of lab are done according to type of experiments being conducted from C1 (minimum containment) to CIV (maximum containment). CIV containment are used to lab involved in biological warfare.

Biological Containment Methods

Host organisms used in recombinant DNA work can be attenuated or crippled so that they cannot survive outside the specialized lab culture conditions.

Combination of physical containment and use of attenuated organisms will reduce the risk of any possible hazards. GMAG and NIH Guidelines should be implemented, and great care should be exercised in this field.

STUDENT'S ACTIVITY

1. Enumerate the features of human genome.
2. What is ENCODE?
3. What do you understand by recombinant DNA technology?
4. List the applications of recombinant DNA technology.
5. Enlist basic tools of DNA cloning.
6. Give a comparison of genomic and cDNA library.

EXERCISE

1. What do you understand by a genetic and physical map?
2. Give an example of map-based DNA cloning using restriction digestion.
3. Describe sequencing.
4. What is DNA library?
5. Discuss advantage of protein array in proteomic research.
6. Discuss various uses of recombinant DNA technology.
7. Describe various blotting techniques.
8. What is gene cloning?

9. What are micro arrays?
10. What is mass spectrometry?
11. Compare genomics and proteomics.
12. What is a vector?
13. Comparing colony and plaque hybridization.
14. What are SSRs? Give its uses?
15. What is genomics?
16. What is EST?
17. Give an account of CpG.
18. What is positional cloning? Enlist its applications.
19. What are candidate genes?
20. What are the two main phases of gene expression? Enlist the techniques of analysis of gene expression?
21. What is a transcriptome? Give techniques for its analysis.
22. What is translational analysis? Give the techniques used for this.
23. Compare MALDI with other methods of MS.

CONCLUSION

In 1988, US National Research Council's special committee formulated a 15-year human genome project, costing some $200 million a year. The final sequence was accomplished in April 2003, with 99.99% sequence accuracy, with no gaps. Of the total 3.2 Gb DNA of the human genome, 2.9 Gb consists of weakly, staining gene-rich euchromatic proteins. By using restriction enzymes, DNA is cut into suitable fragments and then ligated with appropriate fragments to produce a recombinant DNA. 5 main types of commonly used vectors: Plasmid, Bacteriophage, cosmid, bacterial (BAC) and yeast artificial chromosomes (YAC). Following the introduction of foreign DNA fragments into the vector, the recombinant vector is introduced into modified bacterial or yeast host cells, which multiply and produce large quantities of identical copies of the original single target DNA or CLONES. Genes can be directly injected into fruit flies, worms, zebrafish, and mice to create animals carrying integrated genes. Treating human genetic disorders by restoring functional genes through the modification of a mutant gene or by the introduction of a gene by Gene therapy using viral vectors is an alternative strategy. Genomic DNA sequence databases of sequence homology to known genes as well as DNA sequences specific to all genes are available. Those genes which are likely to be involved in the pathogenesis of the inherited disorder are known as candidate genes. In the analysis of gene expression, two main phases of gene expression are transcription and translation. Protein Arrays are emerging as a useful closed system for proteome analysis. These are miniature devices in which proteins or molecules that recognize proteins are arrayed on a surface. Since every human being carries a unique set of genes, novel assemblage of 3 billion base pairs formed into 23 pairs of chromosomes give a unique genetic identity to all individuals. Two Quality management in lab involves specifying the requirements passed by different clinical situations and ensuring that inherent characteristics of laboratory parameters fulfil the specified requirement. This means that the lab parameter is fit for its intended purpose. The safety operations of a lab that focus on biomedical research are difficult. There are numerous aids available for developing safety plans for a biomedical lab. There are extensive governmental regulations focussed on protecting health and safety of lab employees and many governmental and non-governmental organizations provide guidance concerning safety regulations and maintenance of a safe working environment.

CONSENT OF PUBLICATION

Not applicable.

CONFLICT OF INTEREST

No potential conflict of interest is declared by the author. It is also declared the complete work is an individual effort by the author and there was no financial/ administrative/ academic support availed from any individual/ institution /organization.

ACKNOWLEDGMENT

Declared none.

BIBLIOGRAPHY

[1] Molecular Cloning: A Laboratory Manual – Joseph Sambrook and David Russell.
[2] Principles of Gene Manipulation and Genomics – Sandy B. Primrose and Richard Twyman.
[3] Molecular Biotechnology: Principles and applications of recombinant DNA –Bernard R. Glick and Jack J. Pasternak.

CHAPTER 3

Bioinformatics and Application of Computers

LEARNING OBJECTIVES

This chapter gives overview of tools and techniques of Bioinformatics; approaches for studying sequence analysis, protein- protein interactions; approaches in studying evolution of life; signal processing and artificial intelligence in bioinformatics; virtual cell and insilico technology; digital technology and robotics in biotechnology.

Abstract: Bioinformatics applications are effective in generating the vast quantity of inputs. Term simulation is the computation for developing algorithms and software, construction of database and curation, and analysis of gene sequence, functions, and structures. Understanding of genetic control of complex dynamic traits has fundamental importance in research fields of agriculture, evolution, and biomedical genetics. The advances in bioinformatics tools have changed research in both basic and applied biological sciences and these tools are enabling scientists to gain knowledge of complex biological systems. Also, they allow implementation of results towards novel developments in biomedical applications and contribute to promoting both individual and population welfare.

Keywords: Aptamers, Biochips, Data mining, Databases, Genomic, Gene expression array, Phylogenetics, Proteome.

BIOINFORMATICS

INTRODUCTION

It is the science of using information to understand biology. It is conceptualising biology in terms of molecules and applying informatics techniques (computer science, applied mathematics and statistics) to organise their information associated with these molecules.

Thus, bioinformatics is concerned with development and application of computer software and hardware to get, store, analyze and visualize biological information. By providing algorithms, databases, user interfaces and statistical tools, comparison of DNA sequences are possible.

The long-term value of bioinformatics and data mining capabilities does not lie so much in developing tools, as it does in connecting knowledge or information into

Simmi Kharb, Akshat Singh, Abhyuday Singh & Deepa Kharb (Eds.)

products like therapeutics, animal, and plant bioreactors in the Fig. (**1**) form of genetically modified organisms, newly discovered genes, *etc*.

Bioinformatics and data mining are two latest areas of research involving computer-assisted management of data generated for biotechnology applications. The information generated in genomics is enormous and its interpretation requires the use of powerful computers and specific software's.

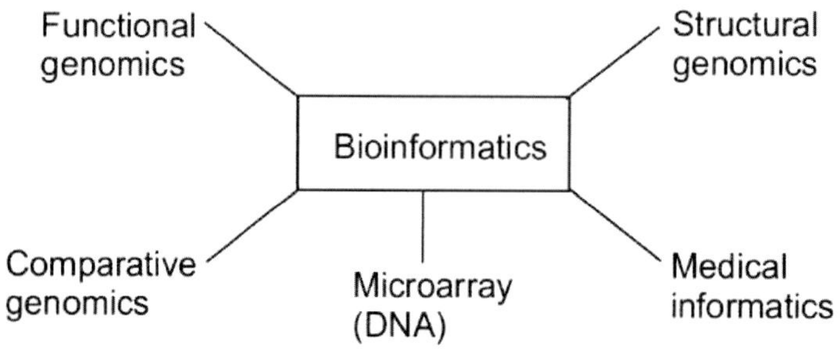

Fig. (1). Recent fields of bioinformatics.

TERMINOLOGY

Genomics

Term genomics has been derived from the word genome, which means haploid DNA content of an organism.

Term *genomics* deals with the genome as a whole and had its origin in the human genome project, which involved determination of the nucleotide sequence of the whole genome.

Today, genomics includes sequencing of genomes, determination of the complete set of proteins encoded by an organism and functioning of genes and metabolic pathways in an organism.

HISTORY OF BIOINFORMATICS

Bioinformatics involves creation, maintenance, and use of databases, to which new data on DNA and protein sequences are constantly added. Bioinformatics came into existence in 1980s after automated DNA and protein sequencing became possible and computers became central repositories that are accessible world-wide. Four years later, bioinformatics proved itself as a foundation of future biotechnology (Table **1**).

Table 1. Chronology of major events in genome sequencing and bioinformatics.

1962	Pauling's theory of molecular evolution
1970	Needleman-Wunsch algorithm
1971	DNA sequencing
1981	Dolittle's concept of sequence motif, Smith-Waterman algorithm
1982	Sequencing of phage lambda genome
1984–1990	Discussion in scientific community for sequencing genome
1985	Sequence database searching algorithm
1986	Human Genome project proposed
1988	Creation of NCBI (National Centre for Biotechnology Information) at NIH/NLM
1990	Human Genome project started
1988	EMBnet: network for database distribution
1990	BLAST

(Table 1) cont.....

1991	EST (Expressed sequence tag) sequencing
1993	Sanger Centre (Hinxton, UK)
1994	EBI (European Bioinformatics Institute) Hinxton, UK
1995	Sequencing of H. influenzae genome
1996	Sequencing of yeast genome (Saccharomyces cerevisiae)
1997	Sequencing of E. coli genome
1998	C. elegans genome sequenced
1999	D. melanogaster genome sequenced
2001	Human genome working draft (Home sapiens) published (90% genome sequenced)

In early 80s, BIONET (Biology Network) was created in Europe to allow use of computers and exchange of software package among its users. This was followed by release of NAPDB (nucleic acid and protein data bank) in 1984 which included of EMBL's nucleotide sequence database and protein data bank of 1200 sequences. NAPDB was renamed as COMSEQ and sold to GENOFIT company which released its first PC compatible version with 33 programs. Intelli-Genetics bought the exclusive rights of COMPSEQ with release of PC/GENE packages with many modified releases, the last version being 6.8.5 version (1995) with 82 programs.

Then come the era of database and their dictionary. The first to be developed was PROSITE in mid 80s to provide database of protein sequences and structures. This database could be used with SEQANALREF software to analyze and compare sequences. Then in 1986, SWISS-PORT protein data bank was developed which is still popular and considered as a valuable resource for protein sequence and structure.

Following emergence of proteomics in 1990s, databases dealing with 2-D Page maps of proteins came into existence, namely, SWISS-2D PAGE, NIH, USA and EMPL, Europe also developed several databases and softwares.

In mid-1990s, networking tools and web servers were made available and networking tools and web the field of bioinformatics and in 21st century, this took off its full bloom.

Thus, bioinformatics has appeared as a scientific discipline encompassing the application of computer science and technology to analyse and manage biological data.

Since sequence data is accumulating rapidly and powerful sequence analysis software and never algorithms are needed to transform the sequence into digital symbols. Only limited alphabet is needed to stand for nucleotide and amino acid monomers (as digital symbols). The data so generated Fig. (**2**) helps to differentiate genetic data from other types of biological data.

THREE LEVELS OF BIOINFORMATICS

1.Analysis of a single gene (protein)

2.Analysis of complete genomes

3.Analysis of genes and genomes with respect to functional data

Analysis of Single Gene

i.Similarity with other known genes

ii.Phylogenetic trees, evolutionary relationships

iii.Identification of well-defined domains in the sequence

iv.Sequence features: Physical properties, binding sites, modification sites

v.Prediction of subcellular localization

vi.Prediction of secondary and tertiary structure of proteins

Analysis of Complete Genome

i.Location of genes on chromosomes, correlation with function or evolution

ii.Expansion/duplication of gene families

iii.Presence or absence of biochemical pathways

iv.Identification of "missing" enzymes

v.Large-scale events in the evolution of organisms

Analysis of Genes and Genomes w.r.t Functional Data

i.Expression analysis, microarray data, an RNA measurement.

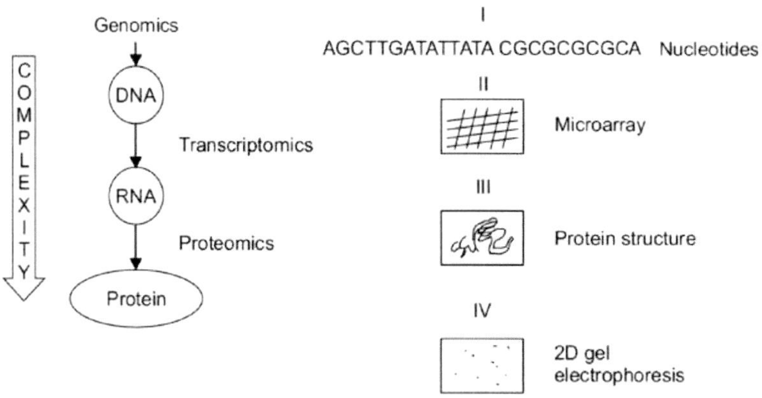

Fig. (2). Complexity of genomic data processing analysis data, interpretation of biological data.

ii.Proteomics

iii.Comparison and analysis of biochemical pathways.

iv.Deletion or mutant genotypes vs phenotypes

v.Identification of essential genes or genes involved in specific processes.

The promise for bioinformatics is that public genome data, mixed with proprietary sequence data, clinical data from earlier drug efforts and other stores of information could unearthen clues about candidates for future drugs.

DATA MINING

It is a tool that allows the user to access multiple data sources and data types, do transforms and other data pre-processing, use a variety of exploratory visualizing tools and application of one or more predictive modelling methods to find an entire solution.

FUNCTIONAL GENOMICS

It assigns functional relevance to genomic information. It is the study of genes, their resulting proteins and the role played by the proteins. Analysis and interpretation of biological data considers information both at level of proteome and transcriptome apart from genome.

Proteomics is analysis of number of proteins (proteome) expressed by a cell.

Transcriptomics is analysis of messenger RNA produced by a cell.

Microarrays: DNA microarray technology can find expression level of genes. It includes genotyping and DNA sequencing.

Gene expression array allows simultaneous analysis of mRNA expression levels of gene in both benign and malignant tumours.

USES OF BIOLOGICAL DATABASES

Databases

Databases are the heart of bioinformatics. There are many types of databases depending on nature of information stored and manner of data storage. These databases are accessible to everyone, and their web addresses can be found in the references 1st issue of Journal Nucleic Acid Research every year (www.nai.oupjournalis.org)

Biological Databases

The data produced by thousands of research teams all over the world are collected and organized in databases specialized for subjects. A biological database is usually associated with computerized software designed to update, query, and retrieve components of data stored within the system. *e.g.*, a record associated with a nucleotide sequence database typically holds information such as contact name, input sequence, description of type of molecule, name of source organism, literature citations associated with the sequence (Figs. **3** - **5**). (Table **2**).

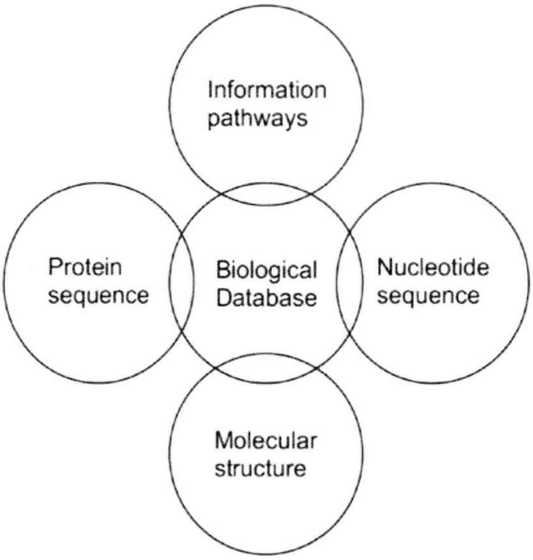

Fig. (3). Biological database.

Database search for a related protein

↓

Design PCR primers using computer program

↓

Isolate total RNA

↓

Amplify transcript using RT-PCR

↓

Derive nucleotide sequence by automated PCR cycle sequence

(Fig. 4) contd.....

↓

Search for homology to nucleic acid sequence

↓

Genetic analysis software

↓

Translation of DNA sequence to protein sequence

↓

Protein analysis and molecular modelling

↓

Putative protein

Fig. (4). Scheme of work using bioinformation to generate protein information.

PRIMARY DATABASES (ARCHIVES)

They stand for experimental results but are not accurated review. They hold information and annotation of DNA and protein sequences, structures, and expression profiles.

Secondary Databases (Curated)

They hold the results of analysis on the primary resources including information on sequence patterns or motifs, variants and mutations and evolutionary relationships.

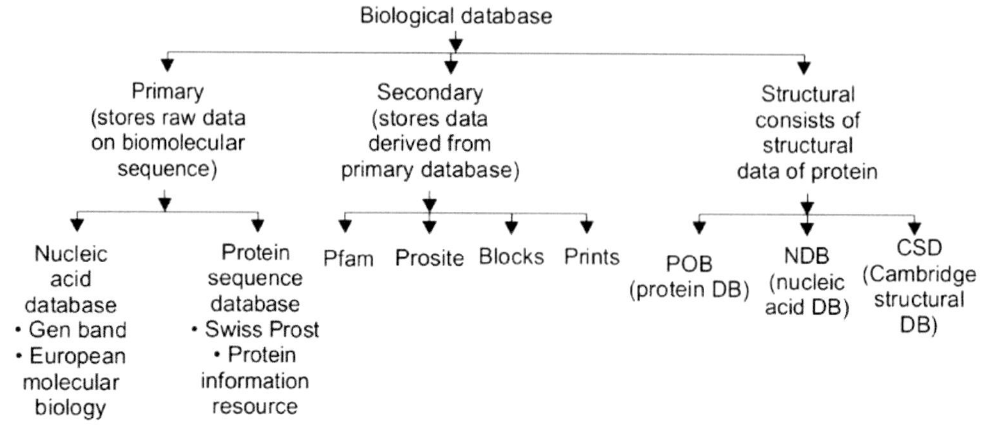

Figure Biological database

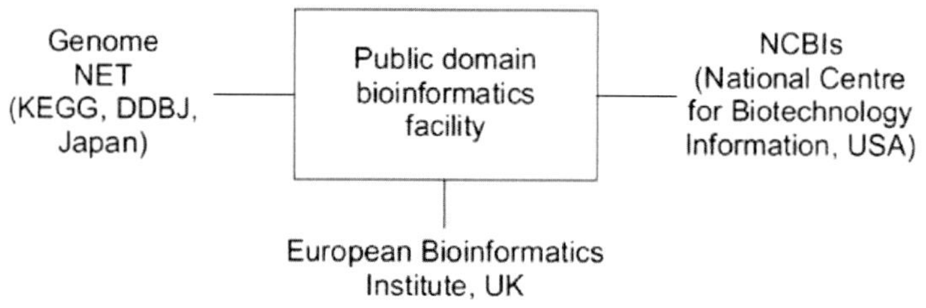

Fig. (5). Major Database for bioinformatics.

Table 2. Characteristics of databases.

	Database	**Characteristics**
1.	Nucleotide Sequence Database	
	Gene bank	www.ncbi.nih.gov/genebank/maintained by National Center for Biotechnology Information (NCBI), USA.

(Table 2) cont.....

	EMBL	www.ebiac.uk/embl European Molecular Biology Lab (EMBL) under aegis of European Bioinformatics Institute (EBI), U.K.
	UniGene	www.ncbi.nih.gov/unigene/
2.	Protein Sequence Database	
	PIR	pir.georgetown.edu Protein Information Resource (PIR) database provided by National Biomedical Research Foundation (NBRF), USA.
	Swiss-PROT	www.expasy.ch/sport
3.	Protein Sequence Motif Database	
	PROSITE	www.expasy.ch/prosite
4.	Macromolecular databases	

(Table 2) cont.....

	PDB	www.rcsb.org/pdp primary database for 3-D structures of biological macromolecules.
5.	Others	
	KEGG	

Table 3. Program.

	Program	Utility/Application	Web link
1.	Gene Mark	• Access coding potential of DNA sequences	www.ebi.ac.uk/genemark
		• 1st tool to be employed for prokaryotic genes	
		• Now exists in separate variants for gene prediction in prokaryotic, eukaryotic, and viral DNA sequences	
2.	Glimmer Gene Locator	• Identify coding and regions	www.tigr.org/softlab
	and Interpolate Markov	• Used as primary gene finder at TIGR.	
	Modeler, John Hopkins tool and TIGR)	•Modified version designed for Plasmodium falciparum: Glimmer M	

(Table 3) cont.....

		• Glimmer HMM for higher organisms	
3.	Grail (Gene recognition assembly internet link, oak ridge National Lab)	• Finds exons, Poly A sites, promoters, CpG Islands, repetitive elements, and frameshift errors in DNA sequences by comparing them with database of known human & mouse sequence elements	http://compbio.ornl.gov
4.	GenScan (Stanford University and MIT)	• Has been used as principal tool for gene prediction in international Human Genome Project	http://genes.mit_edu/ GenScan/html
5.	Gene Builder	• Performs ab initio gene prediction	www.itba.mi.cnr.it/webgene

BIOLOGICAL INFORMATION

Bioinformatics is conceptualizing biology in terms of molecules and then applying "informatics" techniques for understanding and organizing the information concerned with these molecules (Table **3**).

The goal of bioinformatics is to uncover the biological information to get a clearer insight (Figs. **6** and **7**). of fundamental biology of organisms.

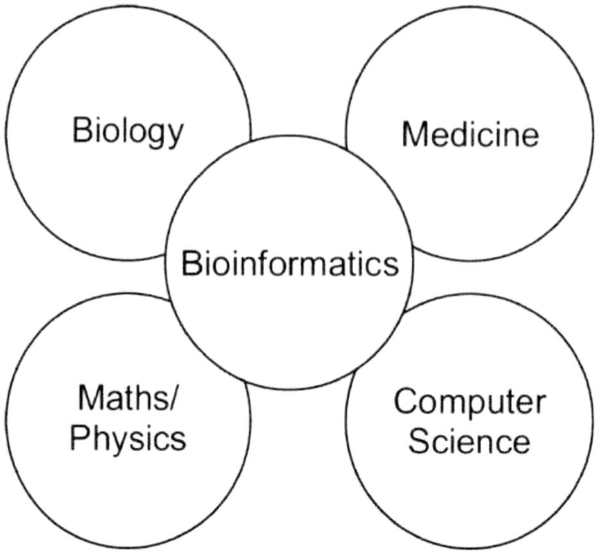

Fig. (6). Interaction of disciplines that contribute to bioinformatics.

The development of bioinformatics not only helped the handling and analysis of sequence data but also, the development of sequencing strategies as well.

Three Components of Bioinformatics

1.Development of new algorithms and statistics to assess relationships among members of data set.

2.Use of these algorithms to analyze and interpret several types of data, *e.g.*, nucleotide sequence, amino acid sequences, protein domain structure and protein interactions.

3.Development and implementation of tools, *i.e.*, databases that allow access and management of several types of information.

COMPUTATIONAL BIOLOGY

It is the process involving analysis of sequence information in bioinformatics. This involves finding of genes in DNA sequences, development of methods to predict structure and/or function of proteins, RNA sequences, clustering protein sequences discovered, and development of protein models, alignment of similar proteins and generation of phylogenetic trees for examining evolutionary relationships.

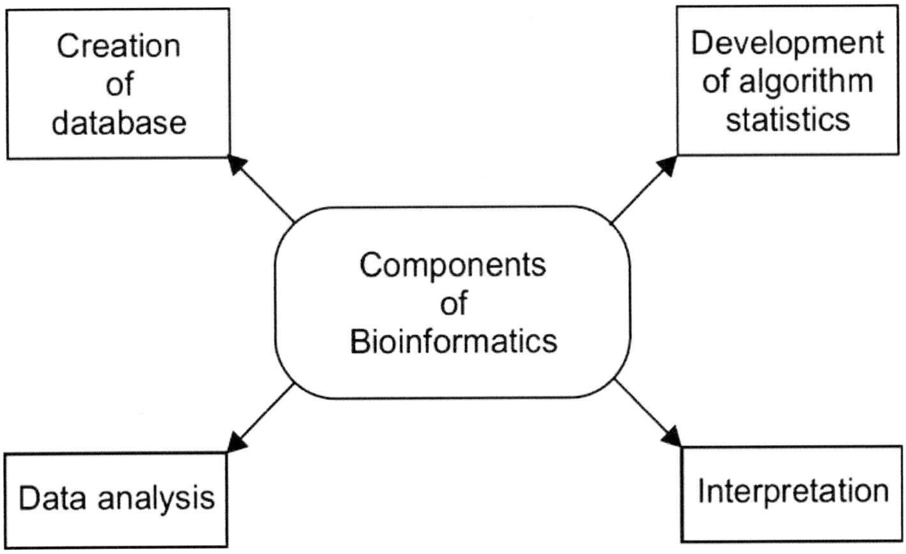

Fig. (7). Components of bioinformatics.

BIOLOGICAL BASIS OF LIFE: OVERVIEW OF ORIGIN AND EVOLUTION OF LIFE

One of the most untraced, mysterious and undissected phenomena is Life. Scientists in contrast to widespread belief of divine origin of life, are bent upon unravelling the mystery of life!

With recent development of biochemical sciences, signal for start of life could be traced down to simple chemical elements (C, H, O, N, P, S, Fe, Cu, *etc.*) that are constituent of all the living organisms It is still not possible to reassemble the chemical elements to constitute a living cell once again. But biochemistry certainly explains the basis of life in organisms.

COMPUTATIONAL BIOLOGY

The primary goal of computational biology is developing algorithms to enable construction of models to study novel biological molecules and processes.

Bioinformatics is focussed on collection and evaluation of existing data. On the other hand, computational biology is purely experimental and exploratory and aims to use knowledge of sequence and structure of well-studied proteins for developing computer algorithms capable of predicting primary sequence, 3D structures and function of novel protein. Also, computer-aided drug designing, and describing of entire range of metabolic activities in a cell with help of computer algorithm are promising. Computational biology promises to accelerate the pace of biomedical research and development of new treatments for human pathologies.

Cell—Fundamental Unit of Organism

Cell is fundamental unit of organism through which life is expressed and is a storehouse of many bio-molecules responsible for actions in the cell. Since the cell is a complex organisation of biomolecules and evidence suggest that a variety of chemical and physical processes occurring on earth, or its atmosphere led to formation of simple biomolecules and finally complex organisation of biomolecules led to origin of life by complex interactions.

Many biomolecules are present in living cells such as carbohydrates (mono-, di-, polysaccharides), proteins, amino acids, enzymes, lipids (fats, oils, fatty acid), nucleotides (nucleic acids, associated histones, acidic proteins) pigments (hemoglobin, chlorophyll), *etc.* Since none of these biomolecules can be expressive of life, it is impossible to pinpoint which biomolecule is living.

The simplest of known living creatures are the versus which represent organisation of protein and RNA/DNA. As viral particle can be stored for exceptionally long time in dormant state, and they multiply only after being injected into a living cell indicating that reproduction is an important expression of life.

Evolution of Macromolecules

Going by organic chemistry, globe can be traced back to four billion years. While decisive phase of biochemistry over past few decades has concentrated on how simple molecules came into being and got organised themselves to express life processes. The direction of origin of biomolecules has begun with non-cellular material to prokaryotic cells (with unorganised genetic material) and finally eukaryotic cell (with an organised genetic material).

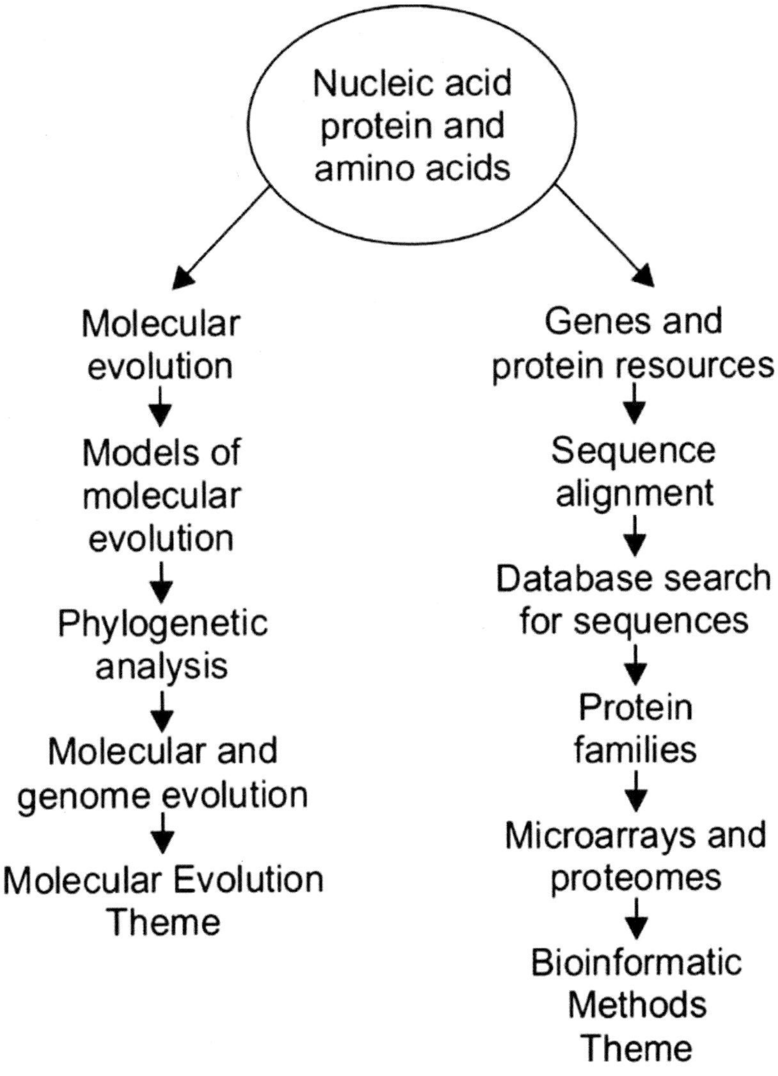

Fig. (8). Bioinformatics and molecular evolution.

Origin of Molecules

About 4.5 billion years ago, earth arised from a dust cloud which underwent condensation due to gravitational forces. At that time, lack of any oxygen producing system in atmosphere of earth along with highly reducing atmosphere along with electric discharge and ultraviolet light from sun aggregated simple molecules to form complex molecules and resulted in formation of ammonia (NH_3) and methane

(CH_4) from reduction of nitrogen and carbon. Also, carbon monoxide and carbon dioxide were present during this prebiotic period. However, origin water is uncertain, though it is present on earth during this period (Figs. **8** - **11**).

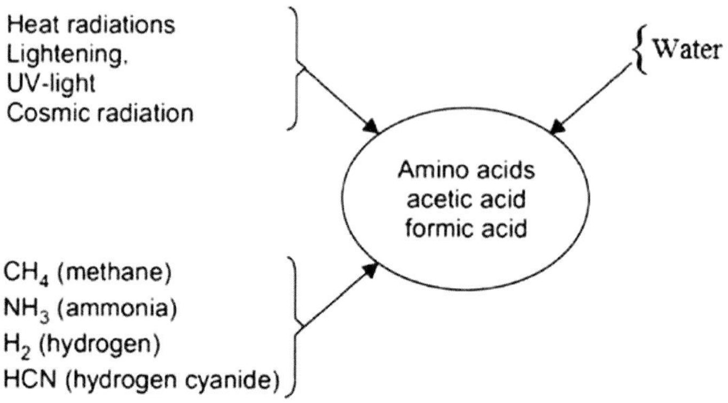

Fig. (9). Origin of macromolecules of cells.

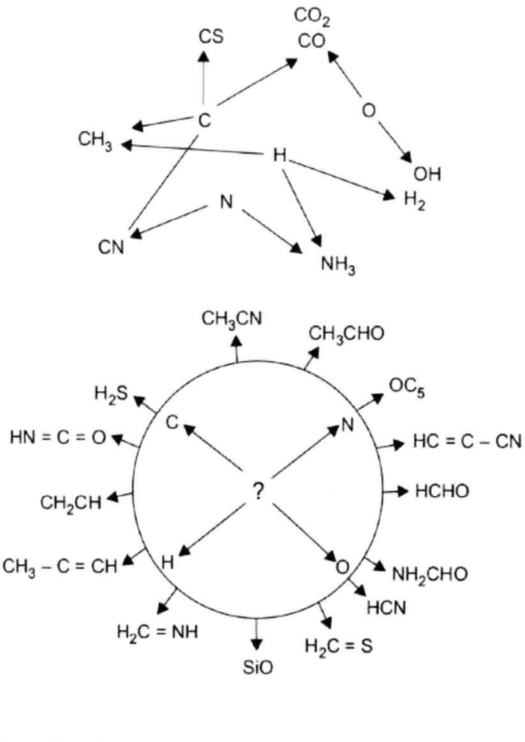

Fig. (10). Precursors of biomolecules.

Ammonia, methane, carbon monoxide and carbon dioxide have been discovered in interstellar space and are precursors of macromolecules such as amino acids and proteins. The latter have been recovered in samples from terrestrial lava as well as from the moon.

The origin of proteinoid molecule is very well-documented and the next step of interaction of such molecules is to form membrane-like structure and finally leading to better evolved cellular characteristic features operational in cells at the right time.

Next major step is flow of energy through development of a catalytic system. No direct evidence about biochemical information of forerunners of enzymes or the genetic signal originated are available. Despite evolution of simple proteinoids or prototypes of nucleic acids, a cell still requires a host of components to be full of life especially a system to extract energy from surroundings and to support energy balance.

Origin of nucleic acid seems to have taken place much earlier than the prototype of living cell evolved. Adenine (6-amino purine) is not only the part of information molecules like DNA and RNA, but also a constituent of energy rich compounds such as NAD and NADP (nicotinamide adenine dinucleotide), FAD (flavin adenine dinucleotide), cAMP (cyclic adenosine 3′, 5′- monophosphate), ADP (Adenosine diphosphate) and ATP (adenosine triphosphate). Also, FAD acts as a coenzyme. Adenine can be easily obtained from hydrogen cyanide; Amination of purine ring would have opened avenues for multiple channels in this prototype of a living cell.

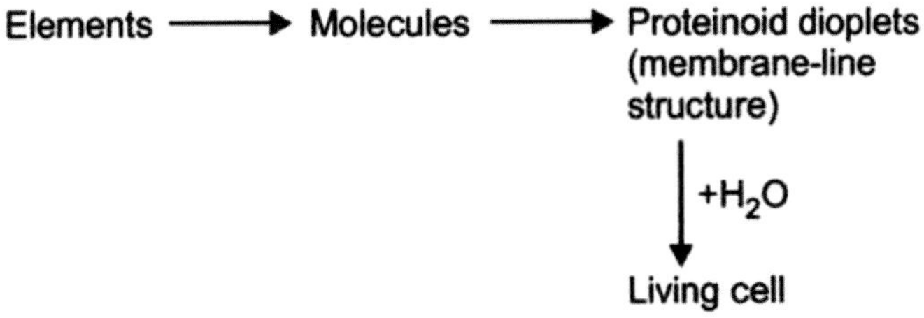

Fig. (11). Molecular assembly organised cell.

Occurrence of errors during duplication of any genetic material resulted in natural selection. These errors usually occur within a single gene and resulting protein may then have one amino acid changed and such changes might be harmful diminishing or destroying the effectiveness of the proteins produced. Also, several new kinds of protein molecules may be formed which did not exist before.

Thus, first animated objective cells formed under prebiotic conditions were anaerobic prokaryotic anaerobes. The precursor enzyme working in these anaerobic prototype living cells under conditions of extremely reducing condition must have been the modern enzyme system including hydrogenase and ferredoxin (iron and sulphur-containing enzymes). The ability of cells to utilize vast resource of light energy from the sun originated at a much later stage.

Formation of pigment system with the heme group was prerequisite to the formation of an autotrophic cells and photosynthesis appeared 2 billion years ago when the earth's atmosphere was anaerobic and reducing. The four most abundant elements C, H, N and O in human body are needed to make living things were also present in sufficient quantities in earth's crust in atmosphere and in ocean.

After cooling of earth, water and various gases on earth's surface were produced. These gases included substantial amount of CO_2 and traces of O_2. From evolutionary point of view, photosynthetic bacteria are most ancient and could use only reducing compounds. While cyanobacteria had both structural and functional changes in photosynthetic machinery were able. It may be added here that photosynthesis occurs in cyanobacteria, chromatophores of purple and green bacteria and in chloroplasts of plants and green algae to evolve oxygen. Even today, the mechanism of splitting of water molecule to release oxygen evolved later is still not clear and cyanobacteria have the credit of owning the responsibility of filling up earth's atmosphere with oxygen.

Biological Diversity

Biological diversity is variability among living organisms from all sources of life forms including terrestrial, marine, aquatic ecosystems, and ecological complexes. It includes diversity within species, between species and of ecosystem Fig. (**12**).

Genetic diversity: It is the variation of genes within genes.

Species diversity: It is variation of species within a region.

Ecosystem diversity: It is the variation in an ecosystem where different landform exists to support different and specific variation.

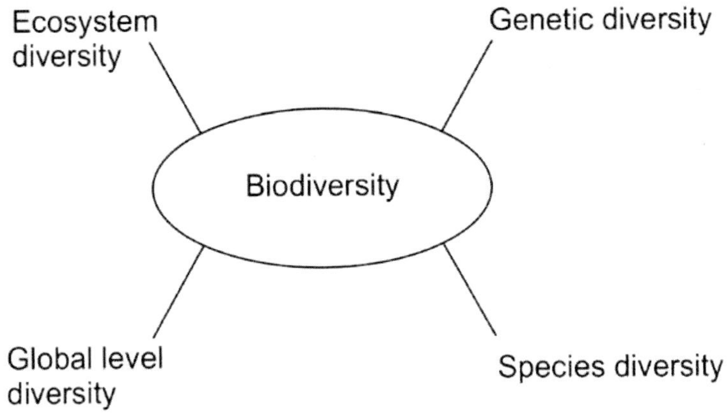

Fig. (12). Diversity of life forms.

Global level diversity: Of the 5–30 million species of life forms existing at global level only 1.5 million have been identified. They include 3,60,000 species of microorganisms, 3 lakh species of green plants and fungi, 8 lakh species of insects and 40,000 species of vertebrates. Tropical forests though cover only 7% of total land surface are the richest in biodiversity, and more than half of the species on earth live in moist tropical forests. The reason for biodiversity in tropical forest being availability of best conditions for evolution and ideal situation for interaction between climate, organisms, soils time and hereditary in tropics. Thus, tropics have low rate of extinction.

Phylogenetic Analysis

Based on the assumption that organisms with more similar genes evolved from a common progenitor than those with more dissimilar genes. Lineage tree shows that archaea and eukaya are thought to have diverged from each other.

Bioinformatic is just not capturing, managing, and presenting data derived from DNA and protein sequencing, but also, it can be used to investigate the evolution of genes and their protein products, and this is termed as molecular phylogeny.

Build models of sequence evolution, two approaches are available:

i)Empirical model

ii)Parametric model

Empirical Models: They are built through comparison of large numbers of observed sequences.

Parametric Models: They are built based on chemical or biological properties of DNA and amino acids.

Parametric approach is favoured for DNA evolution studies using parameters such as base frequency, base exchangeability, and rate heterogeneity.

Base frequency: This parameter describes the frequency of bases (A, G, C & T) averaged over all sequence sites and this is influenced by total GC content.

Base Exchangeability: This parameter describes relative tendency for one base to be substituted for another and purine-purine and pyrimidine-pyrimidine base transitions are expected to be more frequent than base transversions (purine-pyrimidine).

Rate Heterogeneity

This is the variation in mutation rates in a DNA-str*etc*h due to biochemical constraints, structural features, *etc*.

In phylogenetic trees, evolutionary distance is measured in terms of horizontal branch length.

Bioinformatics draws inspiration from a wide variety of quantitative fields including statistics, physics, computer science, engineering to analyze sequence data & protein structure, to metabolic modelling for quantitative analysis of population and ecology. It also supplies tools and computational solutions that are critical for understanding biological problems.

Phylogenetic Analysis

It has been on gross anatomy of species and a phylogenetic tree based on quantitative representation of relationships among species is constructed/drawn. There are certain rules for drawing tree based on quantitative nature of sequence relationships. The tree could be hand-drawn trees of life or modern trees which are binary trees using tree-building algorithms. The modern phylogenetic trees have branching pattern and length of branches can be decided by evolutionary distance.

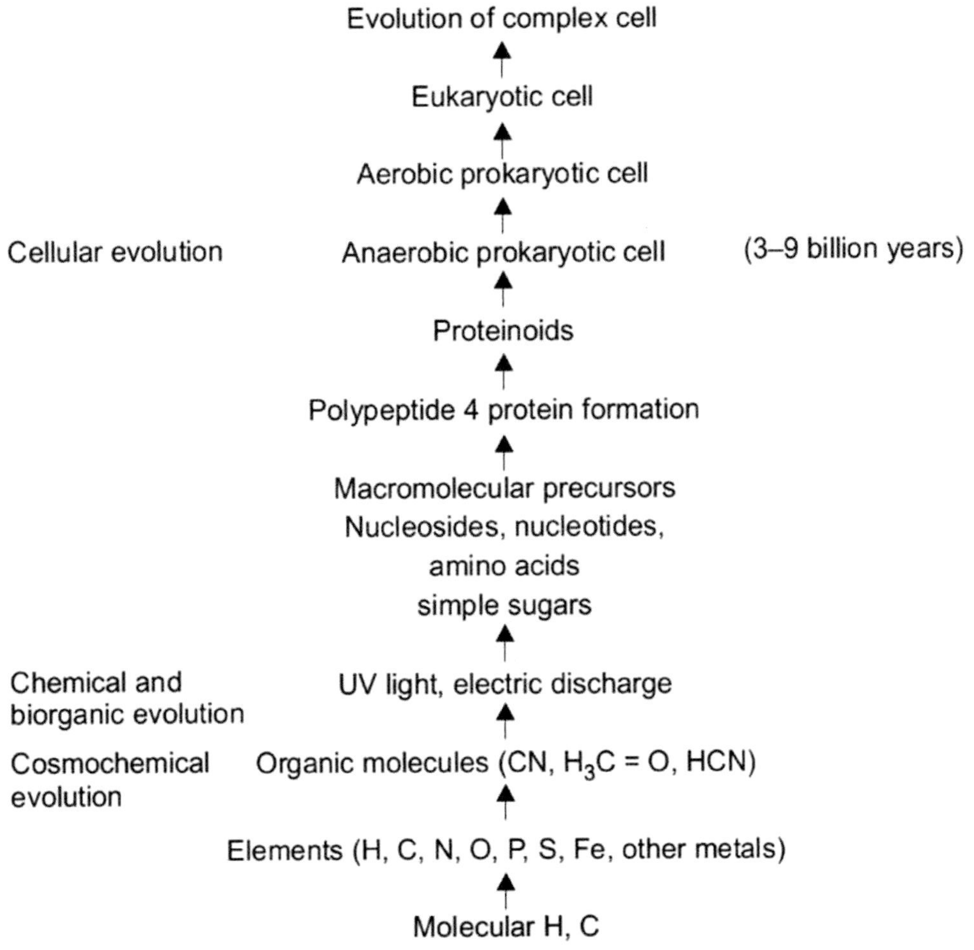

Fig. (13). Evolution of cell.

Phylogeny of species has a root which assumes that all species have a specific common ancestor and phytogenic tree thus derived from sequence data may be rooted or unrooted. However, it is much harder to pinpoint which Figs. (**14** and **15**). sequence or pair of sequence in such a tree is the common ancestor.

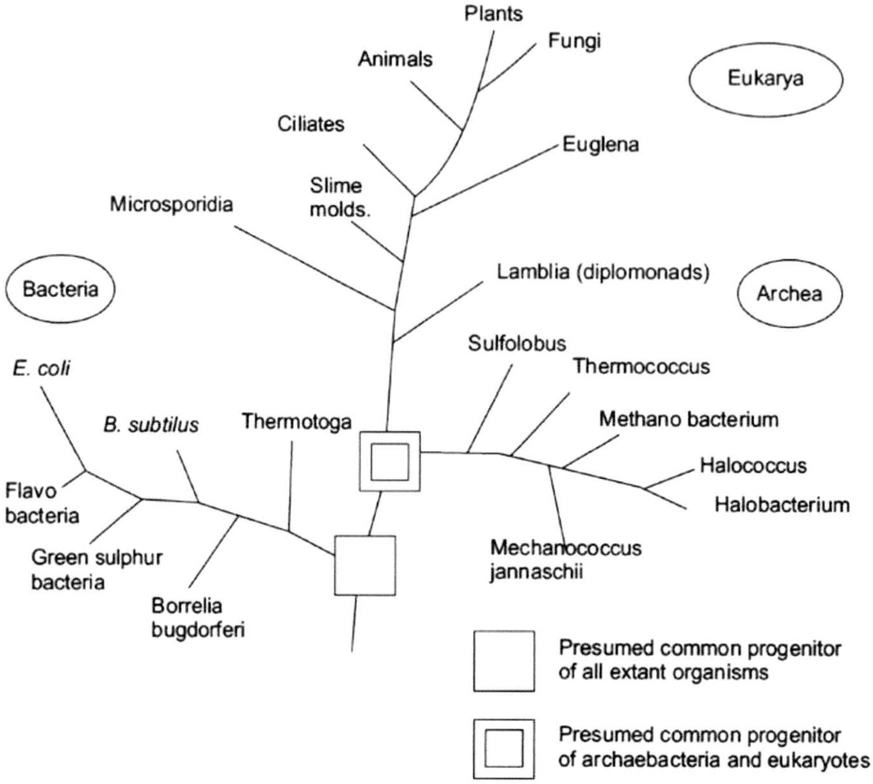

Fig. (14). Three kingdoms of organisms evolved from a single celled progenitor.

Phylogeny inferred from a protein or nucleotide sequence resembles whole-organism tree of life and supply valuable scientifically valid evidence to support the theories of evolutionary history. Phylogenetic analysis of a sequence family is most informative about evolution than that of gene (Table **4**), (Fig. **15**).

Table 4. Properties of tree.

• Root is common ancestor of all taxa
• In case of unrooted tree, prediction is done by uprooted tree
• Genes, species are represented by leaves
• Path from root to node represent an evolutionary path
• Paralogues: genes diverged within same species
• Orthologues: genes diverged with species

Steps in Phylogenetic Analysis

1.Alignment strategy

2.Distribution of substitution method

3.Tree building

4.Tree evaluation.

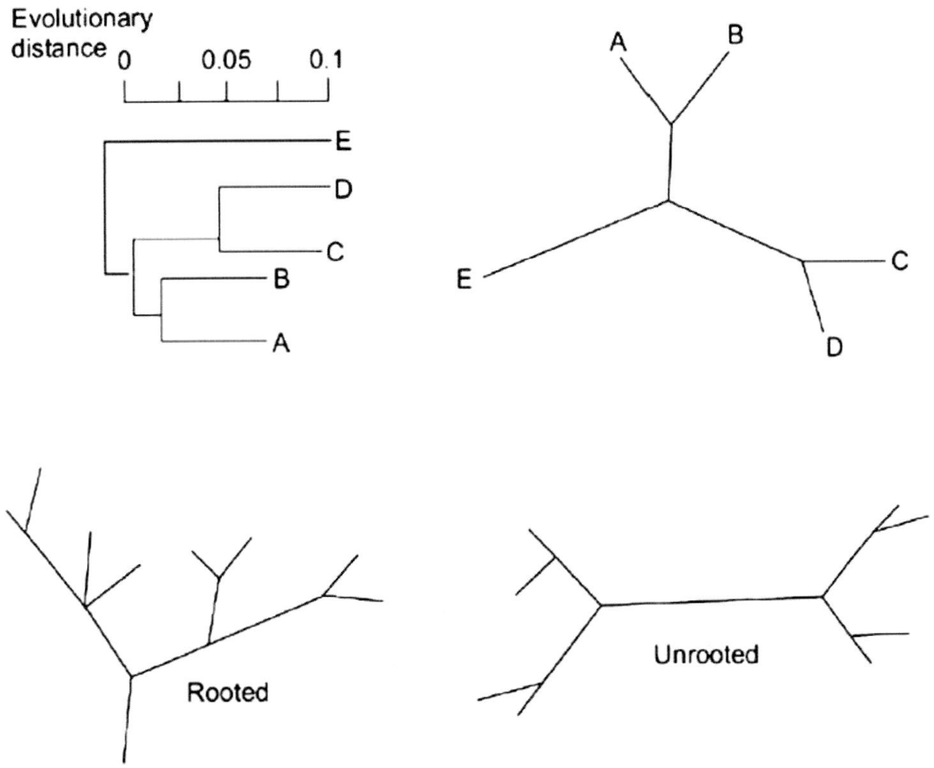

Fig. (15). Types of phylogenetic trees.

Methods

Two main categories of phylogeny methods are:

1. Distance method
2. Character method

1. Distance Method

All pairs of sequences are aligned for determination of most similar or closely related pairs. This alignment supplies genetic distance between the sequences to predict the evolutionary relationship.

2. Character Method

They are of DNA types:

(i)Maximum parsimony method (MP)

(ii)Maximum likelihood method (ML)

MP method: Here multiple sequence alignment is produced to predict corresponding sequence position.

These sequence position will appear in vertical column.

ML method: reliable multiple sequence alignment is obtained and changes in each column in the alignment are examined to find likelihood of a particular tree miscalculated by using expected model of change in sequences.

Distance Matrix Method

In calculation of distance matrices, DNA distance matrices are calculated. Each mismatch between two sequences adds to the distance and each find subtracts from the distance.

Jukes-Cantor Model is simple scoring method in which all nucleotide substitutions are of equal values and each base will have same frequency in DNA sequences.

In case of unequal base frequencies, Kimura method assigns different weights to transition and transversions Typical transversion is weighed as contributing twice the distance of transition. Mutations at different sites in sequence alignment are considered by Kimura and Jukes—Cantor models.

Neighbour-Joining method is one of the simplest distance methods which begins by choosing two most closely related sequences and then adding to next most distance sequences as a third branch to the tree.

Methods of Evaluating Phylogenies

Generate a meaningful tree from data using alignment, scoring methods should be carefully chosen.

Two ways to assess phylogenes are:

1.Jumbling sequence addition order

2.Boot strap and Jacknife replicates.

1. Jumbling Sequence Addition Order

The simplest way to assess a phylogeny is to repeat the analysis several times with different addition orders. All PHYLIP programs and most phylogeny program have JUMBLE option that uses a random number generator to choose which sequence to add at each step.

2. Bootstrap and Jacknife Replicates

Since we are struck with a single set of data, of finite length, there is no way knowing whether the tree inferred from the data is truly representative of the evolutionary history of the gene family.

Bootstrapping is a statistical method based on the assumption that the statistical properties of a sample should be like the statistical properties of the population from which that sample was drawn.

Jacknife resampling assumes that if original sample is large enough, it should also be possible to take smaller samples from the large sample and expect that smaller samples would also keep most of the statistical properties of the original population. In case of phylogenies, if small alignments having only some of the position from the total alignment are created and a tree is constructed using this mini alignment, then one should still get the same tree each time.

Jacknife resampling has been replaced by Bootstrap re-sampling. Bootstrap sampling is typically only practical with distance methods where large numbers of sequences must be used.

SEQUENCE ANALYSIS OF PROTEINS AND NUCLEIC ACID

Finding Genes in DNA Sequence

Genome Sequencing

Genome is completely found DNA sequence of genetic material of an organism.

Sequencing Strategies

Sequence Analysis of Proteins & Nucleic Acids:

The sequencing projects rapidly generate substantial amounts of data which must be mined to extract relevant information.

Terminology

Annotation

It means obtaining biological information from unprocessed sequence data.

Structural Annotation

It means identification of genes and other sequence elements.

Functional Annotation

It means determination of their functional roles in the organism.

Rather than focussing on individual genes, nowadays annotation of entire genomes is undertaken. Raw genomic sequence can be annotated by comparison with database of previously cloned genes and ESTs and sophisticated algorithms.

Annotation is achieved by the application of information technology to the management and analysis of biological data, a field known as bioinformatics.

The Science of Bioinformatics has Three Components

1.Development of new algorithms and statistics for assessing and interpreting large data sets.

2.Using algorithms for analysis and interpretation of nucleotide and amino acid sequences, protein domain structure and protein interacting data.

3. Creation of database that allow efficient access and management of distinct types of information.

Overview of Sequence Analysis

The first task is to show any genes present in a long piece of DNA that has been sequenced.

Once a gene has been shown, the nucleic acid sequence is converted into a protein sequence.

It may be possible to show other proteins with a similar sequence which may help to find its function.

Also, more information about its function can be obtained by sequence comparisons to show motifs in a protein (Figs. **16** - **18**), *e.g.*, ATP binding or DNA binding (Table **5**).

Certain Considerations

1.In prokaryotes, gene density is high, protein coding genes lack introns, so recognition is easy.

2.In eukaryotes, a gene is channel to recognize since it is composed of large no. of exons and introns.

E.g., human genome, exon is 150 bp, intron is several kb, complete gene can be hundreds of kb.

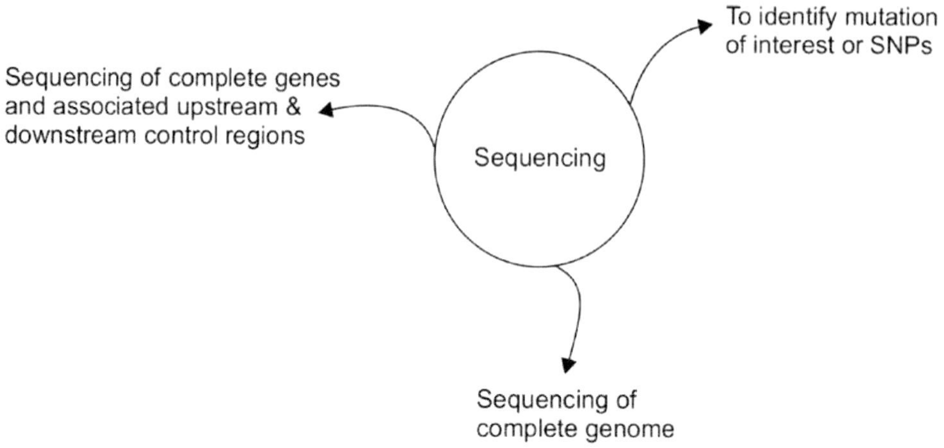

Fig. (16). Application of sequencing.

METHODOLOGY

Includes

1.Detecting open reading frames

2.Exon/Intron boundaries

3.Identification of function of genes (their products.

4.Expression signals

5.Other features of nucleic acid sequences

6.Protein structure

7.Protein motifs and domains.

8. a) Sequence comparisons

   b) Protein comparisons

   c) Protein alignments

   d) Databanks

Table 5. Algorithms used for searching for genes in DNA sequence.

Types of Algorithms	Example
Neural network	GRAIL
Rule-based system	Gene finder
Hidden Markov model Gene Scan	GENIE Gene Mark HMM HMM Gene FGENEH

Table 6: Approaches for data mining.

Influence based data mining
Affinity based data mining
Time-delay based data mining
Trends based data mining
Comparative based data mining
Predictive based data mining

Open Reading Frames (ORF)

This first task during identification of genes in a length of DNA sequence is identification of correct reading frame. Since there are three reading frames on each strand of a DNA molecule. The correct reading frame is assumed to be longest frame interrupted by a stop codon (TGA, TAA, TAG). The longer the ORF, more likely it is to be a gene because long ORFs are unlikely to occur by chance.

5′ end:

i.N-terminal amino acid of a protein usually is methionine so the presence of an ATG codon might show the 5′ end of a gene.

ii.In a mRNA molecule, the start codon may be flanked by a Kozak sequence (CCGCC AUGG) and finding of this sequence helps to find 5’ end of gene.

CpG island: Identification of segments with a much higher than average GC content and higher than average frequency of CpG dinucleotide is indicative of CpGISLAND.

Bias towards G or G as the third base in a codon can also be used as a final aid. Sophisticated computer programs are also available for it.

Software Programs for Finding Genes

Several sophisticated software algorithms have been devised to oversee gene prediction in eukaryotic genomes, namely:

1.Neural network, *e.g*., GRAIL

2.Rule-based systems, *e.g*., Gene finder

3.Hidden Markov method, *e.g*., GENSCAN HMM Gene.

Exon/Intron Boundaries

Human intron/exon boundaries are surrounded by some recurrent motifs and the most obvious and conserved of these is GU-AG motif. Most introns begin with GU (encoded by GT in the sense strand of DNA) and finish with AG. This combination occurs theoretically with frequency of 1:16. Even computer algorithms are available for predicting intron/exon boundaries.

Another evidence can be obtained from screening data banks of ESTs. Also, Gen Bank database can be searched for matching full length cDNA sequence.

Identification of Function of Genes and their Products

The simplest way to show function of new genes is to search homologues in the protein databases.

Blast programs are the fastest sequence alignment tools. Others are SWISS-PORT and Tr EMBL.

Role of Text Mining Technologies

Accelerate Disease-Based Research

Text mining helps scientists (of pharmaceutical and biotechnology industries) who are engaged in disease-based research to review the published literature to confirm their discovery.

Medline

Medline has thousands of journals and over 15 million abstracts (and over 2,000 abstracts added daily). So, it is physically impossible for any scientist to keep current of the research and explore all the areas! Thus, to obtain scientific articles on a topic of interest, special searching softwares are needed that scan fastly for terms identical to the query terms. Sophisticated software programs have been developed that can understand typical language ambiguities to effectively derive key scientific knowledge from biomedical abstracts.

Alma Knowledge Server 2 (AKS2) is a latest text-mining system that examines all abstracts added to Medline, applies statistical and rules-based analyses, to uncover relationships that exist in scientific literature between diseases, symptoms, drugs, genes, proteins, and chemical compounds. It captures formatted data from many sources such as Medline, Entrez Gene, UMLS, PubChem. (Website is www.activemotif.com)

Computational technology of automated text mining available nowadays can help researchers to be more knowledgeable about their disease areas and create more efficient drug discovery processes.

Software Programs for Finding Genes

Computer softwares are available to predict the existence of genes in unprocessed genome sequence data. Also, computer-based prediction has advantage of its speed—annotation can be conducted concurrently with sequencing itself–but it has a disadvantage of inaccuracy particularly in complex genome of higher eukaryotes.

Several sophisticated software algorithms have been devised to oversee gene prediction in eukaryotic genomes (Tables **7** and **8**).

Table 7. Applications of algorithms.

Algorithms	Example	Principle
Rule-based system	Gene Finder	Uses an explicit set of rules to make decisions
Neural Network	GRAIL	Modelled on process of learning in cognitive systems. Uses data training set to build rules for prediction or classification on data sets.
Hidden Markov model	F Geeneh Gene scan Genie Gene Mark HMM HMM Gene	A set of discrete states and transition between those states with associated probability estimate feature.

Many of currently used gene prediction programs incorporate Markov model to distinguish hexamer usage between coding and non-coding DNA. GRAIL is one of the oldest gene prediction programs and can be used with human, mouse, Arabidopsis, Drosophila and E. coli sequence. While GENIE has been trained only on human and drosophila sequences.

Thus, gene-prediction algorithms need to be trained with data or else implanted with a set of rules so that the algorithm can recognize key features that distinguish a gene or exon from noncoding DNA, a feature not identical in all organisms.

Table 8: Gene prediction Software.

Gene Prediction Software	
FGEENEH	Gene Builder
GENEID	Wise 2/Gene wise
GENIE	Blocks.
Gen Scan	
HMM Gene	
Gene Mark HMM	
GRAIL	
GLIMMERM	

Identification of Function a New Gene

It is possible to find the function of new genes or putative genes Table **9**, searching homologues in the protein database. Programs available are:

Blast Tools

BLAST P

PSI-BLAST

FASTA

HMMER

SWISS-PROT

TrEMBL

Blast programs are fastest sequence alignment tools with less sensitivity and FASTA & HMMER are slower but more sensitive.

SWISS-PROT database

It is not just a repository of protein sequence, a collection of confirmed protein sequences annotated with information such as function and biological role of protein, protein family assignment and bibliography.

The data is of remarkably high quality and actively curated (managed). TrEMBL database has entries in the same format as SWISS-PROT and they are derived from translation of all coding sequences in the EMPL nucleotide sequence database. It is easier to compare amino acid sequences than nucleotide sequences due to redundancy in genetic code.

Secondary Protein Databases

Table 9: Features of databases.

Database	Features
BLOCKS	Have conserved protein regions and their multiple alignments
PFAM	Have profiles and alignment for common protein families.
PRINTS	Short protein motif compendium
ProDom	Collection of protein domain
PROSITE	Longer protein signature collection
SMART	Accurated collection of protein domain

These secondary databases have been constructed using different analytical methods, namely, motif recognition, fingerprinting of motifs, domain profiles, hidden Markov models. Inter Pro is cross referencing system that allows screening of protein sequences against each of the secondary databases to extract relevant information.

Gene Ontology enables the relating of protein function to gross cellular or organism function, *e.g.*, central metabolism, cell division, nucleotide replication.

Bioinformatic Tools

(*a*) *Alignment tools*

Local sequence alignment tools

FASTA

Pat Match

Blast

Par Align

Protein Engine

Interpro

Multiple alignment tools

Clustalw

PHYLIP

Bio numeric

Multipurpose analysis tool

Biotechnic 3d

PCR primer designing

Primer

Prima

STS sequence search

Program STS search

SNPs discovery

SNP pipeline

Auto SNP

SEAN

PHRED

PHRAP

CONSED

SSRs mining

TROLL

TANDEM REPEAT FINDER

MSL

(b) Assembly package for large-scale genome sequencing

PHRED

PHRAP

DEMIGLACE

Consed

(c) *EST clustering package*

CORPUS

Paracel EST clustering package

(d) *Gene finder*

GRAIL, GENSCAN, GENEWISE

Gene finder, Glimmer MR

(e) *Gene Ontology Consortium*—known genes in database.

(f) *Central repository* for biological literature

Pub Med.

Global Analysis of Protein Expression

The entire complement of proteins synthesized by a cell or organism is PROTEOME. PROTEOMICS is study of gene products encoded by a genome. Proteomics aims to find the entire complement of proteins elaborated by a cell under diverse conditions, *i.e.*, the protein equivalent of whole genome.

Why to Look at Protein Expression?

Since the ultimate product of most genes is a protein, not an RNA molecule, and proteins conduct the actual function of the gene by interacting with cellular and extracellular environment.

There is no one to-one correspondence between mRNAs and proteins and many genes are under post transcriptional regulation and proteins undergo post-translational modifications which are associated with protein function. Therefore, direct analysis at the protein level is beneficial and desirable.

Currently, the most widely used technology for proteome analysis is protein separation by 2-dimensional gel electrophoresis (2 DGE), followed by annotation using high-throughput mass spectrometry.

Proteome

The entire complement of proteins synthesized by a given cell is termed as PROTEOME and global study of proteins is PROTEOMICS. The term proteome was coined by VC Wasinger in 1995 Fig. (**17a**).

Since proteins cannot be amplified like nucleic acids, analysis of protein expression is challenging. Most widely used technologies for proteome analysis are protein separation by 2-D electrophoresis and/or multidimensional liquid chromatography followed by mass spectrometry.

2-D GEL Electrophoresis (IDGE)

This produces a visual display of the proteome.

IEF Isoelectric Focusing

Electrophoresis is conducted in a pH gradient, allowing protein to migrate to its isoelectric point. Size fractionation is done in second dimension based on molecular mass using SDS (sodium dodecyl sulphate).

After fractionation, staining of gel is conducted by silver nitrate, coomasie brilliant blue dye. For proteomics applications, these agents lack sensitivity to defect scarce proteins and newer sensitive fluorescent stains known as SYPRO dye are available to produce fingerprint of proteins of the cell.

Multiplexed Analysis

Multiplex analysis allows expression of protein profiles on single gels followed by their calculations using algorithms, *e.g.*, Melanie II, CAROL are gel-matching softwares.

Multidimensional Liquid Chromatography

Liquid Chromatography (LC) methods using multidimensional technology have replaced 2DGE. Also, proteins separated in liquid phase. They include SWISS-PROT, WORLD-2DPAGE (www.expasy.ch/ ch2d/2d-index.html). WORLD-2DPAGE site links to further resources that supply lab services, training, and data analysis software relevant to 2DE. Gel matching softwares such as MELANIE II (www.espasy.ch/ch2D/melanie) are freely available programs that work by showing the positions of unambiguous landmark spots and then str*etc*hing, skewing, and rotating parts of the image to match other spots. Another program is Java applet CAROL (http://gelmatching.inf.fuberlin.de/ carol.html). This can be used to compare any two gel images over the internet.

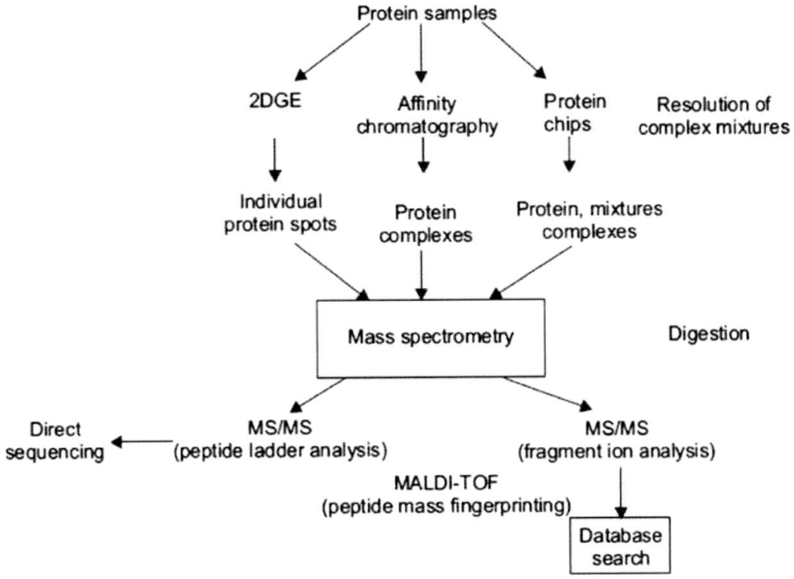

Fig. (17a). Houtes of protein annotation in proteomics.

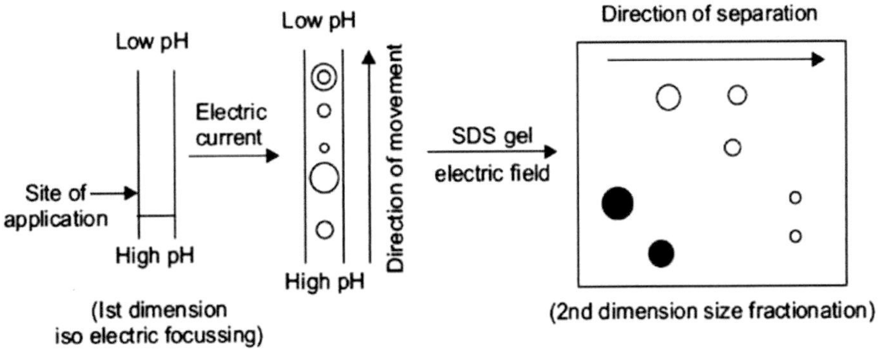

Fig. (17b). 2-D electrophoresis

2DGE technology is workhouse of proteomics and when combined with reverse phase microcapillary liquid chromatography (RPMLC) to it enhances the separation of proteins. Another popular alternative to 2DE is multidimensional chromatography. In case of yeast proteome characterisation, this multidimensional protein technology (Mud PIT) along with tandem mass spectroscopy has helped identification of about 1500 proteins in yeast proteome Fig. (**17**).

Mass Spectrometry (MS)

It helps in high throughput protein annotation. Algorithms have been developed which made possible the searching of protein databases based on their molecular mass.

MS involves separation of charged atoms or molecules according to their mass to charge ratio in a vacuum.

MS Has 3 Components

1.Ionizer converts analyte into gas phase ions

2.Mass analyzer: separates the ions according to their mass: charge ratio (m: z)

3.Ion detector.

The data obtained can be used to search protein databases for finding proteins.

Strategies of Protein Annotation

Two major strategies are:

•Peptide mass fingerprinting

•Fragment ion searching

Peptide Mass Fingerprinting

It is conducted by using MALDI-TOF using gel digestion with a sequence specific protease like trypsin to obtain mass fingerprint using MALDI-TOF.

The fragments generate by protease digestion are analysed by MS for determination of their molecular masses and data thus obtained are used to search protein databases. A number of computer algorithms have been developed to correlate MS determined peptide passes with virtual peptide masses derived from protein databases (Table **10**).

Fragment Ion Searching

Here, fragmentation is achieved by tandem mass spectroscopy (MD/MS) either with quadrupole or TOF analyzers or a mixture, separated by collision cell to induce fragmentation. Then, data of peptide mass and mass of its fragment ions is searched and matched with available databases and ESTs.

Protein Modification—Search

Protein modification can be explored by database searching. Also, post translational modifications can be studied by MS. The commonest modification is phosphorylation of proteins which causes an added mass increment due to phosphor group (80 Da). Other modifications commonly met during routine proteome analysis include acetylation, glycosylation, and N- or C-terminal processing by peptidases. These modifications also cause mass change that can be analyzed by MS.

Also, protein-protein interaction can be exploited for biotechnology applications including therapeutic purposes and drug discovery.

Protein Arrays and Protein Chip

Protein arrays are appearing as a useful closed system for proteome analysis. These are miniature devices in which proteins or molecules that recognize proteins, are arrayed on the surface (Table **11**).

Table 10. Protein identification programs.

Program	Basis
Mascot www.matrix.science.com	Uses MOWSE algorithm
Profound http://prowl.rockfeller.edu	Uses Z-score
Protein Prospector (MS-Fit) http://prospector.ucsf.edu.	Uses MOWSE score
MOWSE: Molecular Weight Search Algorithm.	

Table 11. Mass Spectrometry Sources on Net

Mass Spectrometry Sources on Net
www.expasy.ch/tools/#proteome http://prospector.ucsf.edu www.seqnet.dl.ac.uk/bioinformatics/ www.narrador.embl_heidelberg.de/GroupPages/Pagelink/peptidesearchpage.html

In concept, protein arrays are no different to DNA arrays, but they suffer from several practical limitations (Tables **12** and **13**).

Table 12. Arrays.

	DNA array	Protein Array
Amplification	PCR can amplify nucleic acid sequences	No amplification procedure exists for protein
Sequences	Made up of 4 nucleotides.	No such sequence.
Principle of Molecular Recognization	Hybridization between complementary base pairs, single complex probe used	Recognization parameters vary widely. Same probe cannot be used.
Labelling	Labels are incorporated evenly does not interfere with hybridization	Labels are much more variable. Labelling of protein interfere with protein binding.

Applications of Protein Microarray

Various protein microarrays available are:

1.Antibody (Ab) arrays (microimmoarrays)

2.Antigen (Ag) arrays (reverse microarrays)

3.General protein arrays

4.Arrays of specific capture agents

Table 13. Array types.

Array	**Application**
Ab array	Detection of Ab against bacterial infection cytokines.
Ag array	Used for reverse immunoassay
General protein array	Study protein-protein interactions, protein arrays for yeast proteome, protein functions, *etc.*
Arrays of specific capture agents.	Include aptamers, single stranded nucleotides, molecularly imprint, biochips.

Molecular Imprints

Though they do not fit under umbrella of array but have molecularly imprinted polymers (MIP) which have artificial recognition sites for proteins.

BROAD-Capture Agent Biochips

These devices use broad-specificity capture agents and are marketed as protein chips by Ciphergen Biosystems Inc. which doubles itself as a modified MALDI plate. After washing, this chip is coated with a matrix solution and analyzed by TOF-MS. Also, SELDI (surface—enhanced laser desorption and ionization) supplies more uniform mass spectra than MALDI for protein quantification.

Solution Arrays

This is a microfluidic device and are the next generation of extremely sensitive miniature protein assay platforms.

Approaches for Studying Protein—Protein Interactions

In multidomain proteins, interactions occur between the domains, in stable protein complexes and proteins in transient interactions. Physical contacts between domains are crucial for functioning of cellular machinery.

Approaches

•Experimental

•Theoretical analysis

•Computational

Experimental Approaches

1. Yeast-Two-Hybrid Screens

This system uses transcription of a reporter gene driven by Gal 4 transcription factor. Two chimeric proteins are made, one consists of 'bait' protein (protein A) which is fused to DNA-binding domain of yeast Gal 4 transcription factor (Gal 4-DBD). The second chimeric protein consists of a 'prey' protein (protein B) which is fused to activation domain of Gal 4 transcription factor (Gal 4-AD). When proteins A and B interact, Gal 4-AD will bind upstream (Fig. **18**) of reporter gene Gal 4-AD and reporter gene will be transcribed.

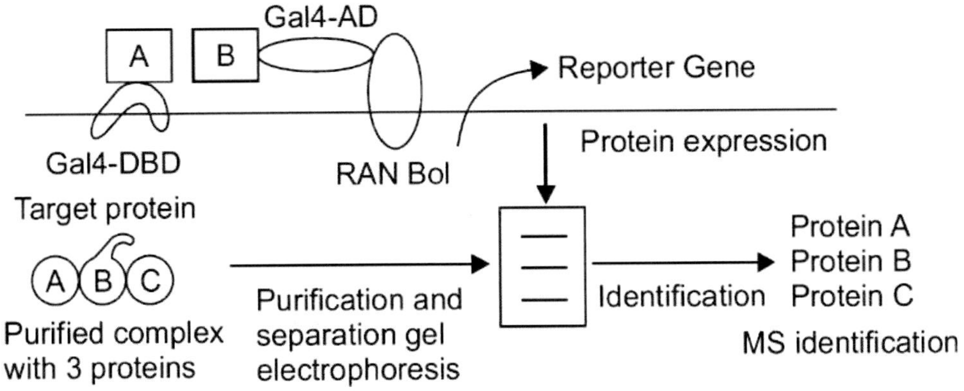

Fig. (18). Yeast-two-hybrid assay.

On large-scale purification of protein complexes, fusion proteins (having tag) are created as well where affinity purification can be conducted (through tag attached to protein) and protein is identified by mass spectrometry (MS). Protein interactions in stable complexes and transient interactions in yeast two-hybrid screens can be found by MALDI-TOF MS.

Micro assay plates of yeast interactions are available where each array element has yeast cells transformed with a particular combination of two plasmids, one carrying the DNA binding domain chimeric protein and other the activation domain chimeric protein.

Disadvantage: Yeast hybrid method

•Only paired interaction evaluated

•Multiple interactions result in high false positive rate

Structural Analysis

In Protein data Bank (PDB), many entries are three-dimensional structures of multiple domains that supply experimental information about interactions between domains at atomic level.

Protein Domain Family Interaction MAPs

Represent interactions of domains in that family and precise information can be extracted by analysis of PDB (protein data bank) entries. Modes of map represent protein families and edges stand for an interaction between at least one of the domains from each of the families. Families can be connected to one, two or more families and network can be constructed based on these interactions (Fig. **19**).

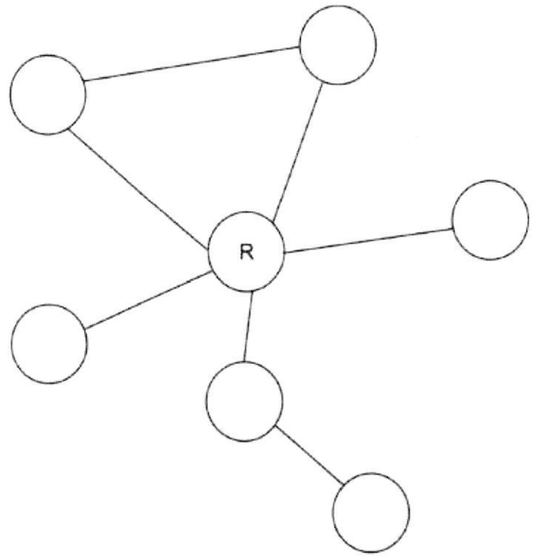

Fig. (19). Protein domain family interaction map.

The family interaction map is a two-dimensional map and does not give any information on three-dimensional geometry of interactions. For this, methods for structure prediction of individual domains can be applied, though less is known about assemblies of domains.

Conservation of Gene Order can be used to predict protein-protein interactions. In prokaryotes, genes are organized into operons of co-regulated and co-expressed groups of genes. Genes that are consistently part of the same operon across different, distantly related genome are likely to be part of same protein complex or functional process across all species. Conservation of gene order across different genomes has been used as a method for predicting protein interaction. For this purpose, it is important to ensure that genes are truly equivalent (orthologs). Conservation of gene order due to operon structure is not applicable to eukaryote genomes, thus interactions for proteins specific to eukaryotes cannot be detected by this method.

Gene Fusion approach can also predict protein interactions by looking for cases across a set of genomes where two or more orthologs are part of the same gene in one genome due to gene fusion. Then, the prediction is applied to orthologs that are on separate genes in the other genomes interact with each other. Members of stable complexes and constitutive enzymes may be involved in gene fusions. However, elements of signal transduction are seldom part of same gene. This method is limited to certain classes of protein-protein interactions due to requirement for coregulation and co-localization.

Use of Phylogeny to predict protein-protein interactions computational methods is another approach. Phylogenetic profile method relies on detection of orthologs (or homologs) in a set of genomes. Presence or absence of orthologous genes is scored across a variety of genome and genes that have same pattern of presence or absence across genomes are predicted to interact.

Predicting Structure of Protein- Biomolecular Interactions

Interactions are key to understanding biological processes as they engage in all regulatory and metabolic processes. For understanding biological processes at the molecular level, determination of structure of the interactions of biomolecules (protein-protein. Protein-DNA and protein-small molecule). Knowledge of three-dimensional structure allows possibility of intervention and manipulation of molecular interactions, structure-based drug design, site-directed mutagenesis, and protein engineering.

Requirements for Studying Structure and Interactions

Atomic resolution structures (atomic coordinates in PDB format)

Computer workstation with high-resolution graphics

Executable version of a docking program

Molecular Complementarity

Molecular complementarity of two proteins can be found using automated computer search and scoring function.

Shape Complementarity

By surface contact or overlap, complementarity between two proteins or a protein and ligand can be found driving force for protein folding and binding is hydrophobic effect that involves free energy gain of removing non-polar surface area from water. Burial of surface area is approximation of this effect.

Property-Based Measures

(i) Hydrophobicity

Hydrophobicity plays a dominant role in folding of proteins and formation of protein-protein or protein-ligand protein-protein interfaces in homodimers and oligomeric proteins. Hydrophobicity is useful as a guide to molecular complementarity in selective protein-protein interactions.

(ii) Electrostatic Complementarity

Burial of charged residues at protein-protein/DNA interfaces is thought to be destabilized effect. On the other hand, hydrophobic effect is the primary driving force. Charge complementarity can play a key role in determining specificity of the interaction and to make a close approach, the protein must have charged residues that complement the negative charges present on the phosphate backbone. Electrostatic complementarity is important in many protein-protein and protein-ligand interactions.

(iii) Amino Acid Conservation

Conservation of residues at the surface of a protein family that may be active site or binding site, is often related to function. This evolutionary information can delineate a functional epitope at times to find the residues important for binding and infer structure-function relationship of proteins.

Molecular Mechanics

Molecular mechanics force-field parameters include equilibrium bind length, bond angles, torsion angles, van der Waals parameters and point charges which are defined by quantum mechanics or experimental observations. These parameters refine or explore the molecular interactions.

Determination of Structure of Two Interacting Proteins is Stilla Problem

Use of six-dimensional search problem with three degrees of rotational freedom (x, y, z axes) and three degrees of translational freedom (x, y, and z axes in cartesian space) for mobile molecule with assumption of one molecule kept stationary is not always or sensible approximation. Also, six-dimensional search is computationally prohibitive for large molecules like proteins. Two widely used methods are:

(i) Constraint- basedMethod

These methods form basis of many proteins' ligand in (small molecule) docking algorithm with the idea of that binding site of receptor molecule can be described by a series of points or vectors.

The search of ligand conformational space is constrained to these points, *i.e.*, a restricted area/ volume of receptor-binding site.

Dock Algorithm

•Define a limited surface area

•Represent cavities on receptors, use clustered spheres

•Complete spheres for every pair of surface points (i and j) that do not intersect the protein surface. Only smallest surface sphere is kept for every surface point i.

•Cluster is defined by a set of overlapping spheres (*i.e.*, i1, i2, i3). Protein can have 10–20 such clusters

•Spheres characterize the molecule/ligand to be docked.

(ii) Matching

Based on similarity in distances between receptor centres (i → j) and ligand centers (k → l), matching is number of matches generated for a given ligand in each cavity is a function of size of both cavity and ligand.

Virtual Screening for Drug Designing

Computer-aided strategies are a key component of modern dry design. For a given experimental protein structure of protein of pharmaceutical interest, identification of small molecules that bind and inhibit/alter activity of target is needed. Computational methods to detect molecular docking or de novo design of ligands by assembly of molecules from small fragments that interact favourably with target are employed.

Conformational Flexibility

Proteins being dynamics undergo conformational change of protein sidechains and loop regions. Protein-ligand docking involve docking of conformational flexible small molecule ligand adapting their shape to fit the receptor-binding pocket. Protein is still treated as a rigid body for studying conformation simulations and multiple conformation rigid-body method and random sampling procedures are applied to search conformation space (Fig. **20**).

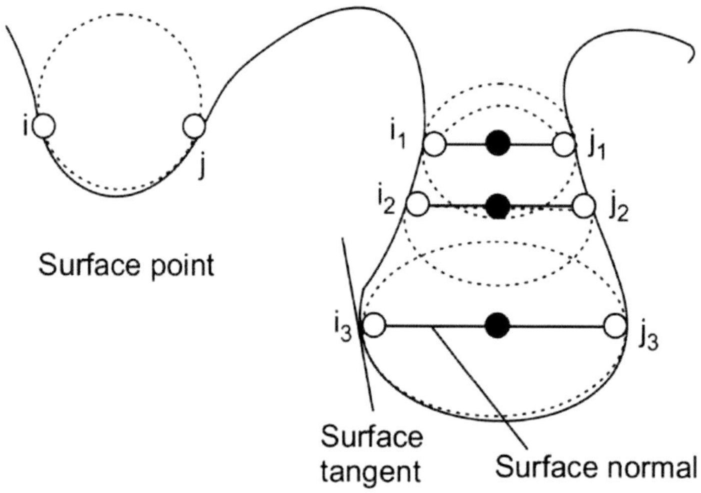

Fig. (20). 2-D representation of protein in molecular surface.

Protein Flexibility

Side-chain flexibility in protein proteins and protein-ligand docking can be predicted by structure prediction methods.

Critical Assessment of Prediction of Interactions (CAPRI)

CAPRI are experiments on comparative evaluation of protein-protein docking for structure prediction conducted by scientific communities to assess various methods.

Challenges to Docking Evaluation

(i)Protein-protein docking, Protein inhibitor systems, Antibody-Antigen Complex.

(ii)Protein-ligand docking CASP2 (Critical Assessment of Structure Prediction 2)

In practice, experimental structure of the complex does not already exist, and hypothetical protein biomolecule complex predict a model of interaction between the two molecules that can be assessed experimentally. Also, validation of evaluation is needed.

Visualization Methods

For viewing molecular properties on molecules, visualization methods are needed.

GRASP program uses rendering of molecular surfaces according to their various properties that can be expressed numerically.

Virtual Reality Modelling Language (VRML) viewers can be used to generate coloured displays. Ras Mol can be used to view molecular properties by assigning these properties to temperature factor column of the PDB file in question.

Web-based interactive exploration of molecules in PDB allow visualization of molecular properties on molecular surfaces and, molecular graphics programs are also available.

EPIDEMIOLOGICAL ANALYSIS

The classical approaches to diseases are being reformulated by epidemiologists with the invent of "omics" areas and molecular biology technologies. Public health and epidemiology scientists are increasingly using various latest molecular epidemiological methodologies and informatics tools along with help from Bioinformatics community for managing genomic information for preparing epidemiological and digital database needed for processing genetic information from pathogens and patients.

New scenarios arisen in molecular epidemiology to analyze the research challenges in biomedical informatics through integration of clinical, environmental, and genetic data in public health. Various integrated medical/biological ontologies and new semantic-based models for managing information would meet the new challenges for research in areas namely, genetic epidemiology, environmental epidemiology, gene environment interactions and the "omics" disciplines, or public health, biomedical research, and healthcare.

RECENT TECHNOLOGIES IN EXPLORING THE EVOLUTION OF LIFE AND EXTRA-TERRESTRIAL / ALIEN LIFE

Recent technologies for exploring the evolution of life and extra-terrestrial/alien life space agencies around the world are exploring the challenge of evolution of life and possibility of extra-terrestrial/alien life by exploring into deep space new emerging technologies such as 3D printer, robotic, artificial intelligence, advanced communication technologies to support both robotic as well as human mission in deep space.

3D Printer

This technology has futuristic applications to support space missions and will be handy in space during emergencies.

Signal Processing, Machine Learning and Artificial Intelligence

Signal processing is key to embedded machine learning and systems designers developing signal processing architectures that can use AI and machine learning for their processing.

A signal is mathematically just a function and signal processing are to convert one signal to another and this is followed by information extraction and interpretation by machine learning. Machine learning has algorithms that automatically detect the patterns in data use the uncovered patterns to predict future data or other outcomes of interest. Signal processing results in data sets with relations of varying, probabilistic strength, and engineers use learning algorithms to figure out these probabilities.

Developments in biotechnology are increasingly producing big data that is generated by modern high-throughput instrumentation technologies, and this is stored in thousands of databases, public and private. A biotechnology researcher needs to master the skills needed to effectively integrate their own contributions with the substantial amounts of information available in these databases. Relations that exist between the fields of big data and biotechnology, including the related technologies of artificial intelligence and machine learning would find how data integration, data exploitation, and process optimization to be done in any future biotechnology project. There are a number of application areas where use of big data will become a key factor, including drug discovery, drug recycling, drug safety, functional and structural genomics, proteomics, and pharmacogenomics, drug discovery, drug recycling, drug safety, and pharmacogenetics. Thus, big data, artificial intelligence, and machine learning will become instrumental in all future biotechnology research. Thus, artificial intelligence is helping biotechnology to get real, and can enhance drug development from candidate screening to trial management and has vast applications in biomedicine, including disease diagnostics, living help, biomedical information processing, and biomedical research.

VIRTUAL CELL, APPLICATIONS OF VIRTUAL LIBRARY AND RESEARCH AVENUES: POTENTIAL OF IN-SILICO TECHNOLOGY

Virtual Life

It is simulation of real life being played in virtual world. Virtual life forms scientists have small pieces of living cells, and the first digital stimulants of entire life form has been created by the scientists.

This will help in better understanding of inner working of living cell and could be used in making nano machines covered by covers simulator to shells of digital living cell.

First virtual virus has been created by the researchers using a million digital atoms and it was brought to digital life for only 50 nanoseconds by advanced computing.

Virtual Cell

Virtual Cell (VCell) is a unique computational environment for the modeling and simulation of cell biology. The National Resource for Cell Analysis and Modeling have specifically designed it to be a tool for a wide range of scientists, from experimental cell biologists to theoretical biophysicists. VCell and other software packages designed for cell biologists supply a variety of tools for modeling a wide range of cell phenomena.

Virtual Embryo

It is a working computer model of mammalian embryo. This can be used for understanding risks posed by environmental chemicals prenatally and predict *in silico* developmental toxicity in such cases.

Virtual Human Embryo

This is an illustrated atlas of human embryology for 8 weeks embryonic period, spanning 14,50 pages continuing digitally reproduced morphology of embryo. Researchers at EMBL have created first complete description of embryo development and this accounts for every single cell of embryo.

This virtual embryo describes the gene expression and morphology of each cell and its fate and future emerging field of developmental genomics.

In Silico Technologies

The experiments and research performed by using computers are termed as *in silico technologies*. Computer modeling and computer simulation are used for various scientific purposes in *in silico technologies*.

Applications

In silico clinical trials are useful in the search for a vaccine for COVID-19. Also, drug discovery and development with the savings in labor, costs, and time t can be achieved with in silico testing and researchers may be able to find and develop drug candidates more quickly in the battle against COVID-19, where time is of the essence.

Develop new drugs that are safe and effective, clinical research has two methodologies in prevalent use namely, first approach is *human organs-on-chips*—microfluidic devices that mimic the functioning of a human organ and disease states for predicting efficacy and toxicity of drugs in development; and second is *in silico*, which is related to harnessing AI for drug discovery.

The term *in silico clinical trials* uses individualized computer simulation for the development or regulatory evaluation of a medical product or intervention, including pharmaceuticals. Even the simulations may involve CT or MRI scans of real patients that can be converted into 3D anatomical shapes and statistical modeling to enhance data for creating anatomy scenarios. This is also known *as computational medicine.*

in silico modeling, simulation, and visualization can help to predict the chances for success of medicinal compounds and drugs being assessed along with possible adverse side effects during the drug discovery process.

Ai-Based Digitalized, Insilico Clinical Trials

In-Silico style in virtual patients are futuristic approaches that are becoming reality. They collect and analyze patient health records to find ideal candidates for clinical trials to analyze the population and perform 'what-if' analyses in real-time, by developing virtual patient cohorts that can be re-named for potential recruitment into clinical trials, automating new drug development from the first identification of biomarkers and therapies through clinical trials' complexities.

ROBOTICS IN BIOTECHNOLOGY

The labs of the future will have humans and robots collaborating with each other, safely and productively. Sensing, collaboration, machine learning, vision, and cloud computing are all big factors to be considered for laboratory automation. Robotic solutions are changing the game of biotechnology at all levels, whether in analysis, biomanufacturing or pharmaceuticals. A robot can also work in a fully closed and sterile environment, and now several robot vendors have approved robots that can be used in class A clean rooms. These robots are even suitable for decontamination processes in vaporized hydrogen peroxide (VHP) environments.

In recent studies, robots are used to stimulate living systems in controlled experimental settings. This research strategy is here called *interactive biorobotics*, to distinguish it from classical biorobotics, in which robots are used to simulate, rather than to stimulate, living system behavior.

Advanced applications of various biological robots (nanobots) fabricated based on bottom-up or top-down approaches are available for making nanotechnology scaffolds. *Nanobots and enzyme-powered nanomotors* being self-propelled vehicles which consume biocompatible fuels. These smart nanostructures are widely used as controlled and targeted drug delivery systems for the efficient treatment of various diseases.

Soft robotics is a sub-field of robotics that deals with construction of robots from highly compliant materials, like those found in living organisms. Soft robots have increased flexibility and adaptability for conducting tasks and improved safety when working around humans.

Soft robotics technology can be combined with tissue engineering to create hybrid systems for medical applications. Soft robots can be implemented in the medical profession, specifically for invasive surgery, soft wearable robots, soft prosthetics, co-robots (assistive robots that cooperate with human partners) to miniaturized robots for field exploration, drug delivery, minimally invasive surgery, and medical implants. Soft robotic technology, computer vision and AI platform have the potential to transform the food industry.

CYBERSECURITY IN BIOTECHNOLOGY: THREATS AND CHALLENGES

Cybersecurity encompasses the protection of computer systems from theft and damage to their hardware, software, or information, as well as from disruption or misdirection of the services they provide. Cyber security is the responsibility of everyone, but passwords are our worst defence, since security of data and cyber security is the responsibility of everyone, not just the "IT department."

Because cybersecurity is a huge concern, there is a major effort to improve the security of manufacturing technology. Without proper attention, business systems, factory systems, machines, tools, and sensors, and engineering systems could be vulnerable to cyberattacks. Companies are using multi-prong approaches to cybersecurity including upgrading to the latest security system, adding endpoint protection for older systems that cannot be upgraded, and locking down firewalls on the factory floor.

Most manufacturing companies today rely on software to automate processes, manage supply chains, and ease research and development, which could increase cyber-crime risk. All stakeholders should be vigilant in implementing cybersecurity measures. The supply chain has become an increasingly attractive target for cyber-criminals. However, attacks against many manufacturing companies tend to be targeted at stealing intellectual property (designs and customer lists), or interrupting operations. Even small- and medium-sized manufacturing businesses should not assume that their size precludes them from threats. Mastering IT security issues supplies a foundation for successful implementation of the digital enterprise.

The US Food and Drug Administration's (FDA) 21 CFR Part 11 regulations require secure access to computer systems. Many companies have invested in two-factor authentication approaches, including biometric finger scans, hand scans, eye scans, and facial recognition.

Cybersecurity in Science and Medicine: Threats and Challenges

Technology offers opportunities to revolutionize medicine and research but can threaten privacy and patient confidentiality. As the scale of patient data explodes, the safety and integrity of medical information are increasingly at stake. We highlight security and privacy issues associated with genomic research, medical devices, and wearable technology.

The advancement of innovative technologies creates new security challenges for businesses that deal in innovative products for consumers. Specifically, the automotive and biotechnology innovations are extremely vulnerable to cybersecurity threats with the creation of new methods to exploit emerging technologies.

Plans against Cyber Threats

Considering the advancements of cybersecurity threats, governments are introducing new regulations and standards to defend systems. For example: European Union has been developing and implementing new cybersecurity regulations in the past few years. The EU plans to introduce the new *ePrivacy* Regulation to enhance the level of confidentiality within electronic communications. Also, the International Organization for Standardization (ISO) is set to roll out new standards about the security and protection of personal information within cloud-based services.

New discipline of ***cyberbiosecurity*** has been created to bring together disparate communities to find and address a complex ecosystem of security vulnerabilities at the interface of the life sciences, information systems, biosecurity, and cybersecurity.

ROLE OF MACHINE LEARNING, DATA MINING AND ARTIFICIAL INTELLIGENCE IN BIOTECHNOLOGY AND BIOINFORMATICS

Biological databases that were once included of sequences and structures of compounds have now advanced into storage of more complex and bulk data.

Unification and standardisation of public data would supply deep and more exact insights in analysis and make it easier and exact for machine to find patterns in data.

Today, how to apply numerous data mining technologies to bioinformatics analysis is a current research hotspot, including data mining architecture, machine learning algorithm development, and new data mining analysis function research suitable for biological information processing. At the same time, the interdisciplinary approach has promoted the development of machine learning. And artificial neural networks, deep learning, and reinforcement learning have made breakthroughs in machine intelligence. Besides, due to the growth of computing power, the acceleration of data storage speed and the reduction of computing costs, scientists in various fields have been able to apply these technologies to biological data. The close integration of machine learning and bioinformatics will result in more meaningful mining results, which will play a positive role in the progress of human society.

Also, scientists use deep learning algorithms to perform classification of cellular images, genome analysis, drug discovery and find out how image data and genome data are link with electronic medical records.

Thus, AI and machine learning are changing the way biologists conduct research, interpret it, and apply it to solve problems. As science grows increasingly interdisciplinary it is only inevitable that biology will continue to borrow from machine learning, or better still, machine learning will lead the way.

DIGITAL TECHNOLOGY

Digital technology stands for technology relying on the use of microprocessors, computers, and applications dependent on computers such as internet, and other devices [video cameras, and mobile devices such as phones and personal-digital assistants (PDAs)].

Digital technology has radically transformed almost every aspect of human life in recent years and enabled immense amounts of information to be compressed on small storage devices that can be easily preserved and transported. Digitization also quickens data transmission speeds.

Digitalization, combined with new manufacturing processes, automation, and therapeutics and personalized medicine have the potential to transform the pharmaceutical and biotechnology industries in new and exciting ways. Digital technology – web and mobile solutions, big and small data, sophisticated analytics, miniaturization, artificial intelligence and machine learning, micro- and nano-technology applications, virtual and augmented reality, blockchain, robotics will change the way research is conducted, trials are designed and executed, products are manufactured, commercialized, and distributed, patients are diagnosed, drugs are delivered, and medicine is hyper-personalized are all within the realm of possibility.

Digital technologies and the life sciences are converging at an incredible pace, creating new opportunities to transform patient care as well as drug discovery and development. Digital technology will transform every part of life sciences in future.

EXERCISES

1. How life evolved on earth?

2. Describe the biological basis of life.

3. Discuss the origin and evolution of macromolecules in the cell.

4. Describe the possible precursors of biomolecules.

5. What is biodiversity?

6. What is bioinformatics?

7. How large-scale molecular biology data are generated?

8. Describe the major historical events in genesis of bioinformatics.

9. What are different tools of bioinformatics?

10. Discuss datamining.

11. Discuss different local and multiple sequence alignment tools used for analysis of a query sequence.

12. Short notes:

1. EMBL Gene finders

2. NCBI

3. Gen bank

4. Pub Med.

13. Describe different nucleic acid and protein databases. How they can be used for data mining for different purposes?

14. What is phytogenic analysis?

15. Describe distance method of predicting phylogenetic analysis.

16. What are the methods of evaluating phylogenies?

CONCLUSION

Bioinformatics is concerned with development and application of computer software and hardware to get, store, analyze and visualize biological information. By supplying algorithms, databases, user interfaces and statistical tools, comparison of DNA sequences are possible. The long-term value of bioinformatics and data mining capabilities does not lie so much in developing tools, as it does in connecting knowledge or information into products like therapeutics, animal, and plant bioreactors in the form of genetically modified organisms, newly discovered genes, *etc*. Databases are the heart of bioinformatics. There are many types of databases depending on nature of information stored and manner of data storage. Three Components of Bioinformatics. (1) Development of new algorithms and statistics to assess relationships among members of data set. (2) Use of these algorithms to analyze and interpret diverse types of data, *e.g.*, nucleotide sequence, amino acid sequences, protein domain structure and protein interactions. (3) Development and implementation of tools, *i.e.*, databases that allow access and management of several types of information.

DECLARATION

It is declared that no material in the book has been reproduced by other sources/publishers.

ACKNOWLEDGMENT & CONFLICT OF INTEREST

No potential conflict of interest is declared by the author. It is also declared the complete work is an individual effort by the author and there was no financial/ administrative/ academic support availed from any individual/ institution /organization.

BIBLOGRAPHY

[1] Hartl DL, Jones EW, Hartl DL, Jones EW. Genetics: principles and analysis. 1998.
[2] Primrose SB. Principles of gene manipulation and genomics by Sandy B Primrose and Richard Twyman.
[3] Brown TA. Genomes 5.
[4] Daniel L. Genetics: Principles and analysis. Sudbury, Massachusetts 2004; p. 854.

CHAPTER 4

Scientific Document

LEARNING OBJECTIVES

After going through this chapter, one should be able to appreciate the following:

- How to plan and organize research?
- What is a good research paper?
- How to write an academic report (thesis/dissertation) /review article/ short - communication/abstract/monograph/ report/book?
- Digital technology platforms for documents.

Abstract: Writing a scientific paper, or research report or presenting research data for oral presentation is an art that comes with practice and experience. This chapter intends to make the reader aware of the basic features of scientific writing and digital technology platforms for documents available

Keywords: Research paper, Report, Abstract, Review of literature.

SCIENTIFIC WRITING

Structures

1.Scientific paper
2.Guidelines for writing a scientific paper
3.Review articles
4.Report
5.Thesis and Dissertation

Types of Scientific Documents

Types of scientific articles include primary articles (original research articles, case reports/case series, and technical notes), *secondary articles* (narrative review articles and systematic reviews), *special articles* (letters to the editor, correspondences, short communications, editorials, commentaries, and pictorial essays), and *tertiary and gray literature* (Reports, Proceedings, Dissertations and theses, Registered trials, White papers, Newsletters, Patents).

Simmi Kharb, Akshat Singh, Abhyuday Singh & Deepa Kharb (Eds.)

Research Paper: its Organization and Writing:

Scientific Paper

A scientific paper is not a technical report or term paper. This is a paper worth writing only if it has general implications for knowledge. One should think of its role as guiding the future efforts of scholars since others will follow with newer data and better models.

Scientists are motivated for writing papers in two ways, namely, to understand the world and to get credit for it. In academic and public sectors, scientific papers are means of expansion of human knowledge. Publish or perish should be the rule for scientists working as individuals for professional survival; if you do not publish, you are out of the field.

Nowadays, the quality of a scientific paper is measured by the citation index. It depends on:

(i)The originality and importance of ideas,
(ii)The effectiveness of communication to flag new ideas,
(iii)The means of communication, the role of advertisement, presentation, communications at meeting, email exchanges, citations, *etc.*

Remember that writing a paper is not merely a description of works, it is the work itself. Suggestions:

(i) Start writing a paper as soon as possible: view it as a tool of your research.

(ii) Write an "introduction" as you engage into your research:

Try to Highlight

•What are you trying to do?
•Why it is important?
•What has been done earlier?

(iii) Write the "methods" when you think they are mature/materialising. Golden rule—Any difficulty in writing means there is a problem with the methods.

(iv) Write "results" and "discussions" after spending enough time on analysing and interpreting results.

(v) Spend a little bit of time daily with your evolving paper. Try to be a critical reader or reviewer to bring the best out of it.

Very few will read your paper in a thorough and deliberate way, from beginning till the end. Remember you must market your paper for casual readers!

1. Title and Abstract—are for search engines and most readers won't go beyond that!
2. Results: Figures + Captions and Table + Footnotes:
(i) Must be self-contained. A lot of readers go through those without reading the text and some look for a brief explanation in the text.
(ii) Make figures attractive.
3. Remember that the take-home message of your paper should be "in your face" *i.e.*, in the abstract, introduction, and conclusions. Make sure that everyone gets the message!

Writing an effective paper is not as easy as an essay. A good rule is to write as if your paper will be read by a person who knows about the field in general but does not already know what you did. You should read some scientific papers that have been written in a format which you plan to use and then plan to write a scientific paper.

Typical Outline of a Paper

Abstract

Introduction

Materials and Methods

Results

Tables and figures

Discussion

Citations

Reference lists

Genetic nomenclature

Format: flow, abbreviations, tense, third person, parenthesis

Proof-reading.

Typically, not more than 100–150 words. The abstract is of course the most important part of the paper— many readers well just read that!

•Try to focus on: What is new—essential idea
•Try to write one fact/idea/per sentence.
•Try to give everything that you want to casual readers to remember!

The abstract must not have a reference. Avoid the use of "in this paper" in the abstract.

In the introduction, let the reader know what this paper is all about?

Points to remember:

•Introduce problem
•Outline solution
•Also, include a clear statement of why the problem is important?

Begin with a mini-review and finish the introduction by explaining the theme and subject of your paper is about.

1st paragraph

•State the problem succinctly.
•Do not encumber with too many references.
•Tell in one sentence what your paper is all about at the end of the 1st para.

2nd and following paragraph:

•You have already told the reader what your paper is about.
•Give = background information

= what people have done before.

•Limitations *etc*. (give references).

In the last paragraph, elaborate on what you will be doing in your paper.

Write this as soon as you think that your methods are mature. The writing process will make you check whether your method is mature. Supply useful references for future modellers to use.

Start by presenting your results and then discuss what they mean. Logically, a linear flow of thoughts is essential. Write one theme per paragraph. 1st sentence lays out the theme and the last one supplies a link to the next paragraph. It should be between 1/2 – 1 page.

Focus on what you can say with confidence.

Comparison of Model (Results) with observations.

Comparison with observation should have a clear purpose in terms of learning.

Most papers need a conclusion section. A default approach is to treat it as an extended abstract. But this is also an opportunity to be reflective about what you have learned, what uncertainties are left, links to other problems, *etc.*

1st para: Focus on what you did.

Following paras: One major finding per para. The 1st sentence states findings, and the following sentence elaborates.

Final para: it should have some forward-looking perspective.

"Please do not let your paper finish on a whimper!"

References

- Be serious about searching and reading papers. Devote a bit of time to this each day.
- Never cite a paper for which you haven't read at least the relevant part.
- Cite papers in a context that makes it clear what the paper did, otherwise the reference is useless.
- If you are not clear on what the cited paper did, then re-read it.
- Do not cite textbooks.
- There is nothing wrong in citing yourself or your group extensively. But do not ignore what others have done.
- References should be helpful to the reader, but, not of historical interest.
- Remember that extensive referencing is the scholarly and ethical thing to do.
- The universal guidelines of citation authority or guidelines of the journal intended for submission.

Avoid the use of *et al.* in a bibliography unless the list is very long (6 or more authors).

•Acknowledge your funding source. List the grant number. Write text like "This work was supported by the National Science Foundation under grant EIA NN-NNNNN."
•Anonymous reviewers don't get acknowledged, unless they really provided an exceptional level of feedback or insight.

1.Avoid too much motivational material, and unnecessary details.
2.Avoid spelling errors:
(i)Spelling checkers are also available.
(ii)Ask your colleague to edit your spelling.
(iii)Consult a dictionary such as Merriam Webster (online)
3.Avoid text in aerial unusual fonts. Use Times Roman.

Review Articles

Review articles are very popular and readers like reviews because they are part of the solution to the problem of keeping up, with the ever-expanding literature.

Most commonly, reviews are written by invitation from the editor of a traditional journal. Sometimes, there are journals and magazines entirely devoted to review articles and again most of them are obtained by invitation.

The reviewer is an expert in the chosen field. However, to produce a good piece of work, considerable time and access to extensive library search are needed.

Usually, subjects are suggested by the person assigning/inviting the review. Sometimes, the author himself approaches an editor for writing a review on his own topic. Authors with a considerable experience and authority must write a review article.

In the days of computer literature searching, it is easier to search the essential references for the article. However, reviewers must visit the library because sometimes related articles that are not revealed by computer search can be picked up. Care should be taken about incorporating unpublished observations and personal communications, since the reader cannot verify these data.

Contents of Review

The review contents should be in the following order:

i.The problem

ii.Background
iii.Basic science
iv.Methodology
v.Animal studies
vi.Human studies
vii.Discussion
viii.Conclusion
ix.Recommendations
x.Prospects

In addition, a review should have a glossary of terms. Also, an abstract or summary is wanted by certain journals.

Layout of Review

While writing a review, one should adhere to instructions for authors of a particular journal. It should be typed on an A4 size paper, double-spaced, and should have 300 words per page.

Also, it should be supported by proper references to address contentious issues using key publications and items. Also, it should be supported by tables and figures. And if tables or figures are to be reproduced from any copyright material, then written permission must be obtained from the copyright holder.

Care should be taken regarding misspellings, and errors in the text. Typeface used should be serif typeface (e g. Times Roman) and most journals accept manuscripts only, by email or computer disk (cd), but still some journals request 2–3 copies of the printed version. Also, one should keep a copy of what is sent to the journal for making changes in the future.

References quoted in the bibliography should be according to the style and format required by requesting journal e.g., Vancouver style.

A good review should help the reader to discern the relevant pros and cons easily and have the key references for confirmation and further information.

Reports: Technical Report, Survey, Report:

Reports

The research report is considered a major part of the research study for the research task. The purpose of research is not well served until the report has been presented and/or written.

1. Logical analysis of the subject matter.
2. Preparation of the final outline.
3. Preparation of a rough draft.
4. Preparation of the final draft out of the rough draft.
5. Preparation of bibliography.
6. Writing the final draft.

It must be kept in mind that every report should be an attempt to solve some intellectual problems and must contribute to the solution of a problem. Also, it should add to the knowledge of both the researchers and the readers.

The aim of writing a research report is that anyone reading the research report must be conveyed enough about the study. It should comprise

(1) Preliminary pages
(2) Main text
(3) End matter

Preliminary pages

- Title date
- Acknowledgments in form of preface (foreword)
- Table of contents
- List of tables and illustrations

Main Text

It provides an outline of research report along with all details.

(i)Introduction: Highlighting why the problem was considered worth investigating along with background and relevant research of others, hypothesis of the study, if any, and the methodology adopted should be explained in detail: how the study was carried out, the basic design of study, the details of experimental manipulation,

instructions/questionnaire if any, details of the sample used: who were the subjects, their no., selection criteria; and statistical analysis adopted. Also the scope of the study should be explained.
(ii)Statement of findings and recommendations.

(iii)Results: Findings of the study should be presented in detail in the form of tables, and charts.

(iv)Implications of results:

a.Inference drawn from the study.

b.Generalizations of their inference.

c.Relevant questions that are still unanswered or few questions by the study along with suggestions for the kind of research that would supply answers for them.

The report should finish with a short conclusion that summarises and recapitulates the main points of the study. Also, a forecast of the probable future of the subject and a sign of the kind of research that needs to be done in that field are also essential.

(v)Summary—Summary in brief about the research problem, major findings and major conclusion drawn.

End Matter

At the end of the report, appendices should be enlisted. Bibliography of sources consulted should also be given.

Results of research investigation can be presented in a no. of ways, viz.,

1.Technical report
2.Popular report
3.Article
4.Monograph
5.Oral presentation

Technical Report

It is used whenever a full written report of the study is needed whether for record-keeping or for public discrimination.

Outline

(i)Summary of results: In 2–3 pages
(ii)Nature of study:
•Objective
•Formulation of problem
•Hypothesis
•Type of analysis data needed
(iii)Methods employed: Details of sample design
(iv)Data:
•Discussion of sources, characteristics, and limitation of data collected.
•In case of survey, the description of details of data collection.
(v)Analysis of data and presentation of findings—in the form of tables and charts.
(vi)Conclusion
(vii)Bibliography
(viii)Technical appendices
(ix)Index

Popular Report

Popular report is used if research results have policy implications. Technical details are minimized. It requires an attractive layout with many subheadings and emphasis on practical aspects and policy implications.

At times, oral presentation of the results of the study is considered effective, particularly in cases where policy recommendations are shown by project results. Slides, wall charts and blackboards are used.

Thus, report-writing is an act that is learnt by practice and experience.

Preparation of Academic Report: Thesis, Dissertation:

Thesis & Dissertation

Students enrolled for an honours degree, a postgraduate degree of a doctoral degree are invariably required to submit a thesis or dissertation. The terms "Thesis" and "Dissertation" are often used interchangeably. However, in Indian University, thesis is considered higher than dissertation since for the Ph.D. degree, the requirement of thesis is imposed; and for the lower degrees of MA/MSc, MEd, M Phil, the requirement is that of a dissertation.

A thesis is divided into three broad sections:

(i)Preliminary section
(ii)Main body
(iii)Reference Section

Reference Section

(i)Introduction
(ii)Review of literature
(iii)Design of study
(iv)Presentation and analysis
(v)Summary
(vi)Conclusion

The reference section includes bibliography, appendices, and index in a proper form.

Before drafting the thesis, a good deal of planning is necessary. It helps thesis writing with proper emphasis on various aspects.

A good thesis must have clarity of both thought as well as language to help the reader grasp the ideas of the researcher easily. The presentation of report is also a vital factor. Thesis should neither be too voluminous nor too concise.

There should be chapters, sections, subsections, headings, subheadings, tables, and diagrams. There is no unique and universally accepted method of authoring the thesis. The thesis must be written in drafts one after the other. Ideas and sentences are to be re-aligned and the material must be carefully re-examined and re-edited.

Summary of Thesis

Along with the thesis, a summary is prepared, softbound separately and sent.

The summary is sent to the evaluators in advance to obtain their consent to examine the full thesis.

A summary is a brief review of all the work that has been performed in the thesis. It is a statement in brief of the theoretical rationale, hypotheses, procedures, and results and is the most widely read part of any thesis.

CONCLUSION

In academic and public sectors, scientific papers are means of expansion of human knowledge. You should read some scientific papers that have been written in a format which you plan to use and then plan to author a scientific paper. Review articles are extremely popular and readers like reviews because they are part of the solution to the problem of keeping up, with the ever-expanding literature. Most commonly, reviews are written by invitation from an editor of a traditional journal. The aim of writing a research report is that anyone reading the research report must be conveyed enough about the study. It should include Preliminary pages, the Main text, and conclusion. Popular report is used if research results have policy implications. Before writing a thesis, a good deal of planning is necessary. A good thesis must have clarity of both thought as well as language to help the reader to grasp the ideas of the researcher easily.

EXERCISE

1. What is a scientific paper?

2. Give details of the style and format of scientific paper.

3. How will your observations be computed?

4. What should be the layout of the report?

5. How to plan and write a dissertation?

6. What is a scientific document?

7. What are the qualities of a good research paper?

8. What is the layout of a review?

9. What are the ways in which results can be computed?

10. What are the different types of reports?

11. Plan a 'research plan' and give the proposed layout of the same.

12. How will you write your research paper?

13. Give an outline of the paper.

14. Suppose you have to subunit a technical report on gene cloning, give the layout of same. v layout of the presentation.

15. Suppose a student is assigned a dissertation on "gene mapping for a genetic disease". Write the headings for the synopsis (research plan).

16. Give an account of the role of computers in research.

BIBLIOGRAPHY

[1] Ranjit K. Research methodology: A step-by-step guide for beginners 2011.

[2] John W. Creswell, J David Creswell Research Design: Qualitative. 5th. Quantitative, and Mixed Methods Approaches 2018.

[3] Booth C, Wayne Colomb G, Gregory Williams M. Joseph The Craft of Research. 3rd. Chicago Guides to Writing, Editing, and Publishing 2008.

[4] Marczyk G, De Matteo D, Festinger D. Essentials of Research Design and Methodology 2005.

CHAPTER 5

Scientific Literature

LEARNING OBJECTIVES

The *Scientific literature* includes abstracts, journals, books and data available on the internet. This unit aims to provide knowledge on different types of scientific literature and different modes of research and use this available literature.

Structure

1. Writing an abstract for a scientific meeting.
2. Using the computer in research.
3. Literature.
4. Methodological references.
5. Computer-based searches and other aids to literature.

The scientific programme includes a limited number of spaces for the presentation of abstracts, either as oral communications or posters.

Abstract: Writing a scientific paper, research report, or presenting research data for oral presentation is an art that comes with practice and experience. This chapter intends to make readers aware of the basic features of scientific writing and digital technology platforms for documents available.

Keywords: Literature, Study design, Data collection, Analysis, Research, Encyclopaedias, Reference works, Publications, Journals, and Bibliography.

TYPES OF SCIENTIFIC LITERATURE

Scientists usually communicate their results of research primarily through the *scientific literature.* Scientific literature is a permanent repository of scientific knowledge and records progress in scientific inquiry. Scientific literature can exist in a variety of physical forms such as print publications in the form of books or journal articles, as electronic documents, such as the data on web sites or as personal communications, *etc.*

There are different types of scientific literature, namely, primary, secondary, tertiary and gray literature.

Primary Literature

It is the first-hand account of new/ original research written and reported by researchers who themselves conducted the research.

Simmi Kharb, Akshat Singh, Abhyuday Singh & Deepa Kharb (Eds.)

A *primary article* is a report of a given study and includes introduction to research, methods used, data and results obtained, a discussion of results, and references related to the literature used in the design and analysis of the research in question. These publications can be found in journals, government, and various institutional research reports, and sometimes referenced in books.

Patents, dissertations, and other documents reporting original research, and journal articles are the most widely used primary sources in the field of science.

Secondary Literature

It is a type of scientific literature that is created when other scientists integrate the information from primary literature into review articles or books; these reviews are termed *secondary literature.* It consists of publications that rely on primary sources for information and includes review journals, monographic books and textbooks, handbooks and manuals. Reviews provide a broad overview of a field or ideas generated by many people. Secondary literature is useful for gaining a broad perspective on a topic or a synthesis of ideas about a topic and to find a bibliography of relevant sources. Thus, secondary literature in the sciences summarizes and synthesizes the primary literature. Examples: literature review articles; books.

Tertiary Literature

It consists of published works based on primary or secondary sources which are aimed both at scientists working in different areas from the subject matter of the publication and interested but lay audiences. They are normally written in a popular style and may include a short bibliography; and do not include references of the primary literature. Thus, tertiary literature presents summaries or condensed versions of materials with references to primary or secondary sources. Examples: textbooks, dictionaries, encyclopedia, and handbooks.

There are many types of scientific documents written for various purposes and a few of the main ones are already described in chapter 4. The remaining types are discussed in this chapter.

COMPUTER, INTERNET, AND WORLD WIDE WEB

Computer & Internet

The computer has become an essential tool in biotechnology research. It may be used for routine jobs of word processing and data collection and analysis. Also, when connected to the Internet, it may be used for searching biomedical (biotechnology) literature, accessing information about nucleic acid and protein sequences, predicting protein structure, seeking research methodology and searching databases of genome programs.

By using computers, one can greatly broaden its use to some of the following:

(i)Searching the biomedical literature for pertinent books and journal articles.
(ii)Accessing biological databases that provide nucleic acid and protein sequences and structures.

Once connected to the Internet, many programs are available as freeware.

One can communicate by e-mail. Messages containing text, files and graphics may be sent to anyone who has a computer with an Internet link and e-mail address.

Communication among scientists is now done primarily by e-mail. Also, one can join several discussion groups such as Use Net.

It has become the most rapidly growing component of the Internet since its launch in 1992. It permits the transfer of data as pages in the multimedia form consisting of texts, graphs, audios and videos. The pages are linked together by hypertext pointers so that data stored on computers in different locations may be retrieved *via* the network by one's computer. To access all the resources on web, one needs a browser (that reads hypertext and displays web pages on the computer) and common web browsers are: Internet Explorer, and Netscape Navigator.

World Wide Web

To access web, a web browser is activated and on-screen home page will be displayed. The dialogue box on this page asks for "address", "net site", "location" or "URL" (Uniform Resource Locator); type in the web page address which is usually in the form http://www.

On the home page, the instructions for the use of the website will be displayed on the screen. One important feature to be noted is that some words on the page are highlighted. If any one of these words are clicked by the used , the computer gets connected to another related web page that provides information on the hyperlink.

Web addresses that are useful for biotechnology research are presented in a Table. Millions of new websites are created every year and to access these new sites, one needs the help of a Search Engine, a searchable directory that organizes web pages by subjected classification. Major search engines include Yahoo, Google, Netscape Search, Sciurus, *etc.* As one "surfs the web", one may find sites of interest. They can be saved and reviewed at a later date.

It is not necessary to have a complete understanding of the Internet in order to tap into its vast resources.

The fundamental concept provided here would allow a junior researcher in biotechnology to take advantage of two essential activities:

(i)Biotechnology and molecular biology literature
(ii)Using web directories and biological databases

The Literature

Researchers do not spend all of their working time in the laboratory. An important component of their research project is the search of biotechnology literature. The library should be considered a tool for experimental biotechnology in the same way as any scientific instrument.

The library is used in all stages of research. Before an investigator can begin experimentation, a research idea must be generated. A research project usually begins in the form of a question to be answered or a problem to be solved.

For an easy solution, a major project can be subdivided into questions that may be answered by experimentation. Before the laboratory work starts, the researchers must have a knowledge of the past and current literature dealing with the research area. Thus, one can reduce the project to two questions:

- What is the current state of knowledge in the area?
- What are the significant unknowns?

Answers to these questions can be achieved only after developing familiarity with the literature.

Not only the knowledge of literature is essential, but also the knowledge of techniques and laboratory procedures is required.

Experimental details can be available in the methods section in well-written books and journals. Finally, while performing experiments, the researcher often needs a lot of information.

ENCYCLOPAEDIA, CONFERENCE PROCEEDINGS AND EXTENDED ABSTRACTS

Writing an Abstract for a Scientific Programme

One should follow the instructions for writing an abstract. It should have the following headings:

(i)Title
(ii)Authors—Name of the author; name and address of the affiliated institution, telephone number, and an email address.
(iii)Background
(iv)Aim of study
(v)Study design
(vi)Results
(vii)Discussion
(viii)Conclusion and implications

Writing an abstract is only the first phase. The next is to convert it into an oral presentation or a poster.

Reference Books & Review Publications

Various handbooks, encyclopaedias, and websites are available for this purpose. The beginner researchers in biotechnology will not be expected to proceed through all of these stages in the design of an experiment. Thus, familiarity with the literature increases the understanding of the experiment and may aid in the development of more effective methods. With this background, when you do begin a research program, you will be able to use the library to the fullest advantage.

The molecular biology literature is massive and rapidly expanding. It is almost a full-time job just to maintain a current awareness of a specialized research area. Since biochemistry, biological sciences, biotechnology, molecular biology, physical sciences and basic medical sciences are overlapping; one should not be hesitant to explore these overlapping literature while planning a research project.

The student's first exposure to biotechnology is probably a lecture course accompanied by reading a general textbook of biotechnology. By providing an in-depth survey of biotechnology, textbooks help in building a strong foundation of important principles and concepts.

More specialized and detailed biotechnology information that is not offered by textbooks, could be available in reference books.

Reference works range from general surveys to specialized series. The best works are multivolume sets that continue the publication of volumes on a periodic basis. Each volume usually covers a specialized area with articles written by recognized authorities in the field. It should be noted that reference articles of interest to biotechnologists are often found in publications that are not strictly related to biotechnology.

The core of the biotechnology literature is research journals. It is essential for a researcher to maintain knowledge of recent advances in his or her research field and related areas.

Scores of research journals are published with the intent of keeping researchers up to date. The expansion of scientific information has generated the need for efficient storage and use of research journals. Many publishers are now providing journals in forms such as micro cards, microfilms, microfiche, floppy and more recently CD-ROM disks and DVDs and online. Nowadays, most journals can be subscribed online, also they provide email alerts for content of tables, or articles of specific interest free-of-cost.

Some research journals have achieved an especially excellent reputation and articles therein are considered to be of the highest quality. A number of citation or indexing authorities index and grade the journals, *e.g.*, Index Medicus, index Copernicus, Excerpta Medica, and the Current Contents, Scopus.

Methodology References

The active researcher has a continuing need for new methods and techniques. Several publications specialize in providing details of research methods and many research methods are non-available on the web.

Some of the useful publications are:

Science (Science now, STKE) www.science.com

Nature (Nature Biotechnology, Nature Reviews, nature Genetics, Nature

Review Genetics) www.nature.com

Genome Research

Bioinformatics

Targets Proc Natl Acad Sco. USA

Am J hum Genet

Hum Hered

Nucleic Acid Research

Blood

NEJM

Cell

Current Opinion Cell Biology

Trends Genetics

Trends Biotechnology Biology Molecular

Trends Biotechnology Medicine

J Mol Biol

Mol Cell Biol

J Clin Invest

A Practical Guide to Molecular Cloning

Methods Enzymology

1.Molecular Cell Biology: Lodish, Baltimore, Darnell (Freeman Publication)
2.Principles of Genetics: Snustad, Simmons (John Wiley and Sons, Inc.)
3.Principles of Genome Analysis and Genomics: Primrose, Teryman (Black Well Publishing)
4.From Genes to Genomes: Dale, Schantz (Wiley)
5.Gene Cloning—an introduction: Brown (Oxford, UK)
6.Molecular Biotechnology Principles and applications of Recombinant DNA (Am. Society for Microbiology, USA)
7.Genes VII–IX:
8.Lowan, B, Oxford University Press, Oxford.

Journals in Biotechnology and Genomics

Annual Review of Biochemistry

Annual Review of Genomics and Human Genetics

Bioinformatics and Genetics

Current Genomics

Current Opinion in Cell

Current Opinion in Biotechnology

Current Opinion in Genetics and Development

Cell

Gene

Genetics

Genomics

Molecular Genetics and Genomics

Nature Biotechnology

Nature Genetics

Nature

Nature Review Genetics

Nucleic Acid Research

PNAS (Proceedings of National Academy of Sciences)

Protein Engineering

Science

Trends in Biotechnology

World Journal of Microbiology and Biotechnology

Biotechnology and Development Monitor

Genetic Engineering News

Genomics and Proteomics

Online mendelian Inheritance in Man (OMIM)

http://www.3.ncbi.nlm.nih.gov/omim/

Genetic interest group

www.gig.org.uk

Genome database

www.gdb.org.

Human Genome Bioinformatics

www.gene.ucl.as.uk.

Human Gene Mutation Database

www.uwcm.ac.uk/uwcm/mg/hgmd 0.html

C. Elegans Genetics and Genomics

http://elegams.swmed.edu/genomes.html

Yeast Genome Projects

http://mips.gsf.de/genre/proj/yeast/index.jsp.

Dolan DNA Learning Centre at cold spring Harbor Lab

www.dnalc.org

Vander Bilt University Medical School

http://peds/mc.vander bilt.edu/VCHWEBI/Medical-Genetics.html

The Human Cytogenetic Database (HCDB)

Schinzel A. Oxford Medical, Oxford University Press, Oxford.

European Bioinformatics Institute

www.ebi-ac-uk

National Centre for Biotechnology Information (NCBI)

www.ncbi.nlm.nih.gov.

DNA Data Bank of Japan

www.ddbj.nig-as-jp/

Swiss Institute of Bioinformatics (SIB)

www.isb-sib.ch/

Sanger Centre

www.Sanger.as.-uk

The Institute for Genomic Research

www.tigr.org

As one studies and works in the field of biotechnology, he/she would often need to complete a thorough literature search on some specialized areas or topics. It is not practical to survey hundreds of books, journals and reports that may contain information related to the topic.

There are a number of publications that provide brief summaries of published articles, reviews and patents, namely, Chemical Abstracts, Biological Abstracts, and Excerpta Medica, and Current Contents give selected titles of articles in relevant fields.

The computer revolution has reached the biomedical literature and most college and university libraries are now getting subscriptions to computer bibliographic search services and online subscriptions for journals. One such service for a bibliography is STN International which allows the direct access to some of the world's largest scientific databases, *e.g.*, BIOSIS Previews/RN (produced by BioSciences Information Services) covers original research articles, reports, reviews, US patents in biology and biomedicine); CA (chemical abstracts service), MEDLINE AND MEDLARS (US National Library of Medicine and Index medicus, respectively) cover all areas of biomedicine. These networks provide online service and their databases can be accessed on the internet.

A wide variety of databases are currently available including genome sequences, bibliography, nucleic acid sequences, protein sequences and structures, metabolic pathways and even useful software programs for exploring new structures and sequences.

Blast (Searching for similar protein and nucleic acid sequences)

Some of these are hyperlinked to the database sites. Several software programs are available

Which are hyperlinked to database sites, namely:

Chime (protein structures on moving 3-D coordinates)

Entrez (NCBI) Cross-referencing database)

Gen Bank (NCBI) (Database of gene sequences)

All these databases are readily available, free of charge on the web.

DIGITAL LIBRARIES IN BIOLOGICAL SCIENCES

Cloud, Web etc.

Digital Libraries in Biological Sciences

Digital Library

A special type of library containing a collection of digital content stored in electronic media formats such as text, digital documents, books, journals, and visual material, and audio & video material. It is a means for data or media files organization, storage, and their retrieval from the library collection. The electronic content may be stored locally, or can be remotely accessed through the internet.

The size and scope of digital libraries vary greatly and they are usually maintained by people, and various organizations. They can be have affiliations with physical library buildings or institutions.

Advantages of the Digital Library

Since the digital library is not confined to a particular location, and rather virtually distributed and accessible on the web throughout the world *via* internet, there is no physical boundary, or time constraints (Round the clock availability). We can have multiple accesses. A digital library has a structured approach to easy data accessibility, having user-friendly interfaces that give access to its resources on a single click. Digital data is preserved and conserved without any degradation of quality and is less costly to manage as compared to the traditional physical library

Disadvantages of the Digital Library

There are risks of computer viruses, lack of standardization for digitized information, quick degradation of digitized material, different display and associated problems, health hazards (radiation from the monitor, *etc.*) along with copyright violation at times. The initial cost of the development of a digital infrastructure is high. They require high bandwidth for the transfer of data.

Biomedical Digital Libraries

BioMed Central is used to publish biomedical digital libraries till 2007, however, all articles published in the journal during this time with BioMed Central are fully searchable. Other biomedical digital libraries store databases of abstracts and citations of peer-reviewed literature: scientific journals, books and conference proceedings and their examples are Scopus; Springer, SClmago, Publons, *etc.*

Cloud computing is the delivery of on-demand computing services -- from applications to storage and processing power -- typically over the internet and it can be paid or have a free access.

Top cloud providers are Microsoft Azure, AWS, Google cloud, *etc.*

VIRTUAL TRAINING

Introduction

Nowadays, people can access high quality education *via* internet and proliferation of internet-based education has occurred in the COVID era, and this has provided easy access to education for wider population through real-time online classes. Plenty of people are advancing their knowledge and skills that they would not have done otherwise due to time, geographical or money constraints. Online learning is the future of education and this has changed the concept of traditional education radically. Since companies allowed their employees to conduct their jobs from their homes using a computer or a smartphone in covid pandemic, and this has given them time for online education.

Importance of Webinars & Online Lectures:

Webinars

Webinars are web-based multimedia lessons, seminars, discussions, and demonstrations that offer the very same advantages as online classes do, and have the ability to reach dozens or hundreds of people all around the world.

Online Training

Online lectures, videos, or screencasts created by an instructor can have a positive impact on students' attitudes towards their learning experience. Students may believe that they comprehend the content better due to hearing their instructor's voice. Students also believe they can work at their own pace because of the ability to replay the recorded video. Flipped learning is, essentially, blended learning. It is a course that utilizes both in-class time and online time for student learning.

Virtual Training for Medical Professionals:

Virtual Training

Virtual training is done in a virtual or simulated environment, wherein the learner and the instructor are at separate locations. Most of the virtual trainings and virtual training environments are designed to simulate the traditional classroom or learning experience.

Virtual training uses the fundamentals of face-to-face training and thus replicates this experience through a virtual platform such as Microsoft Teams or Zoom, and many more. One of the benefits of virtual training is its ability to overcome geographical obstacles.

This allows people to gain access to training that would have otherwise been impossible. This is the power of virtual training; it allows learning for all, no matter where they are in the world. Virtual classrooms are saving on travel costs and thus save a large amount of training budget of many organisations, and this has become the main reason for transitioning to virtual training.

Virtual worlds are rapidly becoming a part of the educational technology landscape and has potential for professional health education. Virtual worlds are promising in new medical education pedagogy for enhancing learning outcomes beyond that provided by more traditional online or face-to-facc postgraduate professional development activities.

Also, emerging changes in healthcare delivery have a significant impact on the structure of healthcare professionals' education. Since medical knowledge doubles every 6-8 years, and new medical procedures are emerging every day and virtual reality represents a promising area with high potential of enhancing the training of healthcare professionals.

Current virtual training applications for healthcare have complex technological/multimedia sophistication requiring various types of skills trained, right from telesurgical applications to interactive simulations of the human body and brain, and to virtual worlds for emergency training. Other interesting applications of virtual reality lie in the development of immersive 3D environments for training psychiatrists and psychologists in the treatment of mental disorders.

This is just the beginning of the digital technological revolution that has potential to completely transform medical training and care systems in current pandemic crisis and the potential of virtual reality is yet to be explored.

Distance Learning:

Various online programs are designed by different universities and groups worldwide for specialization in particular subjects and to pursue further academic study.

Online Portals:

Web Portals

A portal is a web-based platform that collects information from different sources to be fed into a single user interface. It presents the most relevant information to the users. There are several simple web portals that have evolved into portal platforms that support digital customer experience initiatives.

Examples of portals include patient portals, government portals, intra-/extra-/ workplace portals, management portals for knowledge, student portals, *etc*. The basic concept behind each type of portal is personalized access, based on an assigned or assumed user role. With the evolution of advanced digital content management systems, the web portal has transformed into portal platforms

Role of Virtual Reality in Biotechnology

Biotechnology ironically faces many challenges when it comes to teaching and researching. One of the limitations is the abnormally high cost of education as a result of expensive lab equipment, maintenance, and the need for upgrades. Secondly, biotechnology cannot be taught without practical lessons and requires real experiments.

Owing to this, online learning becomes nearly impossible as students are required to be present at laboratories, and at times some of them are high-security enclosures, and deal with dangerous testing. Thirdly, biotechnology is a resource-intensive field, and it is not always possible to have lab equipment; biomaterials (plants and animals) that are necessary to conduct tests and experiments. Also, procuring and storing biomaterials have complications, namely, ethical concerns and ensuring the presence of adequate personnel to continuously monitor it.

Considering the benefits of biotechnology – from finding cures to complex diseases to alleviating food insecurity, it is very important to find ways to overcome these limitations and thankfully, virtual reality (VR) can help.

Virtual Reality (VR)

VR has as yet not alleviated the public preconceptions about biotechnology practices, however, it can play a role in making the field more accessible and overcoming a number of limitations in terms of research.

Virtual reality has already been incorporated into many streams of science and giving highly positive results and generating money. Today, VR has truly changed the way research is done, with many exciting applications in the field of biotechnology.

VR's Benefits to Biotech

Visualize Complex Structures

Genes and cells have complex structures that can be incredibly difficult to comprehend with only 2D images from microscopes. VR allows for these small structures to be visualized in 3D, for a better understanding of their functions.

Create Realistic Simulated Environments

Virtual reality has allowed researchers to create very realistic simulated environments to study brain function and behavior. *e.g.*, the FreemoVR system that includes a "behavioral arena" including walls and floors equipped with computer displays and uses game technology to recreate specific environments, permitting lab animals to behave naturally. Due to this, animals can move freely and explore the environment without any restrictions.

"Virtual and augmented reality is all set to become a huge part of the modern classrooms come 2050".

Creating Virtual Scenarios

Labster virtual labs are based on the concept of "Virtual Scenarios" – one such example being the CSI Lab Simulation. In this simulation, the principles of DNA analysis are explored through the story of a murder mystery and are being used all over the world in partner universities that include Harvard, MIT, and Exeter in the U.K. VR is benefitting biotechnology practices. From making equipment more accessible to aiding in live experimentation, the field of biotechnology has a lot to gain from utilizing VR.

Virtual Textbooks in Classrooms

Virtual and augmented reality is all set to become a huge part of modern classrooms in 2050. It is 2023, and we have already got robots for teaching assistants and virtual reality headgear for learning tools.

Virtual Biotechnology Company

It is a lean, nimble model that is gaining popularity among cash-hungry start-ups. Thus, a growing number of biotechnology companies employ a skeleton crew of managers and outsource hands-on science and no wet labs.

Virtual Pharmaceutical Company

A virtual company can be agile, shifting from drug formulation to toxicity testing without having to build facilities or hire staff. Virtual companies work best when they are developing drugs for an established molecular target, using familiar techniques

How Augmented Reality Strengthens Biotech Manufacturing? Biotech and pharma companies are starting to implement augmented reality technologies at their manufacturing facilities, bringing forth a whole new world of possibilities. The covid-19 pandemic has been a catalyst to embracing new ways of working. Travel restrictions and limited access to facilities have boosted the adoption of technologies that enhance remote work. And augmented reality (AR) is starting a silent revolution in the pharmaceutical and biotech manufacturing field .AR consists of overlaying digital content to your surroundings, adding diverse layers of information into your vision in the form of text, images, videos, or holograms. In pharma and biotech manufacturing, AR is transforming processes, quality monitoring, and training, letting employees virtually collaborate to maintain supply chains and connect with suppliers and partners. “There is a massive surge in its usage during the Covid pandemic as many organizations had to carry out more remote functions than ever before,”. The biggest advantage of AR is that it enables seeing the production process virtually, without the need to be there.

EXERCISE

1. How to write an abstract?

2. Give an account of the role of computers in research.

3. What is an online journal?

4. What are search engines?

6. Prepare a web directory for literature, tools of biomedical science and database.

7. How will you plan an abstract for scientific meeting?

8. How will you write an abstract for oral presentation?

9. Enumerate applications of web in research.

10. List famous search engines for biological research.

11. List the website and clinical database in biomedical fields.

12. What is virtual reality, discuss its role in biotechnology and healthcare.

SUMMARY

The Scientific literature includes abstracts, journals, books, and data available on the net. Computers have become an essential tool in biotechnology research. They may be used for searching biomedical (biotechnology) literature, and accessing information. For ease of solution, a major project can be subdivided into questions that may be answered by experimentation. Before the laboratory work starts, the researchers must have knowledge of the past and current literature dealing with the research area. The core of the biotechnology literature consists of research journals. It is essential for a researcher to maintain knowledge of recent advances in his or her research field and related areas. The active researcher has a continuing need for new methods and techniques. Several publications specialize in providing details of research methods and many research methods are non-available on the web.

BIBLIOGRAPHY

[1] ABD Jones P, Kolloff M, Kolloff F. Humanizing and establishing presence in an online course: The role of introductory videos in distance learning. InE-Learn: World Conference on E-Learning in Corporate, Government, Healthcare, Higher Education 2006 Oct (pp. 1247-1254). Association for the Advancement of Computing in Education (AACE).

[2] Patra C. Digital repository in ceramics: a metadata study. The Electronic Library. 2008 Aug 8; 561-81:(4)26. Available from: http://hdl.handle.net/10603/212642

CHAPTER 6

The Basis for Starting a new Project and Preparing R & D Projects

LEARNING OBJECTIVES

This chapter gives information about science funding organizations along with details of national and international funding agencies for R and D projects.

Abstract: Biological resource centres (BRCs) are an essential part of the infrastructure underpinning life sciences and biotechnology. They consist of service providers and repositories of the living cells, genomes of organisms, and information related to heredity and the functions of biological systems. The growing worldwide demand for biological resources provides good reasons for greatly increasing the number and quality of BRCs. BRCs provide essential expertise for the formulation of government policies on biological resources and for information and assurance to the public.

The establishment of national BRCs can help identify and address existing gaps and take advantage of opportunities not currently met by existing ex-situ collections. They can then improve the quality of services offered and achieve efficiencies and cost savings.

A global BRC network would connect national BRCs and provide the framework within which co-ordination, harmonisation and quality assurance could be provided. BRCs need to provide greater quality assurance than is currently ensured by collections and databases.

Keywords: Literature, Study design, Data collection, Analysis, Research, Encyclopaedias, Reference works, Publications, Journals, Bibliography.

FUNDING AGENCIES

Structure		
1. Science funding organizations		
2. Basis and technology for starting a new project	(i)	Market survey
	(ii)	Marketing strategies for biotech products
	(iii)	Methodology for starting a new project
	(iv)	Technology

Simmi Kharb, Akshat Singh, Abhyuday Singh & Deepa Kharb (Eds.)

Biotechnology companies after reaching a certain size become sufficient enough to get much out of their heavy R & D spending as it was for global pharma. Most biotech companies have achieved their success behind just one or two block-busting drugs that were priced boldly and marketed aggressively. The product life cycles are short and by careful planning after considering the skill to draw funding would help in the survival of a company.

All the knowledge gained from market surveys and planning would help in, achieving and sustaining the success of a biotech company.

INTERNATIONAL FUNDING AGENCIES

Organization	**Funding Offered**
1.Alexander von Humboldt Foundation	Research Fellowship and research awards for scholars and scientists of all nationalities not resident in Germany.
2. Arnold and Mabel Beckman Foundation	Supports basic scientific research in the USA in the fields of chemistry, biochemistry, and medicine.
3.Caledonian Research Foundation	Encourages academic research in biomedicine.
4.Dalmo Giacometti Foundation	Private foundation which supports genetic research and biotechnology.
5.Grants Net	Research funding information from the American Association for the Advancement of Science.
6.Swiss national Science Foundation	Support scientific research at Swiss Universities, awards fellowships to young scientists.
7.US civilian R and D Foundation	Promotes scientific research and technical collaboration between US and countries of the former Soviet Union.
8.Wallace Genetic Foundation	Supports interests including agriculture research, preservation of farmland, ecology, plant genetic research.

cont.....

9.Whitaker Foundation	A private funding source for biomedical engineering research and education in US.

NATIONAL FUNDING AGENCIES

1.ICMR: Indian Council for Medical Research
2.CSIR: Centre for Scientific and Industrial Research
3.DBT: Department of Biotechnology
4.DST: Department of Science and Technology
5.UGC: University Grants Commission

In life science business environment, new product development is swift, competition is fierce, and the marketplace has multiple distribution channels. To make their position, life science companies need reliable information about their markets regarding research activity of competitors and quantification of the impact of business decisions and goals.

New business creation calls for new ways of designing, developing, manufacturing, marketing, or selling a product of service, which disrupt proven ways of running the business and create dilemmas that have to be managed.

PROCESS OF SELECTING VENTURES

One must first understand (Fig. **1**), Why do ventures succeed or fail?

For understanding how to choose ventures:

Satisfy market need?

↓

Sufficient capabilities?

↓

Flexible brand?

Fig. (1). Process of selecting ventures.

Three Main Reasons for Failure are:

(i)Inability to fill a need in the market
(ii)Lack of capabilities
(iii)Misalignment with the brand

So, by examining the venture in terms of market needs, capabilities and branding, the chances of success of the venture can be accessed and thus, the best opportunity can be selected.

The first rule in developing any test of potential ventures is to talk to the customers to explore the market needs.

The key capabilities of a company are typically known as its core competencies. Core competencies consist of skills and resources that a company possesses, and which are superior to those of its competitors. Skills involve people with design abilities, marketing expertise, financial acumen, or customer service experience. Resources are competencies that are inanimate such as product facilities, access to raw materials, financial resources, location and product or service features.

Successful organizations usually have two or three demonstrable superior competencies as compared to their competitors. While evaluating the possible ventures, one must consider whether an organization has the competencies to support the venture. Thus, success requires a blend of old and new organization traits, a subtle mixture of characteristics achieved through balancing acts of skills, resources, and competencies.

Project management is essential to the biotechnology business. Biotechnology companies have a significant challenge ahead of them. They are very much concerned about cost containment and investor confidence, but at the same time, they have to comply with regulations and aggressively pursue quick market entry. Without a solid project management infrastructure, it's unlikely that many companies will be able to address these concerns effectively.

In biotech business environment, new product development is swift, competition is fierce and the marketplace is fragmented with multiple distribution channels. To capture a market leadership position and keep it over the long term, the companies need information regarding the activity of their competitors and impact of business decisions and goals.

It should be kept in mind that biotech companies have unique market circumstances and information needs. Usually, sales representatives in biotech industries promote therapeutic products and constitute companies' most expensive assets.

Not all products entering the consumer's market undergo the same regulatory oversight. Not all the markets are the same—*e.g.*, one can distinguish between domestic and exports, professional users (such as farmers and doctors) and non-professional consumers.

The government enforces standards *e.g.*, food quality, purity of pharmaceuticals, *etc.* that sometimes directly influence the market. When problems are discovered, the government not only wishes to communicate with industry, but, also with consumers.

MARKET SURVEY

The basic components of marketing are (Fig. **2**):

1.Market survey
2.Futuristic estimates
3.Indigenous technology
4.Imported technology

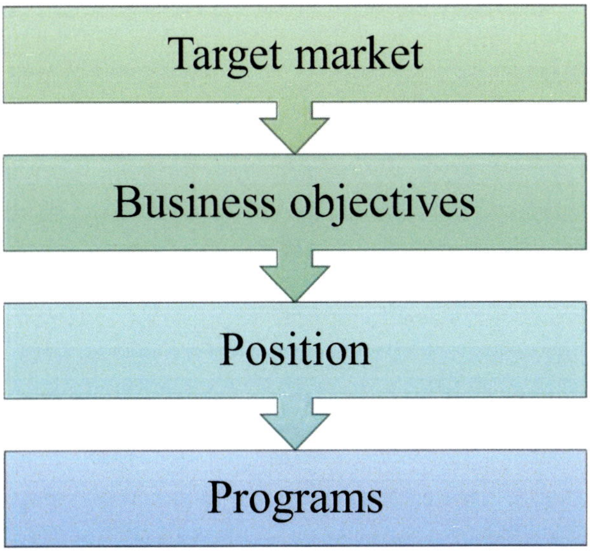

Fig. (2). Components of a marketing strategy.

Implementing Marketing Strategy

Business objectives are what one wants from his business—typically stated as revenue or profits. The programs are the tactics and include advertising, pricing and distribution. The major strategic components of a marketing strategy are “targeting and positioning” which are often ignored!

Targeting consists of selecting the customers in focus. Without customer targets, marketing tactics may be wasted, and the choice of target markets guides the tactics. Also, customer targets help with the setting of prices and distribution. If customer targets are known, distribution will be managed more accurately since you will try to locate near your customer targets.

FOUR KEY QUESTIONS FOR POSITIONING

1.This is the target member of the decision-making unit, be it the family head, or departmental head who may view the benefits of products differently.
2.There are always competitors whom you can choose to fight! They are your target competitors.
3.This idea is very important in marketing. You should concentrate on your communication benefits that you provide more successfully than your competitors to occupy a clearer position in your customer’s mind.
4.For a business to succeed in the long run, it must have capabilities that its competitors do not have.

This requires seven questions to be answered:

(i)Which customer do you want: TARGET MARKET
(ii)What do you want from business: BUSINESS OBJECTIVES
(iii)To whom specifically you must communicate: TARGET-MEMBER OF DECISIONMAKING UNIT.
(iv)What competitor do you need to defeat: TARGET COMPETITOR?
(v)Why should a customer buy from your: BENEFIT ADVANTAGE
(vi)Why will you win: COMPETITIVE ADVANTAGE
(vii)How will you implement your strategy: PROGRAMS?

The first six questions delineate the strategy, and the last question is concerned with how to implement the strategy.

Once the target market and positioning have been determined, one must develop programs to implement the marketing strategy.

MARKETING RESEARCH

Marketing research is defined as the systematic design, collection, analysis and reporting of data and findings relevant to a specific marketing situation facing the company (Fig. **3**).

A company can obtain marketing research in a number of ways. Most large companies/ establishments have their own marketing research departments, which often play crucial roles within the organization.

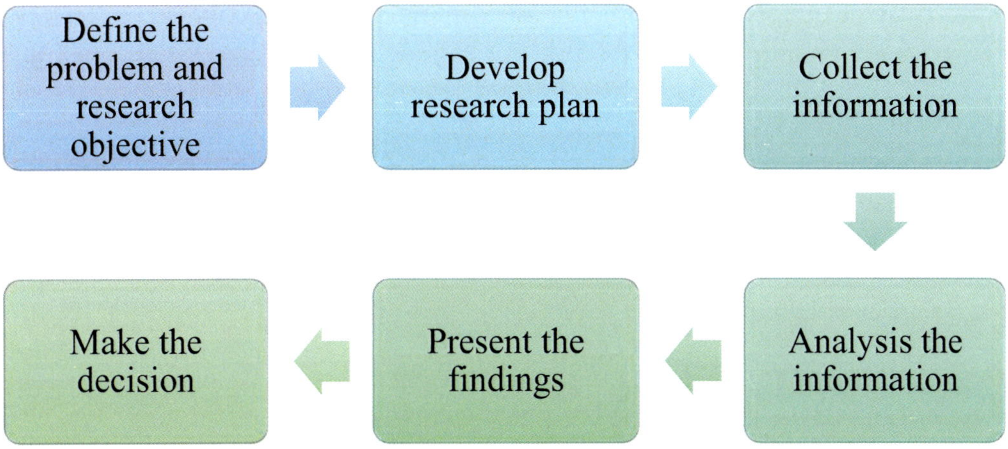

Fig. (3). Marketing Research Process: Flow Chart.

MANAGEMENT OF PROJECTS & MARKETING OF BIOTECHNOLOGY INVENTION

Before starting a new project or as a follow-up approach, surveys are undertaken to learn about people's knowledge, beliefs, preferences, and satisfaction and to measure these magnitudes in the general population. Also, the market for the intended product is surveyed.

Analysis should ensure that the company achieves the sales, profits and other goals established in its plan. The main tools are sales analysis, market share analysis, marketing expense-to-sales analysis and financial analysis of the marketing plan.

Technology is strategic assistance, and it can be developed through R and D activities.

FEATURES OF TECHNOLOGY

It should be

1.Cost-effective
2.Properly located
3.Has low cost of production
4.Ensuring better quality product to meet customer's preferences

Technology acquisition and product development are more critical than ever to biotech product suppliers. Also, predicting accurately which technologies are most viable for development and marketing is challenging. If wrongly identified, this kind of investment may lead to a significant waste to time and resources and can badly injure a company's position in the marketplace. To avoid such a costly misstep, suppliers should establish relationships with national and regional leaders in the research community. So that these relationships can alert a company to scientific trends and establish brand loyalty with this influential group. Relying on ad hoc contacts and research collaborations alone build individual relationships, but, do not give lasting strategic value.

Biotech companies should take lessons from pharmaceuticals who have a long history of building strategic relationships: Continuing education programs (CEPs) and on-hands training programs for physicians, and healthcare professionals should be sponsored to bring together experts of a particular therapeutic field to exchange information and socialize. Also, insights provided by interacting participants are analysed by market research firms to quantify and track opinions and perceptions of key market influences.

Technology is a sort of knowledge or skill used for employing and controlling factors of production.

1.Product Technology: Information that specifies a product feature and uses.
2.Process Technology: Knowledge used in processing or manufacturing of a product.
3.Management Technology: Managerial skills required for running a business.

It is not only the cost involved in R & D, but also how far the cost of product diminishes and how far the quality of the product improves that should be considered. If a new product is designed not keeping in mind the capabilities of the production department, the attempt will be a failure.

Many International Firms have Created Cross-functional Teams that Comprise

R & D department

Production department

Marketing department

In developing countries where funds are too limited to undertake R and D, the import of technology is frequent, although firms are located in industrialised countries to purchase technology.

There are two types of Technology Transfer

i. Point-to-point technology transfer- It is the transfer of technology along with complete secrecy.
ii. Diffusion of technology- In this type, the same technology is transferred to many recipients and secrecy is not maintained.

Biotechnology Entrepreneurship

Since the ultimate objective of biotechnology research is the development of commercial products.

Molecular biotechnology is driven to a greater extent by economics and this unit aims to make reader conversant with biotech product-based life cycles and capital investment.

Structure

1.Commercial potential of biotechnology
2.Cost-estimation of project
3.Biotechnology product-based life cycle.

Biotechnology has unlimited potential due to its capability to generate an unlimited range of useful products/services concerned with virtually every aspect of human existence, *e.g.*, in the mid-90s, over 130 biotechnologically derived pharmaceuticals aimed at everything ranging from haemophilia to AIDS, and from anaemia to leukaemia, were under regulatory review. The contribution of biotechnological products to the global market is rising rapidly and is expected to increase from US $ 100 billion/year in 2000 to further higher.

Also, the biotechnology industry in India is growing rapidly in the wake of liberalization of the economy that fostered alliances between Indian companies and multinationals. In India, the demand for biotechnological products has been estimated at around Rs. 55 billion. (US $ 1.85 billion) in Funding Agencies 161 2000 which doubled by the end of the year 2007. The major share of this demand could be in the areas of human and animal health (72%), followed by industrial products (27%), and agricultural sectors that account for a very small portion (7%) of the demand.

The new biotechnology clearly demands very high expertise and skill and continues heavy funding coupled with a dedicated effort. Therefore, highly industrialized countries have an edge over less industrialized ones and more so, over the developing countries both with regard to research and development (R & D) activities and the exploitation of market potential. This becomes evident when one list of biotechnological products originating from developed countries is compared with those from developing countries; almost all the products are coming from developed countries. Thus, the world trade would become increasingly concentrated on the already highly industrialized and affluent countries, leaving the other countries at a considerable disadvantage. This problem would further aggravate as companies have started to exploit plant genetics to modify "third world crops".

The biotechnology research is both public and private-funded and private sector is increasingly interested in biotechnological research with the aim of making profits. The essence of any biotechnological process is the recovery of the concerned product in a useful form. The efficiency of a product is reflected in terms of product cost and sometimes, the process of product recovery may be either inefficient or costly, preventing the commercial exploitation of the biotechnology process, namely the recovery of insulin, interferon, *etc*. This operation derives inputs from chemistry, chemical engineering, biochemistry, biochemical engineering and biotechnology.

Areas where Biotechnology is Making Marked Contributions

Human Health (Fig. **4**)

Medicine

Animal health

Chemicals and biochemicals

Forensic

Forestry, horticulture

Renewable energy and fuel

Mining

Fisheries

Over the last two decades, biotechnology has also been used for commercial gains and has attracted investments in the stock market, which resulted in closure, merger and acquisition of existing biotechnology companies. This was because the scientists who started biotechnology companies lacked knowledge and experience in business. Also, the businessmen who tried to use biotechnology to make money also failed because they did not have the knowledge of biotechnology. Therefore, it gave rise to a new terminology Biotechnology Entrepreneurship which has now become a specialized subject.

This subject needs the attention of those aspiring to enter biotechnology companies and for sustaining it for commercial gains. To be successful, a variety of skills are also needed apart from research experience degrees. To be a successful, biotechnology entrepreneur, one should possess adaptability, intelligence, confidence, ability to interact with others, modesty, flexibility, and patience. Also, he should have good communication skills, should be persuasive and creative. Also, he should have the basic knowledge of capital investment, and product-based life cycles. Also, he should be able to interpret market surveillance and plan product design, as well as cost estimation and analysis to make appropriate fruitful decisions of capital investment.

Scientific disciplines contributing to molecular biotechnology generate a wide range of commercial products:

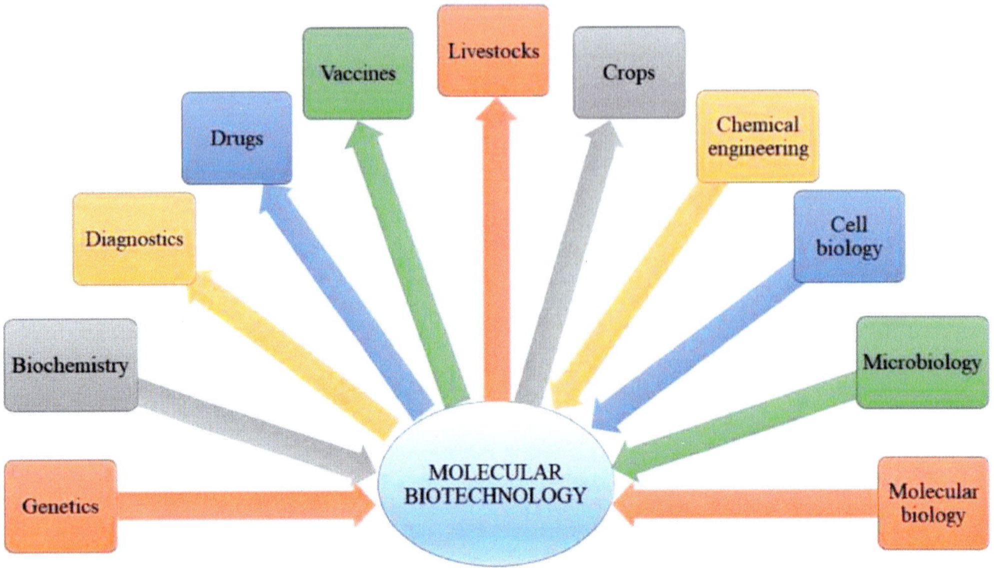

Fig. (4). Inputs and outputs of molecular biotechnology.

The ultimate objective of all biotechnology research is the development of commercial products. Also, molecular biotechnology is driven to a greater extent by economics. Not only does financial investment currently sustain molecular biotechnology, but clearly the expectation of financial gain is responsible for the considerable interest and excitement in its development. Tracing down the history of commercialization, enthusiastic public response to Genetics encouraged others to follow. Between 1980 and 1983, two hundred small biotechnology industries were founded in USA with the help of tax incentives and funding from both stock market speculation and private investment.

Hebert Boyer was the first scientist at the University of California, San Francisco, and then became the Vice President of Genetics. University professors started many of the early companies.

During eighties, rapid proliferation of biotechnology business occurred, and small companies were absorbed by the larger ones, thus strategic merger took place and joint ventures were undertaken.

By mid-nineties, more than a dozen new drugs produced by recombinant DNA technology had been certified for use in humans. By 2000, product sales for molecular biology commodities were US $ 100 billion per year. However, profits for biotechnology companies have been elusive still the continuing enthusiasm of investors for biotechnology indicates, at least in their estimation, that molecular biotechnology will have a persuasive impact on society.

New independent molecular biotechnology companies have always been specialized and tend to stress the use of a particular aspect of recombinant DNA technology that is often reflected in their names, namely, Immunes, Immunogen, Med Immune, ImmuLogic which were formed to produce genetically engineered antibodies for treating infections diseases, cancer and other disorders in humans.

CAPITAL INVESTMENT

Most of the commercial development can be seen in the USA. In other countries, where investment capital is not readily available and where there is less emphasis on entrepreneurial activity, large corporations and governments have taken an active role in creating indigenous molecular biotechnology initiatives. In Japan, biotechnology has been declared a "strategic industry" and made a national priority by the government. In Japan, researchers have acquired necessary expertise by Funding Agencies 163 collaborating with US companies and universities and now major Japanese companies are more directly involved in molecular biotechnology research and product development.

The commercial molecular biology will be exciting in the coming years. Although the specific predications are risky because new technological innovations rapidly replace existing technologies.

Genetic (San Francisco, USA) was the first ever company to be launched in the field of biotechnology and made an initial public offering (IPO) of $ 35 million at the rate of $ 35 per share that soared to $88 per share and closed at $ 56 per share at the end of the day, giving a valuation of $ 400 million.

PRICING POLICY

Demand sets a ceiling on the price the company can charge for its product. The company wants to charge a price that covers its cost of producing, distributing, and selling the product, including a fair return for its effort and risk. Net result is not always profitability when companies price products to cover full costs.

Thc costs are of two forms, variable and fixed. Fixed costs include rent, heat, interest, salaries, *etc*. Variable costs vary directly with the level of production and their costs tend to be constant per unit produced.

While setting the pricing policy, the following six-step procedure is followed by the companies:

1.Selecting its pricing objective.
2.Estimating the demand curve.
3.Estimating how its costs vary at different levels of output.
4.Examining competitors' costs, prices and offers.
5.Selecting a pricing method.
6.Selecting the final price.

Companies do not usually set a single price, but rather a pricing structure that varies according to the geographical demand, market segment requirements, *etc*.

After developing pricing strategies, firms often face situations where they need to change prices in response to declining market share, a desire to dominate the market, and in response to competitors' price change.

In the life cycle of a product, nine steps have been identified where biotechnology ethics are applied:

1.Framework setting, proposal, funding, communication.
2.Early research and patenting.
3.Product design, development and testing.
4.Product assessment, regulation, registration, communication.
5.Market launch (including labels and communication).
6.Market surveillance, enforcement, communication, user education.
7.Product re-evaluation.
8.Evaluate the performance of ethics evaluation.
9.Improve governance of ethics evaluation.

The most important are ethical issues that arise during formulation of ideas, goals and research proposals. Issues may be specific to a planned research proposal or they may open the need to reflect on broader issues such as re-evaluation of the framework within which funding is taking place, *e.g*., broad issue-type would be related to ethics, political philosophy and governance issues in a research using embryonic stem-cells.

• How should researchers and society deal with projects that are described as "playing God" by some observers?

• Is it sufficient to announce a research, "I will be able to create such-and-such (*e.g.*, artificial life, cloned humans, *etc.*):

INTERNATIONAL ORGANIZATIONS:

FAO

Biological Research Centres and Bioresources

Biological resource centres (BRCs) are comprised of service providers and the repositories of living cells, and genomes of organisms. They contain information regarding heredity and various functions of biological systems. BRCs have collections of culturable organisms (micro-organisms, plant, animal, and human cells) ; viable but not yet culturable organisms, cells and tissues (*e.g.* genomes, plasmids, viruses, cDNAs), and databases with their molecular, physiological and structural information and related bioinformatics of these collections.

Biological resource centres are an essential component of infrastructure for R&D in the fields of life sciences, environment, agriculture, and human health, and are important for the commercialization of biotechnology. They have many crucial roles namely,

i. To preserve and provide biological resources for scientific, industrial, agricultural, environmental, and medical R&D and applications.

ii. For the performance of R&D of these biological resources.

iii. To conserve biodiversity.

iv. To prepare repositories of biological resources so as to protect their intellectual property.

v. Serve as a resource of public information and policy formulation.

Need For Biological Resource Centres

Biological resources (living organisms, cells, genes, and related information) are responsible for preserving and distributing biological materials and information. The recent advances in molecular biology was aided by the feasibility and ease of accessibility, procurement and modification of these biological resources will be benefitting the human beings. Gene sequencing and associated functional analysis for a growing number of genomes will have an unprecedented effect on the use of biological resources and their accessibility. Both governments and industry are making large investments to recover biological resources from nature and explore and engineer these recovered resources, especially human genome to reap scientific, economic and medical benefits in long run. A global network of biological resource centres came into being nearly two decades back and this has encouraged the establishment of National BRCs and an accreditation system. Most international frameworks and organisations have linked their resource centres into networks to reach these specific goals more efficiently rather than acting alone. Also, the global Biodiversity Information Facility (GBIF) network linking biodiversity databases began operating in 2001 for making the databases universally accessible.

EXERCISE

1. What are biological resource centres?

2. What are the roles of BRCs?

3. What are the challenges faced by BRCs?

4. Give functions of Biological Resources Centres.

5. Why are BRCs needed and explain their essential functions?

6. Explain in detail the sources for financial support to BRCs.

7. Give a detailed discussion on the Responsibilities of BRCs.

8. What are the ways to enhance access to biological resources?

CONCLUSION

The product life cycles are short and careful planning after taking into account the skill to draw funding would help in the survival of a company. So, by examining the venture in terms of market needs, capabilities and branding, chances of success of the ventures can be accessed and thus, the best opportunity can be selected. Business objectives are what one wants from his business—typically stated as revenue or profits. The programs are the tactics and include advertising, pricing, and distribution. The major strategic components of a marketing strategy are "targeting and positioning". Once the target market and positioning have been determined, one must develop programs to implement the marketing strategy.

In developing countries where funds are too limited to undertake R and D, the import of technology is frequent. Biotechnology research is both public and private-funded and the private sector is increasingly interested in biotechnological research with the aim of making profits. Over the last two decades, biotechnology has also been used for commercial gains and has attracted investments in the stock market, which resulted in the closure, merger and acquisition of existing biotechnology companies.

BIBLIOGRAPHY

[1] Rapley R. Molecular biology, bioinformatics and basic techniques.Principles and Techniques of Biochemistry and Molecular Biology. Cambridge: Cambridge University Press 2010; pp. 138-94. http://dx.doi.org/10.1017/CBO9780511841477.006

[2] Sambrook J, Russell DW. (David William), 1957- and Cold Spring Harbor Laboratory Molecular cloning: a laboratory manual / Joseph Sambrook, David W. N.Y.: Russell Cold Spring Harbor Laboratory Cold Spring Harbor 2001.

[3] Primrose SB, Twyman RM. Principles of Gene Manipulation and Genomics. 7th. Malden, MA, Oxford: Blackwell Pub 2006.

[4] Vijayashree PP, Alagamma M. Entrepreneurial Development and Small Business Management. Markham Publications 2010.

[5] Khatoon N. Entrepreneurial Development. Himalaya Publishing House 2023.

[6] Glick B, Patten C. Molecular Biotechnology: Principles and Applications of Recombinant DNA. 5th. ASM Books 2017.

[7] Morrison A. Biotechnology Law: A Primer for Scientists. Columbia University Press 2020. http://dx.doi.org/10.7312/morr17938

[8] Rogers S, Makonnen R. Entrepreneurial Finance: Finance and Business Strategies for the Serious Entrepreneur. 3rd. New York: McGraw-Hill Education 2014.

[9] Creswell JW, Creswell JD. Research Design: Qualitative, Quantitative, and Mixed Methods Approaches. 5th. Los Angeles, CA: SAGE 2018.

CHAPTER 7

Intellectual Property Rights

LEARNING OBJECTIVES

This chapter gives an overview of intellectual Property (IP), its categories, benefits and management; intellectual property rights (IPR) and filing of patents.

Abstract: Intellectual Property (IP) is the intangible creation arising from the application of human intellect and its legal characterization is intellectual property right (IPR). With the emergence of modern biotechnology, the era of patents, copyright, and IPR have come into being. One needs to be conversant about IPRs and patent systems to protect, license, trade, and market his research and inventions. This chapter aims to prepare oneself to face the legal and ethical challenges of research and trade. IPR appears to play an important role in facilitating production and exchange in certain input markets.

Keywords: Intellectual Property, Patent, Trade secret, Copyright, Trademark.

INTELLECTUAL PROPERTY (IP)

IP is created through the application of intellect and ingenuity and is usually in the form of an idea, concept, design, process, *etc.* to generate a product ultimately. With the emergence of modern technology, intellectual property is the legal characterization and treatment of trade-related biotechnological processes and products.

Under biotechnology, important examples of intellectual property are processes and products that result from the development of genetic engineering techniques (using restriction enzymes) to create recombinant DNA. These IPs can be copied and used by others, thereby reducing the benefits of original inventors.

The right of any individual to derive from intellectual property and to exclude others from doing so is referred to as Intellectual Property Rights. Utility Patents for genetic materials (both plants and animals) that have been allowed in some countries so that patented material cannot be used for further breeding or cultivation (in case of seeds) without paying a fee to the patent holder.

These IPRs affect (both favourably as well as unfavourably) the conservation, availability and use of plant and animal genetic resources (PGR & AGR).

Simmi Kharb, Akshat Singh, Abhyuday Singh & Deepa Kharb (Eds.)

Also, IPRs may adversely affect:

- food security
- use of evolved agricultural practices
- biological diversity
- ecological balance

CATEGORIES OF IPRs

There are four major types of IPRs application in biotechnology:

1.Trade secret
2.Patent
3.Copyright
4.Trademark

Trade Secret

Trade secrets include private proprietary information or physical material that allows a definite Commercial advantage to the owner over his competitors. A trade secret may protect a formula, production process, microbial strain or cell line, *etc.* However, a manuscript, design, product, *etc.* cannot be protected as a trade secret.

Trade secrets in biotechnology include:

- cell lines
- hybridization condition
- merchandising (corporate) plans
- customer lists

Duration

Trade secrets have an unlimited duration and the process is simpler as compared to patents.

Disclosure of Trade Secret

Disclosure and unauthorised use of a disclosure of a trade secret are punishable by law and the owner may be allowed compensation. Secrecy is ensured through non-disclosure/confidentially agreements.

Advantages of Trade Secret

1.Unlimited duration whereas IPRs are for a limited duration.
2.Easy to obtain - lack of legal formalities and requirements. While a patent is granted in 2-3 years after the application is filed.
3.Involve reduced risk of someone improving upon the process/for mutation, *etc.*
4.Does not require the filing of applications, or paying fees for renewal every year.
5.Does not require contesting and enforcing IPR.

Limitations

1.Its maintenance is costly.
2.It has no protection from independent innovation/invention.
3.It cannot be applied to many IPs.
4.Since it involves non-disclosure, this delays and hampers scientific/ technological progress and further innovations.
5.The title cannot be restored to the owner once secrecy is lost. Does not give rights against public at large unlike IPRs. If secrecy is breached, it becomes open and free to use for all.

Copyright

Copyright is associated with the expression of any idea or information by the author in any tangible form. These IPs include books (authored and edited), computer programs, paintings, sculptures, audio and video cassettes and cinematographic films. A work of copyright cannot be reproduced, in part or total, translated or distributed to the public without the permission of the person holding the copyright (author, editor, publisher, producer).

Copyright is possible only on expressed material (printed, painted, tape/video/computer recorder expressed in any other form).

Copyright rules are modified from time to time. They are territorial in nature and application and there are divergent rules in different jurisdictions. In the case of biotechnology, copyright may cover DNA sequences, computer databases, and DNA instruction manuals. However, the protection of copyright is limited, *e.g.*, ideas given in print can be used for any other purposes though photocopy that may not be allowed.

Trademark

It is a symbol or a word used by a manufacturer or an agent to identify and distinguish his goods and services from those of others. For example in biotechnology, laboratory equipment bear trademarks, certain vectors used in recombinant research are known by their trademarks. Trademarks are silent advertisers of the quality and performance of the goods and services associated with the mark. The proprietor is the owner of the trademark and does not allow others to use trademarks identical or similar to his. These trademarks are also used for advertising, packaging or in any other way like trade name, logo, *etc.* The rules against such use are available under trademark law and passing off under common law.

Patents

A patent is a grant of right to exclude others from making, using or selling and importing an invention for a limited period *i.e.* 20 years. A patent is valid in a country that has granted it, but, one can apply for the same in 2 or more countries through convention or PCT application route. Patents are granted for— an invention, improvement/innovation., - it may be granted with respect to a product or the process of producing a product.

RELEVANCE OF IPR

Benefits of IPR

Biotechnological products can be protected under any of the 4 IPRs (patent, trade secret, copyright, and trademark).

These rights can be held, bought, sold and licenced like any property, though for a limited duration. Time durations are different different types of IP rights, for example in patients, it is 20 years, and life time plus sixty years for copyright.

Factors affecting the selection of the most appropriate of mode of protection.

1. **Pace of technological development**: In case of rapid technological growth, trade secret approach may be preferred.
2. **Cost-effectiveness of obtaining a patent**: One has to decide between the cost of secrecy (trade secret) and cost of obtaining and enforcing a patent.
3. **Security**: If it is impossible and expansive to prevent disclosure of a trade secret, one may prefer rights other than secrecy.

4. **Need to show patents to investors**: For the purpose of showing inventions to investors, patents may have to be shown.

Also, the need for protection depends on the nature of the subject matter that needs to be protected, *e.g.*, an instruction manual can be subjected to copyright or protected as trade secret, but cannot be protected as a patent.

Benefits of IPR

1.IPR encourages and safeguards intellectual and artistic creations.
2.It promotes a quick spread of newer ideas and technologies widely by disclosure of patents.
3.It encourages investment in R & D efforts and funding.
4.It leads to overall economic development.

Requirements for Award of a Patent

1.Novelty
2.Inventiveness
3.Industrial application and usefulness
4.Patentability of subject matters
5.Disclosure

Procedure

The details of patent requirements will be discussed in next chapter.

1.The preparation of an application for a patent according to the prescribed format.
2.Filing of application with patents office of the country. International filing under PCT (Patent Cooperation Treaty) route for 2 or more countries may be done in addition to the basic/national application.
3.Scrutiny of application by a competent person at patent office and if found suitable for patenting, it is published.
4.Objections can be raised by the patenting authority or anyone who challenges the application file. Appeals and challenges are decided by competent authorities.
5.Grant/award of the patent to the applicant.

MANAGEMENT OF IPR

IPR is acquired by IP owners for anticipated profits on commercialization of concerned IP. This further requires R & D efforts which involve:

1.The transfer of IPR to generate maximum profit from IP.
2.Collaborations with business establishments to facilitate the commercialization of IPRs.
3.Monitoring of infringements of IPRs.
4.Renewal of patents and designs periodically
5.Evaluation of royalty for further periodic renewal in the country of interest.

PROBLEMS OF IPR

1.IPR encourages monopoly, market power and lead to industrial rivalry and takeovers. In case of broad patents, IPR will work only for financially powerful corporations/nations.

2.This will be detrimental to scientific and technological progress in the field of biotechnology and would pose a threat for global food security. Also, it will further increase the gap between developing and developed countries in terms of economic status and quantum of innovations (IPR holdings).

3. It may adversely affect the biological diversity and ecological balance.

4.Developing countries should undertake well-planned programmes to promote innovations and inventions to boost their IPR holdings for their overall economic and scientific growth and development.

SELF-ASSESSMENT ACTIVITY

1.How will you exercise your choice to protect an intellectual property?
2.How IP differs from patents?
3.Prepare a list of benefits of IPR.
4.Make a list of mode of IP protection.
5.What is the concept of trade secret in biotechnology?
6.Prepare a list of items coming under copyright.
7.Prepare a list of requirements for awarding a patent.
8.Enumerate problems of IPR.

EXERCISE

1. What is IP and what are the rights available to protect it?

2. Enlist the advantages and limitations of trade secrets.

3. How is the IPR managed?

CONCLUSION

With the emergence of modern biotechnology, era of patents, copyright and IPR have come into being. One needs to be conversant about IPRs and patent systems to protect, licence, trade and market his research and inventions. The need for protection depends on the nature of subject matter that needs to be protected. There are four major types of IPRs application in biotechnology, namely Trade secret, Patent, Copyright, and Trademark.

BIBLOGRAPHY

[1] Morrison A. Biotechnology Law: A Primer for Scientists. Columbia University Press 2020. http://dx.doi.org/10.7312/morr17938

[2] Karp G. Cell and Molecular Biology: Concepts and Experiments. 5th. Chichester: John Wiley 2008.

[3] Daniel L. Hartl, Elizabeth W Jones Jones and Bartlett. Sudbury, Massachusetts: Publishers 2004.

[4] Sambrook J, Russell DW. (David William), 1957- and Cold Spring Harbor Laboratory Molecular cloning: a laboratory manual / Joseph Sambrook, David W. N.Y.: Russell Cold Spring Harbor Laboratory Cold Spring Harbor 2001.

[5] Primrose SB, Twyman RM. Principles of Gene Manipulation and Genomics. 7th. Malden, MA, Oxford: Blackwell Pub 2006.

[6] Creswell JW, Creswell JD. Research Design: Qualitative, Quantitative, and Mixed Methods Approaches. 4th. Newbury Park: Sage 2017.

CHAPTER 8

Biotechnology Regulations

LEARNING OBJECTIVES

This chapter gives an overview of the existing patent regime and its application to the field of biotechnology. It also analyses the legal and social implications arising from the interface of biotechnology with IPRs.

Abstract: This chapter introduces patenting and fundamental research, copyrights, trademarks, biotechnological patents, current issues in patenting, Indian response to patent upheaval and bioprospecting along with the existing risk-analysis system for biotechnology products, surveying agency authorities. Regulations in biotechnology apply to the production, sale and use of biotech products and genetically modified organisms and regulatory agencies conduct their functions to protect public health, safety, and the environment.

Keywords: Intellectual property rights, Patent, Economic incentive, Innovative, Bioprospecting, Erythropoietin, Hybridoma, Biopirates.

PATENTING AND FUNDAMENTAL RESEARCH

INTRODUCTION

From the very outset of its use, biotechnology has raised some concerns which led the countries to recognize the need for regulation to ensure the safety of human, animal and plant health and the environment. Regulations apply from the stage of production to sale and the use of biotechnological products and genetically modified microorganisms which are tested and documented before the products enter the market for being used. Medical products and foods are regulated by the government and these regulations have profound effects on the biotechnology workplace. The National Institute of Health (NIH) was the first regulatory body over biotechnology in the USA and from 1984, biotechnology research has become a joint responsibility of NIH, USDA (US Department of Agriculture) and EPA (Environment Protection Agency). USDA makes sure a given organism is safe to grow, EPA makes it certain that it is safe for environment and FDA determines its safety for consumption.

In India, Recombinant DNA Safety Guidelines, 1990 (revised in 1994) were released by the DBT (Department of Biotechnology) which cover areas of research

Simmi Kharb, Akshat Singh, Abhyuday Singh & Deepa Kharb (Eds.)

involving genetically engineered organisms and these guidelines were further revised in 1994. The Biotechnology Regulatory Authority of India Bill was introduced in 2013 for setting up an independent Biotechnology Regulatory Authority of India (BRAI) to regulate organisms and products of modern biotechnology and it is yet to be passed by the parliament. GEAC (Genetic Engineering Approval Committee) under the Ministry of Environment, Forests and Climate Change (India) is responsible for the approval of genetically engineered products in India.

Intellectual Property Rights

According to the official interpretation of the World Intellectual Property Organisation (WIPO), IPR comprises those legal rights, by which the products of intellectual activity over a range of endeavours are defined.

Intellectual Property Rights are property rights over intangible things/products derived from human intellectual activity in the form of innovations and creations. There are awarded for a limited duration (time limited rights) creating the legal right of exclusivity to reward the creator/innovator and help the public at large *via* access and use of such creations/inventions. These are statutory rights, and their extent and scope are defined by the statute and cannot extend beyond that. IPRs apply to all fields of technology and arts.

Biotechnology and IPRs

Biotechnology is the result of the application of human intelligence and knowledge to the biological process. The conjugation between biotechnology and IPRs is not of new origin. Biotechnological research was earlier restricted to academic research only. After biotechnology started giving out commercially viable innovations, it became a matter of necessity to protect its products and creations under IPRs.

The principal objective of modern biotechnology, through the collaboration of academic labs with industry labs or otherwise, is to produce commercial products for economic gain. Investors will be hesitant to invest in high-cost biotechnology ventures if legal protection against unauthorized use by competitors is lacking as the level of uncertainty is very high. Also, society is encouraging industrial innovation. It is for the government to grant exclusive rights to inventors for novel products and processes they develop. These sanctioned privileges are collectively termed as Intellectual Property Rights.

COPYRIGHTS AND TRADEMARKS

Different types of IPRs

Though there are around 7 types of intellectual property rights recognised at the international level, for biotechnology-related inventions and creations, the following types of IPRs are relevant and discussed briefly:

1.Trade secrets
2.Copyrights
3.Trademarks and
4.Patents

Trade Secrets

It comprises confidential information about specific technical procedures and formulations of commercial value that a company wishes to protect from others. The right is automatic, and they are not registered with any government or regulatory body, but the owner takes reasonable security measures to protect the secrecy.

Copyrights

Copyrights protect authorship and ownership of different forms of published work i.e., literary, artistic, musical, dramatic, sound recordings, and cinematographic films from their unauthorized access.

Trademark

It can be either symbols or words that are distinctive and identify a particular service or product of a company.

Patent

For biotechnology, patents form the most important part of intellectual property. A patent is a legal document that provides exclusive rights to the patent holder for implementing the invention commercially.

Though biotechnological products can have connections with copyright, trademarks, and designs, this chapter exclusively discusses the concept of patenting. Patents are critical for the protection of biotechnology inventions. Since the principal objective of biotechnology is the production of commercial products for economic gains and society is also encouraging industrial innovation, patents offer a viable option in this regard. The commercial viability of biotech inventions has led the inclusion of subject matters like DNA sequences, microorganisms, etc. in the existing patent systems because of the high economic incentive attached.

Features of Patent

1.Patent is an exclusive right granted for an invention-a product or the process of making a product.
2.Extent and scope of patent is based on the construction of claims in the patent application.
3.Patent is a public document containing a detailed description of invention shared as *quid pro quo* for the right granted.
4.It also informs about nature and limits of invention, allowing people to start/continue working in a particular direction.
5.Also, they have the right to sell/license right to use their invention to their competitors/licensees for developing a product based on it.

INTERNATIONAL TREATIES AND BODIES ON PATENTS

Treaties

1.Paris Convention for the Protection of Industrial Property,1883
2.Patent Cooperation Treaty,1970 (PCT)
3.European Patent Convention,1973 (EPC)
4.Trade Related Intellectual Property Rights (TRIPs),1994

International Bodies Regulating Patents

1.World Intellectual Property Organization (WIPO)
2.World Trade Organization (WTO)

Prior to coming of TRIPS Agreement in 1994, Patent decisions and law varied from country to country:

1.In the US, the duration of exclusion rights of a patent was 17 years after it was officially awarded. In Canada, and many European countries, it is 20 years from the date of filing the patent application.

2.In India, it was 14 years for product patents and 7 years for process patents in drugs, foods and pharmaceuticals. Now it is minimum 20 years from the date of filing the patent application for all types of patents- products or processes.

After the TRIPS Agreement, there was an attempt to harmonize patent laws across countries. However, despite stipulating minimum standards with respect to patentability, the rights of owners and enforcement, laws and interpretations are still country-specific or territorial.

FUNDAMENTAL REQUIREMENTS FOR PATENTING

1.The invention after having been shown to work must be "novel".
2.The invention must contain an inventive step/technical advancement over existing knowledge.
3.The invention must have industrial application and is useful in the same way.
4.Every patent application must contain enough description of the invention so that a person is knowledgeable in the same field and capable of working/implementing his invention.
5.Subject matter not excluded by law.

SUBJECT MATTERS NOT PATENTABLE

Certain inventions and discoveries are not patentable, namely:

1.Natural laws.
2.Product of Nature- found naturally in nature.
3.Against public order or morality.
4.Abstract Ideas *e.g.*, scientific theories, mathematical methods, aesthetic creations.
5.Therapeutic treatments of humans or animals (Discretionary- allowed in US).

APPLYING FOR A PATENT

The process of filing is a technical process. Filing must be done by the inventor or his assignee or legal representative (after death). The application has a standard format and must be prepared by an expert (technical and legal both) and organized in a definite pattern:

The application must have

✓A title
✓An abstract
✓A section on the background of invention-prior art, drawbacks in prior art, efforts to remove drawbacks
✓A comprehensive summary of invention with relevant figures, schematic representations, biological content if used and information on its origin.
✓Detailed description of the invention- account of nature of invention how it works.
✓List of claims about the invention, what it covers and what it does not and what all needs to be protected.

Then the application is submitted to the patent and trademark office. It is then reviewed for novelty, utility, acceptability, non-obviousness, and feasibility of invention. The application is examined by the examiner, an expert from the field of invention and if it meets all the criteria for patentability, then a patent is awarded. It usually takes 2 to 5 years in different jurisdictions following the filing of the initial patent application before it is granted. The patent is available for 20 years from the date of filing till it is either surrendered by the owner or quashed by the court of law if proved to be contrary to public order, morality, and patent regulations.

REMEDIES AVAILABLE AGAINST THE DECISION OF THE PATENT OFFICE

If a patent application is rejected by an examiner, the applicant can appeal the decision with the patent appeals board/ judicial court having jurisdiction as provided under the patent law of the country.

Types of Patents

Major categories of patent: Common types of patent categories:

1.Product Patents
2.Process Patents

	Categories	**Example**
1.	*Product Patents:*	
	Substance	Cloned genes, recombinant proteins, monoclonal Ab, plasmid, vectors
	Composition of matter	Vaccines, pharmaceutical, mixtures, microorganisms, and transgenic organisms
	Devices	DNA sequences, pulsed-field gel electrophoresis.
2.	*Process Patents:*	
	Process of preparation	DNA isolation, PCR applications, purification of recombinant protein, vector-insert construction
	Methodologies	Nucleic acid hybridization assay, diagnostic assay, PCR-based detection systems.
	Actual use	Non-therapeutic animal treatment systems, fermentation of genetically modified organisms

BIOTECHNOLOGICAL PATENTS

Patenting in Biotechnology

Biotechnology deals with the isolation, augmentation, and practical applications of biomolecules and other features of living things. Under biotechnology, processes and products resulting from genetic engineering techniques (using restriction enzymes for creating recombinant DNA) are examples of intellectual property (IP) created. Also, this biotechnological IP encourages the creation of research & development (R&D) units, the raising of funds, and the commercial production of marketable items.

Business models of most biotech companies rely heavily upon Intellectual Property Rights. A patent is the most important form of intellectual property rights (IPRs) in biotechnology. It provides a viable option for economic exploitation giving economic incentives required for any startup/ technology industry. However, the growth has not been the same as in other fields of technology. Constant challenges to subject matters like DNA sequences, microorganisms, plants, and animals on moral, ethical, and legal grounds are treating biotechnology at par with other older technologies in terms of interpreting the subject matter and the three-pronged patentability criteria- novelty, inventive step and industrial application/utility are big concerns. Anything 'found naturally' or the creation of nature like genes was held not patentable in the US after the Myriad Lab BRCA gene decision by the Supreme Court. The court held that a naturally occurring DNA segment is a product of nature and hence not patent eligible just because it has been identified and isolated. However, when there is a gene manipulation to create something which is not free-flowing, and not found in nature, it could be eligible for patent protection or the process maybe patented. This has changed the entire discourse of the patentability of life forms in humans and animals. Modern biotechnology differs significantly from chemical inventions and what may be the criteria for novelty and inventiveness for other technologies may sound an obvious variant of naturally occurring products especially for GMOs, tissues, and cells. Many legal and public policies of biotechnological research have been challenged and modified. The need of the hour is to make research scientists and university/institute administrators to increase the pace of research for the development of technologies in biotechnology.

CURRENT ISSUES IN PATENTING

Patenting and Fundamental Research

Patenting has an impact on how university-based biotechnology research is conducted. Traditionally, science, especially university-based research, has been an open system with a free exchange of ideas and materials through publications and personal communications. However, the scientific community has begun to feel that the integrity of traditional scientific inquiry has become secondary to self-interest, where public recognition and financial gain from primary innovations are the prime motivations for conducting scientific research. Now scientists are advised by patent lawyers to keep their work secret until a patent is filed. Consequently, the lure of patenting has made many scientists reluctant to talk about their work, until the patent has been filed.

Also, due to the shortage of funds available to researchers, licensing fees and royalties from patents can be the source of new income. Massachusetts Institute of Technology files more than 100 patents annually in all research fields, generating $5.5 million per year from licensing patent rights.

To sum up, due to enthusiasm for patenting and patent protection, traditional science may become hostage to patent holdings and research will become less fruitful. On the other hand, the traditional way of doing science is an outdated, inefficient, and indulged exercise and driving patent ownership will spur new discoveries.

With the development of molecular biotechnology, the question arises regarding allowing the private industries to own or patent genetically engineered organisms.

Fundamental Requirement of Patent Law for Inventions Related to Biotechnology

1.An inventor should describe the invention fully in the application. Every country has different disclosure requirements.
2.The inventor must obtain prior approval from the biodiversity authority of the source country of the biological resource plant/animal before filing for the patent.
3.The inventor must conform to the mandatory requirements of signing Access and Benefit Sharing (ABS) Agreements with the local/indigenous communities as provided under the Convention on Biodiversity (CBD) and Nagoya Protocol and national law of the country (US is not signatory of this Convention and Protocol but India and most European countries are).
4.Biological content used in the invention with the patent filing form must be deposited in the national patent office.

Categories of Biotechnological Inventions that are Patentable

1.Methods/processes that generate useful products.
2.Production of biologicals *e.g.*, antibiotics, antibodies, vitamins.
3.Application of various processes/products: *e.g.*, using a promoter sequence for regulating the action of gene.
4.Methods to obtain streams of microorganisms, cell lines.
5.DNA sequences (in EU, Australia not in US).
6.Methods for genetic modification of organisms.

Patenting Multi-cellular Organisms

The patenting of multi-cellular organisms continues to raise ethical and social concerns. To date, a transgenic mouse (onco mouse) carrying an activable gene that makes it susceptible to tumor formation has been patented in both US and Europe. Also, genetically manipulated plants have been accepted as patentable inventions.

Patenting transgenic animals will be a challenge on moral grounds. Danish parliament has passed a statute that exempts animals from becoming an intellectual property. They are not subject to patent protection.

Patenting of Genes and DNA Sequences

Artificially synthesized genes normally fulfill the requirements of patent and are patentable. In the US, EU and Australia, the requirement of practical applicability of a gene is relaxed, *e.g.*, in the case of isolated genes (not in the US post 2013 USSC Myriad Lab judgment), vectors, transformed cells expressing hormone angiogenesis factor A (GF), *e.g.*, gene aroA (confers glyphosate resistance isolated from mutant bacterium was patented in USA. On the other hand, in UK and India, isolated natural genes are not patentable.

Gene Patent and Genetic Resources

Developed countries are technologically rich but gene poor. On the other hand, developing countries are technologically poor, but they are rich in genes. Developed countries have made extensive collections of germplasms of all important crops of developing countries and are using them to develop superior varieties which are sold to developing countries to generate huge profits.

BROAD PATENTS IN BIOTECHNOLOGY

Broad patents granted in the USA for plant traits and technological processes are as follows:

1. For Technology

(a) Antisense RNA technology:	EnzoBioChem Inc.
(b) Gene gun method of genetic engineering of soyabean:	WR Grace & Co.

2. For Specific Traits

(a) Transgenic plants:	Pioneer Hi-Bred with increase lysine

cont.....

(b) Sunflower with low saturated FA:	Dekalb Genetic Corp.

3. For plants

(a) All transgenic	
(i) Cotton	
(ii) All Transgenic Soya bean	WR Grace and Co.
(b) All transgenic Brassica:	Calgene Inc.

However, patent for transgenic cotton has been challenged in the USA and revoked.

These broad patents are morally unacceptable and fundamentally inequitable. If such protections are allowed, IPR will work only for financially powerful corporations/nation's leading to their monopoly control over biotechnological modifications which would be detrimental to scientific and technological progress.

ISSUES RELATED TO PATENTING LIFE FORMS

Points Favoring Patenting Genetically Modified Life Forms

1. Their production requires large financial, technical, and innovative inputs.
2. They perform novel and useful functions.
3. They generate economic benefits for the nation.
4. They provide financial returns to the inventor.
5. Assured returns from inventions promote R & D and thus inventiveness.

Main Objections

They are based on moral, ethical, and religious grounds:

1. Life forms are products of nature.
2. Their genetic modification does not mean their invention.
3. Biotechnological innovation cause cruelty to animals.
4. Biopiracy; and
5. Access and Benefit Sharing Issues in Bioprospecting.

Current Issues in Patenting

The most current issue is "when can live forms be patented?"

The human genomic project has elucidated almost the entire sequence of the human genome, besides identifying the genes. Patenting of DNA sequences and genes has become a debatable issue. So far, no patents have been granted for genes.

Patent law makes a distinction between invention and discovery and does not allow patents for discovery. However, if a natural substance has been first isolated, then the process developed to isolate this may be patentable. Similarly, antibiotics and other microbial metabolites are patentable substances.

Other Examples are

(i)Pure vitamin B12
(ii)E. coli in which human genes have been incorporated for the production of human insulin, human GH, and human tissue plasminogen activator (tPA) has been recognized for a patent.

Cases Dealing with Patents of Products of Nature Contested in USA

Factor VIII

Protein VIIIC was purified by Scripps Clinic and Research Foundation (USA). Gene Tech later produced VIII:C by a recombinant method and it was used by Sripps for the re-infringement of their re-issued patent.

Erythropoietin

Amgen Inc held a US patent for preparing erythropoietin. However, Genetics Institute Inc. obtained a broad product claim for erythropoietin.

tPA

UK patent claim for recombinant tPA was allowed to Genetech which later failed on legal grounds to US patent.

Human Nerve Growth Factor (βNGF)

A patent application for recombinant βNGF was rejected by the US patent office based on the absence of evidence that the recombinant product was significantly different from natural materials or has any novel properties.

Hybridoma Technology

Wister Institute's application to US Patent Office for producing viral antibodies by hybridoma technology was rejected. But the use of monoclonal antibodies was later allowed by the High Court of Appeals in the USA.

INDIAN RESPONSE TO PATENT UPHEAVAL

Patenting of Life Forms in India

Life forms are not patentable in India. By the implication of Sec. 3(j), genetically modified multi-cellular organisms, including plants, animals and human beings, their parts and essential biological processes for the production and propagation of plants and animals are not patentable in India. According to the Examiner Guidelines issued under the Patent Manual in 2005 and in 2019, biological materials, such as recombinant DNA, plasmids and processes of manufacturing thereof are patentable if they are produced by substantive human intervention. Gene sequences and DNA sequences with disclosed function are considered patentable in India subject to section 3(k).

In some developed countries, naturally occurring microorganisms are not patentable, however, modified microorganisms by employing more ingenious techniques such as genetic engineering are now patentable. USA and Japan allowed patents on non-naturally occurring, non-human multi-cellular organisms. European Union allows patents on genetically modified microorganisms, plants, and animals. Such patents are not allowed in India. So far patents have not been granted for genes owing to the reason that genes are natural, universal, inherent, biological function units of all life forms. However, in 2019, the Indian Supreme Court in *Monsanto Technology LLC* v. *Nuziveedu Seeds Ltd.* allowed a patent on the genetically-modified seed.

BIO PROSPECTING

Biopiracy

According to the concise Oxford Dictionary, piracy means a practice or an act of robbery of ships; hijacking; infringement of copyright. To "pirate" means to appropriate or reproduce (the work or ideas, etc. of others) without permission from the rightful owner for one's own benefit. *Biopiracy* is the unauthorized extraction of biological resources and/or associated traditional knowledge from developing countries, or the patenting of spurious inventions based on such knowledge or resources without compensation. The traditional knowledge is the knowledge system which is held by indigenous people often relating to their surrounding environment.

Biopiracy has emerged as a term to describe the ways that corporations (of the developed world) claim ownership of or take unfair advantage of genetic resources and traditional knowledge and technologies of the developing world. "*Bio pirates*" are those individuals and companies that carry out the following acts:

(i)Theft, misappropriation of or unfair free-riding on, genetic resources and/or traditional knowledge through the patent system.
(ii)Unauthorized and uncompensated collection for commercial ends of genetic resources and/or traditional knowledge.

Biopiracy cannot be considered merely as a matter of law, but also, as morality and fairness. For this, we need to know where to draw lines between the acts of biopiracy and legitimate practice. This is difficult to draw owing to the vagueness of the way in which the term is applied. In the following paragraph, a list of actions that have been labelled as acts of biopiracy is given:

TRADITIONAL KNOWLEDGE BIOPIRACY

Collection and Use

(a) Unauthorized Use of

i.Common traditional knowledge (TK).
ii.TK/associated knowledge found among the indigenous group who have preserved or possessed the knowledge for a very long time for generations at times.

iii.TK acquired by deception or failure to fully disclose the commercial motive behind the acquisition.
iv.TK acquired on the basis of exploitative transaction.
v.TK acquired on the basis of a conviction that transactions are inherently exploitative ("all bioprospecting is biopiracy").

(b) Commercial Use of TK on the Basis of a Literature Search

Patenting

i.Patent claims TK in the form in which it was acquired.
ii.Patent covers refinement of TK.
iii.Patent covers an invention based on TK and other knowledge.

GENETIC RESOURCE BIOPIRACY

Collection and use

(a) Unauthorized extraction and use/export of:

i.Widespread resources.
ii.Resources that can be formed in one location.
iii.Resource in the breach of ABS regulations of relevant country.
iv.Resources in countries lacking ABC regulations.

(b) Authorized extraction of resources based on:

i.A transaction deemed to be exploitative.
ii.A conviction that all such transactions are inherently exploitative.

Patenting

i.A patent claims the resource itself excluding its usage even by the indigenous people.
ii.A patent claims a purified version of the resource.
iii.A patent covers a derivative of the resource and/or is based on more than one resource.

WHAT TO DO ABOUT BIOPIRACY

The rhetoric and strategic vagueness behind biopiracy raise the problem of what one should agree on and how to measure it. One extreme view is that all bioprospecting is biopiracy and it should be banned out rightly. Other, majorly developed countries and corporates from developed countries hold that such a ban should not be enforced at all as it hinders research in the biotechnology field. Where it is being used for the common good like the production of some lifesaving drugs or high-yielding crops helping food scarcity issue, the ban is not justified. If biopiracy causes demonstrable economic and/or cultural harm, then the ban should be enforced. However, the developing countries which hold such rich biodiversity assert on the regulation of access to genetic resources, exerting their sovereign right over natural resources of their country. Payment of compensation (monetary or non-monetary) to the indigenous communities as per the ABS rules agreed under the CBD & Nagoya Protocol of 2014 based on benefits earned/to be earned should be enforceable against such a big corporate. Stringent laws on ABS agreements and their enforcement are required.

BIOPROSPECTING AND ISSUE OF ABS (ACCESS AND BENEFIT SHARING)

Bioprospecting describes the systematic search for and the development of new sources of chemical compounds, genes, micro- and macro-organisms, and other valuable products from nature. Bioprospecting refers to the search for biological products with characteristics interesting to humankind. Earlier, bioprospecting focused on the quest for new chemical compounds with medicinal or anti-microbial properties.

If bioprospecting leads to a successful commercial product, it is likely that the company will protect its intellectual property rights on that product. The question of acknowledging or rewarding the communities or country for using their beneficial natural resource arises and the patent filed by the company prohibits the use or sale of the natural resource by indigenous groups.

These questions and issues are now getting even more complex, as advances in biochemistry and molecular biology make their own genetic material of living organism easy and exploit it for commercial use of their products. Thus, the future of bioprospecting ties in the search for genes rather than for chemical compounds. At present, it seems difficult to bridge the gap between the people who discovered a product through trial and errors of the course of their culture history and a biotech company. When land is used for mining purposes, indigenous communities get financial compensation and logically communities should get a share of benefits resulting from the use or exploration of their genetic resources. Unfortunately, current patent laws clearly favor 'Western Science' and innovative economies. As a result, many civil society groups and activists describe bioprospecting as a form of piracy, since bioprospecting leads to a loss of power of indigenous people over their own resources. Countries like India are establishing national gene banks and legislation for plant genetic resources forbidding open access to gene banks. Unfortunately, many of the developing countries do not have the economic power or political commitment to put similar national protective measures. WTO (World Trade Organization) has brought about an international agreement on intellectual property rights, the TRIPS Agreement that supports the idea than government control of resources is an obstacle to economic growth and should be avoided. The treaty imposes no requirement for bioprospecting parties to obtain approval from local communities to proceed with biological resource hunting and benefits obtained for commercialization of a product obtained by bioprospecting do not have to be shared with indigenous communities. Despite these controversial aspects, all WTO member countries are under great pressure to sign this agreement or face trade sanctions. However, those countries who are signatory to Convention on Biodiversity (CBD) and Nagoya Protocol have introduced the concept of access based on PIC (Prior Informed Consent) and MAT (Mutually Agreed Terms) requiring prior approval conditioned under their domestic patent laws and signing of ABS contracts and their enforceability. In India, section 10 of Patent Act introduced the mandatory requirement of prior approval of NBA (National Biodiversity Authority) before filing for a patent in India if the invention uses genetic resource from India. It is required to be filed with the patent application, failing which the application maybe rejected. The US has not signed the CBD therefore such condition is not applicable under their patent law.

Bioprospecting is also beginning to foster a renewal of awareness toward the conservation of biodiversity. Also, bioprospecting has potential to bring not only hope to human health, but also to social justice and environment protection.

GOALS

Bioprospecting Incorporates Two Fundamental Goals

1.Sustainable use through biotechnology of biological resources and their conservation.
2.Scientific and socioeconomic development of source countries and local communities.

In recent years, bioprospecting has acquired increased attention as countries seek to conserve their biodiversity and share the benefits from bioprospecting. In theory, bioprospecting offers a potentially interesting approach for linking biodiversity conservation with the biotechnology sector, its success in practice will depend upon the ability of these efforts to isolate useful compounds at a cost comparable to other techniques for drug development. There continues to be great interest in bioprospecting programs to data.

Bioprospecting is fundamentally tied to scientific interest and commercial success of natural product derivatives.

EXAMPLE OF BIOPROSPECTING AND BENEFIT SHAVING

A well-known documented example is Kani-TBGRI-model in Kerala. The team of TBGRI (Tropical Botanical Garden and Research Institute) undertook ethno-medical information on wild plant *Trichophuszeylanicus* (local name: "Arigyapacha). Kani is a tribal community in South-Western Ghat region of Kerala. The team convinced Kani men that the information about this plant would not be misused and if marketable drugs/products got developed, benefits accrued would be shared with the tribe. The result was "Jeevni" Ayurvedic medicine license fees and loyalty which is shared between TBGRI and the Trust of Kani Community (1:1).

SELF-ASSESSMENT ACTIVITY

1.Prepare a list of features of patent.
2.Give an account of patent laws in various countries.
3.Discuss treaties regarding patenting.
4.Prepare a list of subject matters that can be patented and those which cannot be patented.
5.Discuss the current issues in patenting.

EXERCISE

1. How can one apply for a patent?
2. What are broad patents granted in biotech?
3. What are WTO GATT and TRIPS?
4. Give an account of cases dealing with patents for producing natural products.

CONCLUSION

Due to enthusiasm for patenting and patent protection, traditional science may become hostage to patent holding and research will be less fruitful. With the development of molecular technology, fundamental issues are arising regarding what to patent, how to patent and how to derive benefits from patent. A biotechnologist needs to be conversant with IPRs, patent laws, mandatory regulations related to it under Biodiversity laws, Environment laws as well as ethical and moral issues related to it.

BIBLIOGRAPHY

[1] Karp G. Cell and Molecular Biology: Concepts and Experiments. 5th. Chichester: John Wiley 2008.

[2] Daniel L. Genetics: Principles and analysis. Sudbury, Massachusetts 2004; p. 854.

[3] Sambrook J, Russell DW. (David William), 1957- and Cold Spring Harbor Laboratory Molecular cloning: a laboratory manual / Joseph Sambrook, David W. N.Y.: Russell Cold Spring Harbor Laboratory Cold Spring Harbor 2001.

[4] Glick B, Patten C. Molecular Biotechnology: Principles and Applications of Recombinant DNA. 5th. ASM Books 2017.

[5] EOP. Modernizing the Regulatory System for Biotechnology Products: An Update to the Coordinated Framework for the Regulation of Biotechnology. 2017. Available from: https://obamawhitehouse.archives.gov/sites/default/files/microsites/ostp/2017_coordinated_framework_update.pdf [January 30, 2017].

CHAPTER 9

Genomics and Proteomics

LEARNING OBJECTIVES

This chapter gives an overview of genome sequencing, gene mapping, sequence analysis, DNA sequencing, microarrays, genomics in drug discovery, translational medicine era of 'omics'– single-cell multi-omics, metabolic engineering, epigenetics, protein products and protein expression systems, and microbiome.

Abstract: Genomics is the science of mapping sequences and analysing genomes. This chapter gives an overview of techniques of genome sequencing, gene mapping, sequence analysis, DNA sequencing and microarrays. Genomics offers sequencing, mapping, and analysis of a genome. With the help of computer-based techniques, a human genome was sequenced. Now it is possible to identify the function of genes from protein databases. Since proteins cannot be amplified like nucleic acid, the analysis of protein expression is challenging 2 DGE; MS and protein chips are the most widely used technologies for proteome analysis.

Keywords: Genomics, Proteomics, Metabolomics, Transcriptome, Metabolome Database, Protein expression, Heterologous proteins.

TERMINOLOGY

Bioinformatics	A branch of biology that deals with in silico processing and analysis of DNA, RNA, and protein sequence data.
Genomics	Study of structure and function of genome.
Comparative genomics	Uses sequence similarity and comparative gene order for determining gene function and phylogeny.
Functional genomics	Determines the function of a gene product.
Structural genomics	Determines structural motifs and complete protein structures and their relationship in terms of structure and function.
Proteomics	Study of proteome, *i.e.* the full complement of proteins made by a cell.
Transcriptomics	A study of transcriptome, *i.e.*, all the RNA molecules made by a cell, tissue organism.

Simmi Kharb, Akshat Singh, Abhyuday Singh & Deepa Kharb (Eds.)

cont.....

Metabolomics	Uses genome sequence analysis to determine the capability of cell, tissue or organism to synthesize small molecules.

COMPARISON

Table 1. Comparison of omics.

	Description	Time dependence	Manipulation in cell	Measurement in cell
Genome	Complete DNA sequence of organism	First approximation: none	Genetic manipulation; site directed mutagenesis Genetic screens	Routine high accuracy end complete
Transcriptome	Complete set mRNA transcripts in a cell or a tissue	Reflect the state of gene expression	Indirectly *via* genetic manipulation	Routine cDNA, microarrays SAGE, Northern Blot Quantification, inaccurate, approximate completeness
Proteome	Complete set of proteins present in a cell or tissues	Responsive to all manner of influences throughout life cycle	Indirectly *via* genetic manipulations	Not routine, 2-D-gels with MS. Fusion with reporter proteins (GFP)
Metabolome	All metabolites and their concentrations Defined as organic small molecules, not protein RNA or DNA	Responsive to all manner of influences throughout life cycle	Difficult	Difficult, completeness far away.Net routine, NMR, MS a few other methods. Quantification and resolution difficult.

GENOMICS IN DRUG DISCOVERY

Medical genomics pinpoints the normal and abnormal functions of individual genes and uses the information for the diagnosis and treatment of disease. Functional genomics is the process of determining the function of genes to find those genes that are good targets for drug discovery. Newer proteins discovered through genomics may serve as drugs themselves and they can be proteins or hormones or growth-factors that are under/overexpressed in disease states. Diseases linked to defective, misfolded, and misregulated proteins are good candidates for drug discovery.

A drug target could be a single gene or protein or an entire interacting pathway of proteins. Once a suitable target and compound are identified, the target is validated and the compound is altered so as to improve its efficiency and minimize any side effects, finally generating the compound for clinical trial and approval for their usage.

Functional genomics is becoming increasingly important for genome-based drug discovery.

TRANSLATIONAL MEDICINE

Translational medicine is the integrated application of innovative pharmacology tools, biomarkers, clinical methods, clinical technologies and study designs to improve disease understanding, confidence in human drug targets and increase confidence in drug candidates.

Translational research provides the knowledge necessary to draw important conclusions from clinical testing of diseases and the viability of novel drug mechanisms.

Pathway Analysis

Analysis of metabolic pathways in humans helps to recognize how proteins and other biological molecules are connected to each other and which biological processes they regulate or represent.

How pathways and molecular interactions are explored?

Tools for Analysis

Tools for analysis can be open source, *e.g.*, Cytoscape available on web or commercially available tools such as Ingenuity, Gene GO, Pathway Studio, Pathway Architect. These information databases help in text-mining and in determining the duration of biological information (Figs. **1** and **2**).

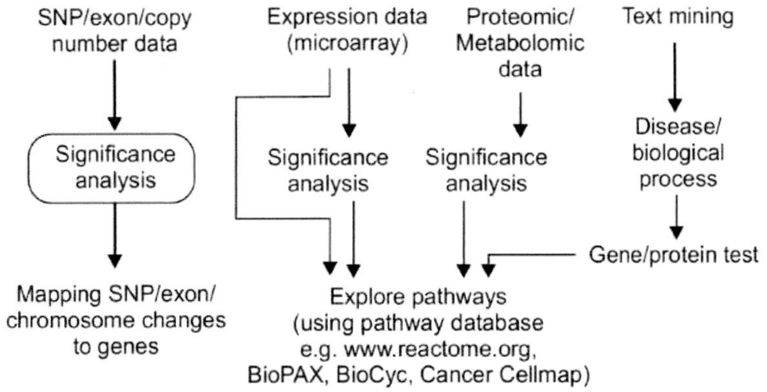

Fig. (1). Tools for analysis.

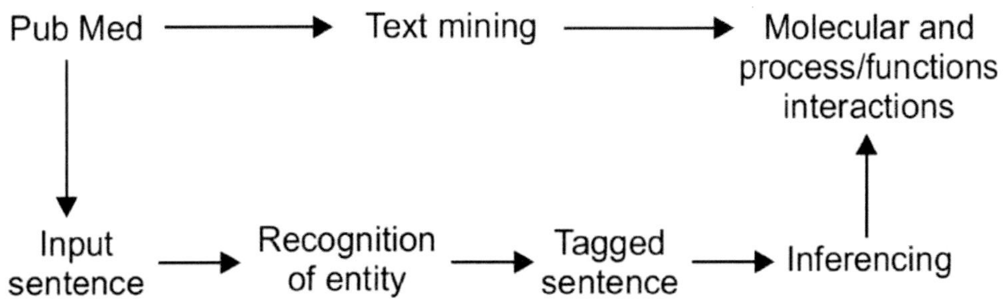

Fig. (2). Data mining.

Pathway Architect

A number of open and commercial sources are available for creating interactions.

PArch: It is one of the largest databases with 2 million facts, large number of filters and statistical algorithms to create networks. It is fully integrated with KEGG, Reactome and other pathway databases.

Metabolic Networks

Metabolism is the process involved in the maintenance of life. It is comprised of a vast repertoire of enzymatic reactions and transport processes that convert thousands of organic compounds into various molecules necessary to support life. Metabolic pathway is a subnetwork of the complete network of metabolic reactions. Metabolic pathways help in better understanding of cellular physiology and vulnerabilities of its metabolism.

Points to be considered while constructing a model:

1.Biological networks are dynamic in nature and

2.Abstraction resolution depends on the building blocks of a network, *e.g.*, low resolution is required by metabolites and enzymes, pathways, and special pathways.

Methods of biotechnology produce a huge amount of data that must be stored and analyzed for which different database systems and software tools are available. Moreover, for the analysis of metabolic networks, models and simulation environments are available.

Molecular Information Systems

The molecular data must be stored and analyzed. Different database systems for genes and proteins (EMBL, JDDB, GENBANK, PIR) are available to analyze metabolic processes in quantitative and qualitative terms.

Molecular information systems allow access to molecular data and knowledge and implement and integrate powerful interactive information systems that can support the progress of biotechnology and molecular diagnostic processes.

ERA OF 'OMICS'– SINGLE CELL MULTI-OMICS

Metabolomics

Metabolomics is a field of life science research that uses high throughput technologies to identify and/or characterize all the metabolites in a given cell, tissue or organism (*i.e.*, the metabolome). The rapidly emerging field of metabolomics combines strategies to identify and quantify cellular metabolites using sophisticated analytical technologies with the application of statistical and multivariant methods for information extraction and data interpretation.

Metabolomics is a concept that has been defined as the science of comprehensive monitoring of the metabolic compartment in biological systems. Metabolomics provides information about biological systems that cannot be obtained by the classical 'omics' approaches transcriptomics, genomics and proteomics (Figs. **3** and **4**).

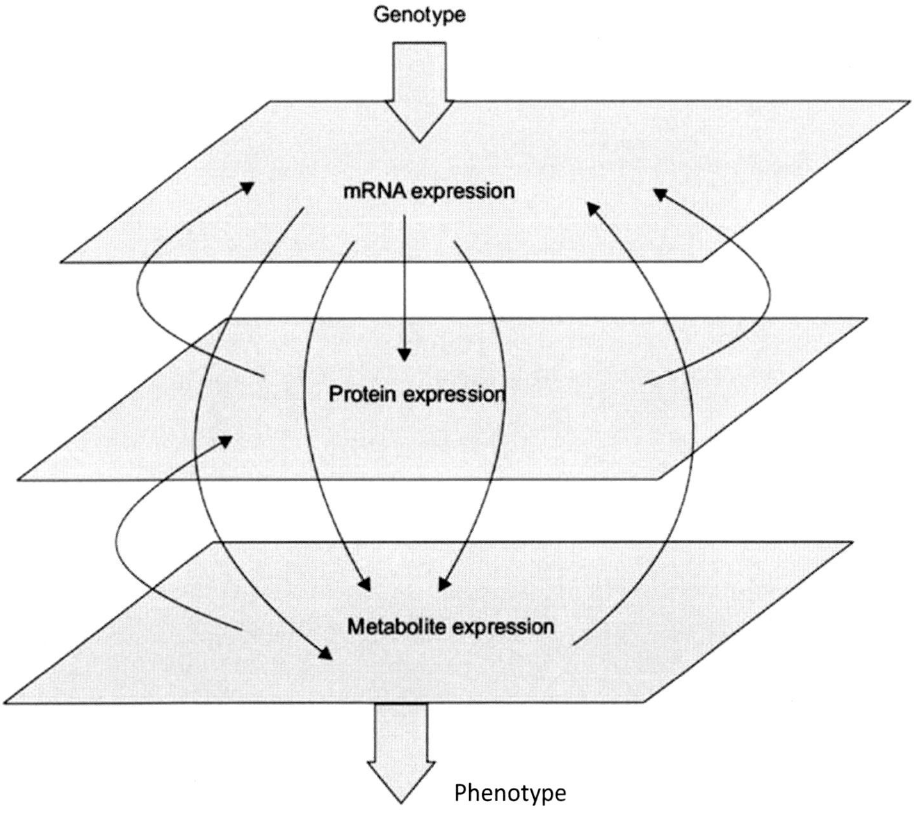

Fig. (3). Expression pathway.

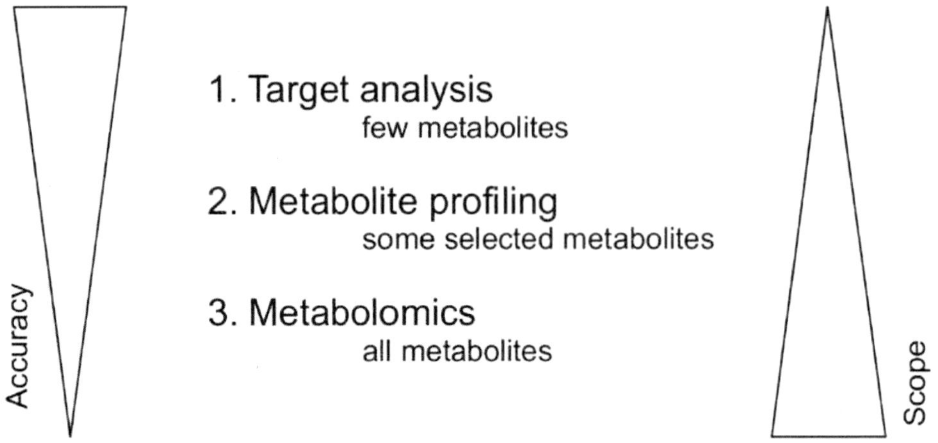

Fig. (4). Metabolomics: Detect the unexpected.

Understanding the biochemical pathways that comprise human metabolism represents one of the major achievements of research in the biological sciences over the past 100 years. The enzymes, cofactors, substrates, products and intermediates throughout the multitude of molecular pathways are more completely understood as compared to any other aspects of human biology.

The human genome initiative has established a vision for future research and the application of this knowledge resource includes a challenge of establishing a relationship between phenotypes and genomics. Since metabolism is a key aspect of phenotype, the next logical step is the description of the distribution of metabolites to elaborate functional genomics. Individual metabolite analyses have been pursued for decades as a part of the search for biomarkers of health and disease and with the help of modern analytical technologies, it monitors many analytes simultaneously generating the concept of 'personalized metabolic profiling'.

What is a Metabolite?

•Any organic molecule detectable in the body with MW < 1500 Da

•Includes: peptides, oligonucleotides, sugars, nucleosides, organic acids, ketones, aldehydes, amines, amino acids, lipids, steroids, alkaloids, food additives, pollutants/toxins and drugs.

•Includes, endogenous, exogenous, primary and secondary metabolites.

What one can do with Metabolomics?

Generate metabolic signatures

•Monitor/measure metabolite flux.

•Monitor enzyme/pathway kinetics.

•Assess/identify phenotypes.

•Monitor gene/environment interactions.

•Track effects from toxins/ perturbant.

•Monitor consequences of gene knockout.

•Identify functions of unknown genes.

Technologies for metabolomics

UPLC, HPLC

CE/microfluidics

LC-MS

FT-MS

QqQ-MS

•NMR spectroscopy

•X-ray crystallography

•GCMS

•LIF detection

Metabolome

The quantitative collection of all the low molecular weight molecules present in cells in a particular physiological or developmental state (Figs. **5** and **6**).

Applications of Metabolomics

•Toxicology testing

•Clinical trial testing

•Fermentation monitoring

•Food and beverage tests

•Nutraceutical analysis

•Drug phenotyping

•Waste quality testing

•Petrochemical analysis

•Genetic disease tests

•Nutritional analysis

•Clinical blood analysis

•Clinical urine analysis
•Cholesterol testing
•Drug compliance
•Transplant monitoring
•MRS and/MRI

Advantages of Metabolomics

•Identification of a target organ, severity, onset, duration and reversal of the effects.
•Classify sample as 'normal' vs 'abnormal'.
•Determine mechanisms of action within the organ.
•Potential for identifying novel biomarkers of toxic effect.
•Non-invasive.
•No prior decisions about sample need be made.
•No sample processing necessary other than cold collection.
•Complete time course data can readily be obtained.
•Minimization of compound requirements.
•Relatively fast analysis (200–300 samples day)

•Useful tool for modelling physiological variation and exposure conditions in animals and humans.

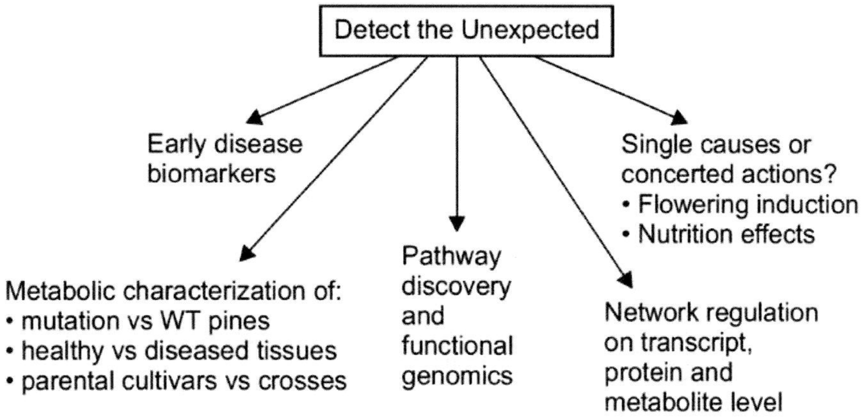

Fig. (5). Use of Metabolomic approaches.

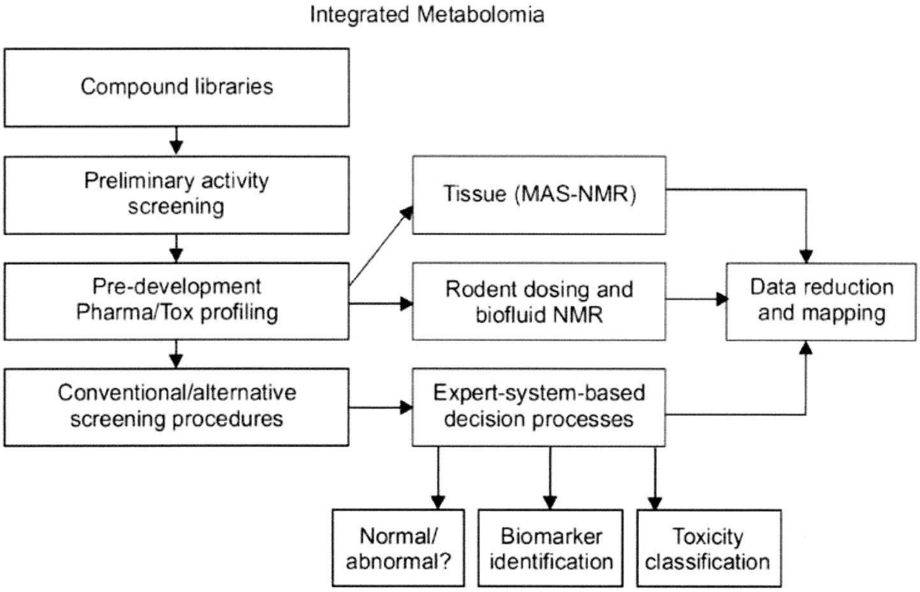

Fig. (6). Integrated metabolome.

Metabolomics

It is a quantitative measurement of dynamic multiparametric metabolic response of living systems to pathophysiological stimuli or genetic modification. Metabolomics is more associated with NMR spectroscopy and extends metabolic profiling to include information about perturbations of metabolism caused by environmental factors, and disease processes. Metabolomics with mass spectrometry-based techniques places greater emphasis on metabolic profiling at the cellular or organ level and is primarily concerned with normal endogenous metabolism.

In practice, there is still a large overlap in the way both terms are used.

Metabolome Database

The Human Metabolome Database (HMDB, www.hmdb.ca) has been a richly annotated resource for metabolomics since 2007. Now the recent release of HMDB (version 2.0) has been significantly expanded and data on fully annotated metabolite entries and the number of metabolites with biofluid or tissue concentration has expanded. Also, algorithms for spectral searching and matching, chemical substructure searches, faster text searching software and pathway searching tools and metabolic maps have been added to this database.

Currently, there are five types of databases used in metabolomics research:

(i)Metabolic pathway databases, *e.g.*, KEGG, Cys, Reactome.

(ii)Compound specific databases, *e.g.*, Lipid Maps, KEGG Glycan, Drug Bank, Ch EBI, PubChem.

(iii)Spectral databases, *e.g.*, BMRB, MMCD, Massbank, Golm, Metabolome database, Metlin

(iv)Disease physiology databases, *e.g.*, OMIM, Metagene, OMMBID.

(v)Comprehensive organism-specific databases *e.g.* BiGG, systonomas, HMDB.

HMDB is designed to be a comprehensive, Web-accessible metabolomics database that brings together quantitative, chemical, physical, clinical and biological data about all experimentally proven or experimentally detected human metabolites.

Personalized Metabolic Assessment

There is a need for assessment technologies for personalized and presentation focussed strategies such as a single biomarker-based diagnostic for metabolism-based diseases. Metabolomics is better suited for determining individual metabolic context, which is an integration of individual genetic, nutritional, pharmacological and environmental status.

ANALYTICAL TECHNOLOGIES

The main objective of metabolomics is to measure all or a substantial fraction of all metabolites within a biological sample and to quantify each. Gene transcription analysis (transcriptomics) and gene product analysis (proteomics) are working on the task of simultaneously identifying and quantifying their respective classes of biomolecules mRNAs and proteins on respective single platforms. Even though complete sets of metabolites in animals and humans are fewer in absolute number than either transcripts or proteins. Also, metabolites span a much wider distribution of molecular compositions and physical properties within single biological samples.

At present, there is no single technological platform capable of measuring and identifying all metabolites in a single sample simultaneously. Comprehensive metabolomic data from different platforms must be assembled.

Techniques available at present are NMR spectroscopy and bottom-up tactics using MS or chromato-graphic techniques to analyze discreet metabolites and resemble the complete metabolite database.

The technological developments in metabolomics will be significant in the near future and pharmacometabolomic data is also imaging that will pave way for personalized medicine.

METABOLIC ENGINEERING

To be discussed in chapter 12.

EPIGENETICS

Already discussed in chapter 2, and to be discussed in chapter 10 & 12.

PROTEINS AS PRODUCTS: PROTEIN EXPRESSION SYSTEM

Applications of proteins are as numerous as the proteins themselves. A protein structure initiative, $600 million project, was launched by NIH in 2000 to further understand the structure of proteins. Its public database holds more than 33,000 protein sequences. In this chapter, we will start with a quick survey of applications of proteins, process of protein folding and protein expression method followed by purification, analysis and verification of the final product.

Proteins Produced by Biotechnology

Food processing:

•Beer brewing

•Winemaking

•Cheese-making

Hormones

Antibodies

Therapeutic proteins:

•Monoclonal antibodies

•Blood proteins

•Enzymes

Textile and leather goods

Detergents

Paper manufacturing and recycling

Adhesives

Pharmaceutical products: Recombinant proteins

•Erythropoietin

•Interleukin: IL1, 2, 3, 4

•Interferons (α, β γ)

•Monoclonal antibodies

•Colony-stimulating factors

•Coagulation factors

•Human growth factors

•Epidermal growth factors

•Insulin

•IGF (insulin-like growth factor)

•Tissue plasminogen factor

•Tumor necrosis factor

•Vaccines: hepatitis B, herpes

How drugs are produced by biotechnology? The relevant therapeutic protein is identified and its gene sequence is determined. Then method for producing biotech drug is determined. Then host cells are transformed to contain therapeutic genes in carefully controlled conditions (temperature, oxygen, acidity, etc.) in a bioreactor and cells are stimulated to produce target proteins. After an appropriate time, proteins are isolated, purified and formulated into pharmaceutically active products.

Protein Folding

The structure and function of a protein depend on its folding, *i.e.*, how different strands of amino acids take their shapes. Protein misfolding results in the loss of the desired function of a protein and even diseases, *e.g.*

Sickle cell anemia: protein misfolding due to a single amino acid replacement;

•Alzheimer's disease: misfolded proteins accumulate as plague.

•Cystic fibrosis, mad cow disease (bovine & spongiform encephalitis, BSE), certain cancers have been linked to clumps of incorrectly folded proteins.

Protein folding occurs naturally, and understanding and controlling the folding of proteins is the biggest challenge in biotechnology processing.

Points to Remember

•A hydrogen atom is attached to electronegative 'N' and 'O' that pull away hydrogen atom's electron cloud leaving it positively charged resulting in H-bonding.

•In alpha helix, right-handed spirals are formed ad H-bonds stabilize the structure.

•In the beta-sheet, 'H'-bonds also link 'N' and 'O' atoms, however, atoms belong to amino acid chains that run side beside.

•Hydrogen bonds can be broken easily, damaging a valuable protein.

Glycosylation

More than a hundred posttranslational modifications occur after a protein is synthesized on the ribosome and glycosylation being the most common.

Glycosylation has a significant effect on the activity of a protein, namely, increased solubility orientation of proteins into membranes and extension of active life of proteins.

Protein Expression

Over 90% of all proteins whose structures have been determined and coordinates deposited in Protein Data Bank (PDB) have been expressed in *Escherichia coli.*

Directed Molecular Evolution Technology

A technique of introducing specific changes in the nucleotide sequences of a particular gene results in the generation of a diverse group of novel gene sequences. The gene product is screened for its properties and the process is repeated until the maximum function is obtained (Fig. 7).

In addition to naturally occurring and mutation-induced proteins, biotechnology is creating entirely new protein molecules.

Pool of cells

↓

Induce mutations

↓

Screen gene product

↓

Product with specific enhancement

Fig. (7). Directed molecular evolution.

POINTS TO CONSIDER BEFORE STARTING A NEW PROTEIN EXPRESSION PROJECT

Questions to be answered:

• *What is the target protein, what are its properties?*

Examine the properties such as:

– Molecular weight

– Presence of:

a.signal peptides

b.transmembrane domains

c.multiple disulfide bridges

d.post-translational modification sites

– Domain structure

– Presence of low complexity or disordered regions

• *Source of organisms from which protein will be derived*

• *Natural cellular location of protein*:

a.Nuclear

b.Cytoplasmic

c.Organelle

d.Extracellular

• *Protein expressed previously*

• *What is protein to be used for and how much is required?*

Expression of Previously Expressed Proteins

If a protein has not been expressed or had its structure solved by X-ray crystallography or NMR, then structural databases should be searched to check whether a homologous protein has been studied and its structural domain boundaries can be inferred by multiple sequence alignment or else, literature search can be carried out *via* Pub Med search engine.

For a large protein (750 kDa), consider the use of a eukaryotic expression system or truncate the protein to a smaller size for soluble expression in E. coli. Uniport, Pfam, and SMART (Single Modular Architecture Research Tool) are employed to map the proteins. Perl script can predict disordered regions of proteins and can be mapped into linear sequences as a fold index score. Prediction methods are available for identifying signal peptides, transmembrane domains, sites of glycosylphosphatidylinositol, lipid anchoring, prenylation, and N-myristylation. Following the mapping of a target protein sequence, one can decide on the expression strategy.

1st Phase of Protein Expression

This includes the selection of cells to be used as a protein source. Microorganisms, fungi, plant cells and animal cells can be used as expression systems.

Microorganism

A number of recombinant DNA technology methods can be used, namely, additional copies of a relevant gene can be introduced to the host cell; introduction of the relevant gene for gene expression. E. coli is the most common species used to produce genetically engineered proteins.

Advantages of Microorganisms as Protein Source

•The fermentation process is well-understood.

•Can be cultured in large quantities in a short time hence, product on large-scale can be generated.

•Relatively easy to alter genetically: recombinant DNA technology.

Disadvantages of Microbial Protein Expression System

•Protein contained in intracellular inclusion bodies (insoluble clumps) that must be purified.

•Protein folding needed for many active proteins in mammalian systems cannot be achieved.

•Certain proteins can only be produced by the eukaryotic system because certain post-translational modifications such as glycosylation do not occur in prokaryotes.

•Some proteins are inactive in humans.

For the desired protein, a foreign gene (cDNA) is treated directly to complete or partial E. coli gene and the desired protein is produced in the form of a fusion protein (target protein fused to the bacterial protein).

The fusion protein is broken away from the target protein by a fused bacterial protein (usually an enzyme attached to a purification column) and the target protein is thus purified.

Nowadays, the entire process of protein expression from genetically engineered microorganisms is conducted in bioreactors.

Bioreactor

Bioreactor is a self-contained, closed (sterile) system of large-volume cell culture containing sterile ports through which pH, gas concentrations, temperature and other variables can be controlled by workers. Also, cell growth is monitored carefully and accordingly proteins are taken out in the phase of growth when the yield is the highest (Fig. **8**).

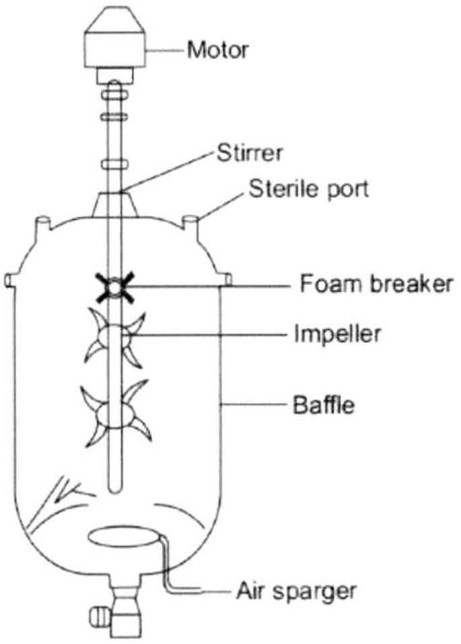

Fig. (8). Bioreactor.

STEPS OF PROTEIN EXPRESSION IN *E-COLI*

Owing to the easy handling, low cost and fast growth of E. coli, the E. coli expression system has become the system of choice.

Cloning of PCR Products

i. Preparation of insert

ii. Preparation of vector

iii. Formation of hybrid products:

•Vector and insert are incubated to produce hybrid products which are then transformed.

iv. Transformation into the expression vector:

•Transformation of constructs into E. coli expression host and plated onto selective media.

Small Scale Expression

Two to four colonies of transformed E. coli expression host are selected and grown into auto-inducing medium. Cells are grown in a 96 deep well plate overnight, spun down, resuspended and disrupted by mechanical lysis (sonication) or protein extraction reagent. The lysate is analyzed by the SDS-PAGE. This whole process of PCR for 96 targets to analyse the level of expression of targets is automated and achieved in 3–4 days.

Cell Paste Growth

Clones showing the highest level of soluble expression of the target protein of correct molecular weight are selected and plasmid DNA is prepared and sequenced and overnight incubation of cells is carried out.

Clear Lysate Preparation

Frozen cell paste is resuspended in lysis buffer (based on pI of the protein) and a protease inhibitor is added to prevent proteolysis of the target.

Purification of Protein

By affinity chromatography methods, having specific affinity tags, proteins are purified. Protein purification has also become automated nowadays.

For checking the expression of constructs, a negative control is included. Try expression in different media and different temperatures in parallel. Always sequence the expression constructs and perform MS after purification to ensure that that molecular mass matches the calculated mass.

PLANT CELLS FOR PROTEIN EXPRESSION

85% of current drugs can be found in plants and plants are an important source of biologically active molecules.

Advantage of Plants as Expression System

•Plants produce enzymes that can be used for future drug production.
•Can be genetically modified to produce desired proteins that do not occur naturally.
•Rapid growth and reproduction rates of plants: a single plant can produce upto a million of seeds.

Disadvantages

•Not all proteins can be expressed in plants.
•Due to tough cell walls of plant cells, extraction of proteins can be tough and time-consuming.
•The glycosylation of proteins by plant cells is different from what occurs in animal cells.

FUNGI AS EXPRESSION SYSTEM

Naturally occurring proteins found in some fungi are nutritious and used as a food source. Fungi are eukaryotic and capable of some post-translational modifications and protein folding.

Table 2. Recombinant proteins from fungi.

Fungi	Protein
Aspartic proteinase	A. oryzae
Bovine chymosin	A. niger, A. nidulans
Human interferon	A. niger, A. nidulans
Human lactoferrin	A. oryzae, A. niger
Triglyceride lipase	A. oryzae

MAMMALIAN CELL EXPRESSION SYSTEMS

The animal cell culture has complex nutritional requirements and is a very complex process. Animal cells grow slowly, require a large number of cells to seed bioreactors and require a sterile environment. In many cases, animal cell cultures are still the best.

INSECT SYSTEMS AS PROTEIN PRODUCERS

Baculoviruses (viruses that infect insects) are used as vehicles to insert DNA to produce desired proteins. However, at times, post-translational modifications are slightly different.

WHOLE ANIMAL PRODUCTION SYSTEMS

Living animals are also protein producers and have been used to harvest monoclonal antibodies for therapeutic and diagnostic applications. *e.g.*, mice are injected with an antigen to secrete desired antibodies, or the antibody-producing tissue from mouse is fused with cancer cells.

Whole animal protein production makes use of milk or eggs from transgenic animals as a source of proteins from a recombinant gene that was introduced into transgenic animals.

EUKARYOTIC EXPRESSION SYSTEM

Saccharomyces Cerevisiae

S. cerevisiae is widely recognized and a robust host for recombinant protein expression.

Fact File

Recombinant proteins are expressed as:

•Intracellular (soluble or membrane-bound)

•Extracellular

•Eukaryotic expression system.

•Post-translation modifications possible.

•Produces active and functional proteins for

– Enzymatic assay

– Functional assay

– Structural biology

– Commercial use

Advantages

•Allows easy scaling up of production.

•Genetic tools are available that allow fast and convenient construction of customized host stains.

•Allow both integrative and plasmid-based expression.

•Offers a whole range of constitutive and regulated promoters.

•Can modify protein post-translationally by glycosylation, phosphorylation, and methylation.

•Used as a model to understand the function and properties of many mammalian proteins, g-protein coupled pathway.

Vectors and Promoters

The most commonly used vectors are E. coli/yeast multicopy shuttle plasmid. Also, autonomously replicating sequences and integrative transformation vector system are available.

The integration of foreign DNA into a genome gives high stability to stain, especially when more than one heterologous gene has to be introduced in one strain.

Fact File: S. Cerevisiae Strain

• 2 μm DNA is 6318 bp plasmid.

• Carries a plasmid at a copy number of about 60 per cell.

• The plasmid exhibits high transformation rate, high meiotic and meiotic stability.

• The plasmids lacking foreign DNA are extremely stable and employed in industries, *e.g*., to yield human albumin upto 5 g/l and human α1-antitryspin at 40% (w/v) of total proteins.

• Secretion leader of alpha mating type factor has proved to be the most robust and versatile sequence for the heterologous protein.

The expression of recombinant proteins is designed as constitutive or regulated by induction. Also, promoter selection markers and selection leader sequence (to direct protein to be expressed by selection machinery and its release into growth media finally) are present in expression vectors.

Strains

Standard host strains for most expression solutions are available in strain collections: Yeast Genetic Stock Center at ATCC (American Type Culture Collection, DSMZ (German Collection of Microprograms and Cell Cultures). Choosing the right strain for the target protein influences high expression yield and quality.

Proteases in Yeast

• Wild-type S. cerevisiae cells contain vacuolar proteases:

– aspartic endoproteinase A (PrA)

– serine protease (protease B or PrB)

• Also, proteases are located in other cellular compartments.

• Vacuolar proteases degrade endogenous yeast and heterologous proteins.

• If certain vacuolar proteases are deficient then the problem of proteolysis arises.

• A PEP 4 gene encoding proteinase A stabilizes the production of many heterologous proteins and reduce their degradation significantly.

Analysis of Expression

The expression of a transformed gene has to be induced and assayed after establishment and confirmation of colonies (by PCR). Various assay procedures are immunoblotting, enzymatic, function and the most common strategy in recent years is immunoblotting using antibodies directed against a fused 'tag'.

Tags

•Tags are short epitope tags or fusion proteins.

•Use of tags may interfere with either the expression yield (positively or negatively) or actively and correct folding of proteins.

•Tags are fused to N or C terminus.

•Tags can be placed at both ends to verify and select full-length gene products.

•Tags may be chosen to work both for detection and amplification by affinity chromatography.

Recombinant proteins if required in milligram amounts for functional or structural analysis, then *S. cerevisiae* is a favoured expression system.

Expression of Proteins in Pichia Pastoris

P. pastoris is methylotrophic (utilizes methanol as a sole source of carbon) and many enzymes required for methanol metabolism are present at high levels.

When cells grow on methanol Alcohol oxidase (AOX), the first enzyme in the methanol utilization pathway gets induced when cells are shifted to methanol. AOX1 is responsible for the gene product.

Plasmid

All expression vectors are E. coli/P. pastoris shuttle vectors, containing an origin of replication for plasmid maintenance in E. coli; expression cassette. Consisting of multiple cloning sites for insertion of a foreign coding sequence, flanked by the promoter.

AOX1 promoter is one of the strongest promoters known. Other promoters are the GAP gene promoter (which can be used in glucose and other carbon sources), glutathione-dependent for an aldehyde dehydrogenase promotor.

Strain

All *P. pastoris* is derived from a wild-type strain Y-11430. Strain X-33 is also wild-type, and is GS115 (his 4) transformed with P. pastoris H1S4 gene.

Advantages

•Relative case of genetic manipulation.

•Its ability to produce proteins and high levels either extracellularly or intracellularly.

•Its capability to perform many eukaryotic post-translation modifications: glycosylation disulfide bond formation, proteolytic processing, and folding.

•Ability to scale up for large-scale shake flask culturing and grow to extremely high concentrations 'Even its kits are available (*e.g.*, from Invitrogen).

Pichia Pastoris Fact File

•Yeast, used successfully for the production of over 550 heterologous proteins since 1984.

•An excellent source of single cell protein.

•Originally developed as a high-protein animal feed, but later shifted to the recombinant protein expression.

•Yield ranges from a few mg to over 10 g/l of P. close pastoris culture.

•Often termed as 'program-made protein machine' (Table **3**).

Table 3. Strains of P. pastoris that are commonly used.

Strain	Genotype
Wild type	
Y-11430	Wild type
X-33	Wild type (GS115::4154)

(Table 3) cont.....

Autotrophic strain	
GS115	his 4
GS190	arg 4
S5200	arg 4 his 4
fc301	ade1 arg 4 his 4
YJN165	ura 5
Methanol utilization strains	
KM71	his 4 arg 4 aoc 1 Δ::ScARG 4
MC100-3	his 4 arg 4 aoc 1Δ: ScARG4 aoc 2 Δ::hr Pphis 4
Protease-deficient strains	
SMD1168	his 4 Δ pep4::URA3 ura 3
SMD1165	prb1 his 4
Other strains	
GS241	fld1.

Methodology Steps

1.*Transformation:* Construction of a plasmid and its introduction into P. pastoris genome.
2.*Screening of transformants*: To identify the best expressers. Spot Western blot will identify the most productive strains.
3.*Optimization:* Optimization of several culturing factors for optimal expression is important for the quality of expression.
4.*Small-scale purification:* Recombinant proteins can be isolated with size exclusion, and affinity chromatography. Or else, heterologous proteins are expressed as a fusion protein to some types of peptide bag).

5.*Purification:* P. pastoris does not like to format and prefers respiratory growth (requires cultures to be well a aerated) and culture volume should never exceed 1/5 of volume of the flask.

Dialysis or ammonium sulphate precipitation prior to the concentration of expressed protein prevents clogging to concentrators. In the case of recreated proteins, proteins may be glycosylated and require digestion with peptide: N-glycosidase F. This sample should be resolved by SDS-PAGE.

Baculovirus Expression System

Baculovirus expression system produces high yields of structurally, functionally and antigenically authentic foreign proteins in insect cells.

Flash BAC

Flash BAC system is a new platform technology for the production of recombinant baculoviruses. It is based on the AcMNPV genome.

Fact File

•A well-established and popular method for the production of foreign proteins in insect cells.
•The virus genome (Autographa californica multinucleopoly retrovirus AcMNPV) and transfer vector are introduced into host insect cells resulting in the recombinant virus genome.
•Bacterial artificial chromosomes (BACs) have been incorporated into the baculovirus genome to allow recombinant virus construction in E. coli.
•Commercial bacmid-based systems are available.

Insect Cell Culture Requirement

A septic technique must be used when working with insect cells. Culturing should be carried out in a laminar flow cabinet or around a flame. The most commonly used insect cells are sf21 cells (derived from pupal ovarian cells of Spodoptera frugiperda) sfq cells (clonal isolate of sf21); and High Five cells (BTI-TN-5B1-4: clonal isolate of Trichoplusia ni) ovarian cell line TN-368).

Nowadays, workstations automated for the production of recombinant baculoviruses and their screening of recombinant proteins are available.

Fact File for Culture Requirements

Temperature	:	27–28°C
Culture medium	:	Phosphate buffering system
CO_2 incubators	:	not required
Serum	:	May or may not be required nowadays serum free conditions are applied.
Precaution	:	Handle one cell line at a time.

Protein Purification Methods

Once the proteins are produced, they must be harvested. In case of the intracellular protein, the entire cell is harvested, however, if it is extracellular, the protein excreted into culture media is collected.

Then the protein is purified after separating the target protein from a complex mixture of biological molecules and it is desirable that the sample is composed of 99.99% of the target protein after purification.

Separation of proteins from all other cellular contents and isolation of the target protein from other proteins are not easy. In the coming section, commonly followed steps for protein isolation and purification are covered.

Preparation of Extract

For intracellular proteins, cell lysis (disruption of cell wall to release protein) is carried out by various methods, namely, freezing and throwing of cells, detergents, ultrasonics or grinding with tiny glass leads. The disruption process releases the protein of interest along with the entire intracellular content of the cell.

Stabilization of Proteins

After the preparation of the mixture, proteins must be stabilized to protect and maintain their biological activity.

Threats to Protein

1.Temperature: Heat as moderate as room temperature limits the lifespan of proteins.

Precaution	:	Avoid outright freezing and freeze-thaw cycle to prevent the destruction of proteins.
Remedy	:	Do purification barely above freezing.

2.Nature proteases: They can digest the target proteins.

Remedy	:	Add protease inhibitors and antimicrobials.
Precaution	:	Addition of protease is inhibited by FΔA since it can lead to degradation and harmful reactions.

3. Mechanical destruction of protein by foaming or shearing of proteins.

Remedy: Add additives to prevent foaming and shearing.

These additives must be removed later in the purification process.

Separation of Proteins from Extract

(i) Protein Precipitation

Salts (most commonly, ammonium sulphate) can be added to the protein mixture to precipitate the proteins. Protein precipitation separates the proteins away from non-proteins in a stable from.

•Precipitating agents
•Ethanol
•Isopropanol
•Acetone
•Diethyl ether

(ii) Filtration

Molecules can be separated based on their size and density in various ways:

Filtration Methods

Centrifugation:

•Small-volume centrifuges (few litres each run).
•Large reactions: industrial-scale centrifugation (continuous flow centrifuges).

Filters:

•Membrane filtration using thin membranes of nylon or other engineered substances.
•Microfiltration: for precipitates and bacteria.
•Ultrafiltration: to catch proteins and nucleic acids.
•Diafiltration
•Dialysis based on the equilibrium of chemicals.

(iii) Chromatography

Chromatography methods allow sorting out proteins by their size.

Chromatography technique

•*Size exclusion chromatography (SEC):* uses gel beads of various pore sizes.
•*Ion change (IonX) chromatography:* extremely useful protein purification and concentration method based on the electrostatic change.
•Affinity chromatography: based on the ability of proteins to bind specifically and reversibly to uniquely shaped compounds (ligands).
•Hydrophobic interaction chromatography: based on sorting of proteins on the basis of their repulsion of water.
•Iso-electric focusing: based on the unique isoelectric point (IEP) of each protein, isoelectric focusing can be used to separate proteins in the first dimension of two-dimensional electrophoresis.

Two-dimensional electrophoresis: to separate proteins based on their electrical charge and size.

Analysis

HPLC systems separate proteins under great pressure through a column in a shorter time. Less protein is separated by this technique and it is useful in analytical situations.

Mass spectrometry (Mass spec.) is a highly sensitive method to identify trace elements (even picogram : 1 billionth of a gram) based on mass-to-charge ratios.

Verification

At each step of the purification process, it is important to verify that the target protein is not lost and concentration efforts are successful.

Methods for Verification

SDS-PAGE: Sodium dodecyl sulphate (detergent) is added to a sample of protein mixture and heated to distribute sulphate charges evenly along the denatured protein for the separation of the protein sample (loaded on PAGE after denaturation) of form a single band.

Method for Section of Protein Separated by SDS-PAGE:

•Staining with Coomassie stain
•Western blotting: transfer of a protein from gel to nitrocellulose membrane and detection by specific antibody tagged to an enzyme to convert the fluorescent substrate.
•ELISA (enzyme-linked immunosorbent assay): requires two antibodies: one to capture protein and the second attached to an enzyme to produce a colour reaction.

Preservation of Proteins

Following isolation and collection of target protein, protein needs to be saved until it can be used.

Lyophilization or *freeze* drying is used to preserve proteins by applying a vacuum to liquid products to hasten the evaporation of water (ice crystals sublimate to water vapour directly without melting from the fluid, leaving behind dried proteins). Lyophilization maintains the protein structure and these proteins may be stored at room temperature for prolonged proteins.

Post Purification Analysis

Following protein purification, the molecular structure of proteins is determined or its structure is changed to change its function.

Automated protein sequences using the current mass spec method can identify many proteins in a matter of minutes.

Also, X-ray crystallography can be used to determine the tertiary and quaternary structure of proteins using a pure protein. "Ribbon" diagrams can be generated by computer analysis and potential modifications of proteins to improve their function can be planned.

Proteomics

Proteomics is dedicated to the understanding of complex relationships between diseases and protein expressions.

Proteomes (Protein complement to a genome) are compared under healthy and disease states and variations in the protein expression can be correlated to the onset or progression of a specific disease. Thus, protein markers can be discovered to be used as diagnostic methods and drug targets.

Proteomics has been discussed in detail in Chapter 2. Protein microarrays can detect proteins and functional protein microarrays have been applied to study protein-protein, protein-lipid, protein- DNA, protein-drug and protein-protein interactions.

Microbiome

Microbiome describes the genome of all microorganisms living in and on all vertebrates. The gut microbiome is comprised of the collective genome of microbes inhabiting the gut namely, bacteria, archaea, viruses, and fungi. More details will be discussed in chapter 10.

EXERCISE

1.Provide examples of medical applications of proteins

2.Give uses of biotechnologically produced enzymes in the industry.

3.Microbial, fungi, plant and animal sources for protein expression.

4.Protein expression system, protein purification processes.

5.Explain proteomics

CONCLUSION

Medical genomics pinpoints the normal and abnormal functions of individual genes and uses this information for the diagnosis and treatment of the disease. Newer proteins discovered through genomics may serve as drugs themselves and they can be proteins or hormones or growth factors that are under/over-expressed in disease states. Functional genomics is becoming increasingly important for genome-based drug discovery. Translational research provides the knowledge necessary to draw important conclusions from the clinical testing of the disease and the viability of novel drug mechanisms. Metabolomics is a concept that has been defined as the science of comprehensive monitoring of the metabolic processes in biological systems. Since metabolism is a key aspect of a phenotype, the next logical step is the description of the distribution of metabolites to elaborate functional genomics. Proteomics is dedicated to the understanding of complex relationships between diseases and the protein expression.

BIBLIOGRAPHY

[1] Wilson K, Hofmann A, Walker JM, Clokie S, Eds. Wilson and Walker's principles and techniques of biochemistry and molecular biology. Cambridge university press 2018.

[2] Karp G. Cell and molecular biology: concepts and experiments. John Wiley & Sons 2009.

[3] Hartl DL, Jones EW, Hartl DL, Jones EW. Genetics: principles and analysis. 1998.

[4] Sambrook J, Russell DW. Molecular Cloning Laboratory Manual (Volume). Beijing: Science Press 2002; pp. 69-71.

[5] Primrose SB. Principles of gene manipulation and genomics by Sandy B Primrose and Richard Twyman.

[6] Glick BR, Pasternak JJ. Principles and applications of recombinant DNA. Washington, DC: ASM 1998; p. 683.

CHAPTER 10

Newer Technologies in Molecular Biology

LEARNING OBJECTIVES

This chapter gives an overview of antisense RNA technology and gene silencing; mRNA surveillance; using biotechnology against bioweapons; molecular cytogenetics; mutation detection, detection of genomic duplications and deletion, mutation database & analysis of human splicing defects;, molecular techniques for DNA methylation studies, pharmacogenetics, pharmacogenomics and nutrigenomics; preimplantation genetic diagnosis and prenatal diagnosis; next-generation DNA sequencing techniques (NGS); single cell biopsy; CRISPR, gene editing; transformative advances in regenerative medicine; Encode, exomic studies, ancestry studies.

Abstract: Technical advances began with the advent of array comparative genomic hybridization and single nucleotide polymorphism arrays and are enabling researchers to identify disease-associated genetic variants by virtually scanning the entire genome. With the help of these technologies, it is now possible to screen for common genetic variants and even rare small deletions and duplications *i.e.*, microdeletions and microduplications. This has led to a virtual explosion of gene identifications. This chapter aims to provide an overview of new technologies.

Keywords: Antisense RNA, Antisense therapy, Gene silencing, Jumping gene, Bioterrorism, Bioweapons, cytogenetic, DNA methylation, Pharmacogenetics, Pharmacogenomics, Nutrigenomics.

ANTISENSE TECHNOLOGY

Antisense RNAs

Antisense RNA is an RNA molecule that is complementary to mRNA and binds to mRNA, preventing its translation. Antisense RNA is occasionally used in gene regulation both by bacteria and eukaryotes.

The antisense RNA approach is designed to specifically interfere with the virus replication. A complementary DNA strand of a gene can be inserted in reverse orientation ($3' \rightarrow 5'$) and is termed as an antisense gene. The antisense gene produces mRNA complementary to mRNA synthesized by the normal gene. Both of these mRNAs hybridize, blocking the normal translation of mRNAs. Antisense approach can be useful in both single-stranded RNA viruses and DNA viruses.

Simmi Kharb, Akshat Singh, Abhyuday Singh & Deepa Kharb (Eds.)

Antisense Therapy

This refers to the inhibition of translation by using a single-stranded nucleotide (antisense oligonucleotide). Also, it is possible to inhibit both transcription and translation Figs. (**1** and **2**).

For Cancer Therapy

Antisense RNA molecules are more frequently used in cancer therapy.

Two Ways of Inhibition of Translation by Antisense RNA

(i) Antisense cDNA is cloned and transfected into cells to synthesize antisense mRNA. This antisense mRNA binds with the specific mRNA and block translation.

(ii) Antisense RNA is directly introduced into the cells which hybridize with target mRNA and blocks translation.

For HIV Prevention

Antisense therapy can prevent HIV infection. Target cells for HIV infection are genetically engineered to contain a gene that can express a complimentary copy of the HIV genome and antisense RNA. When cells with antisense RNA are infected with HIV, a double-stranded RNA hybrid molecule is formed that cannot be used by the enzyme reverse transcriptase.

Antisense technology in conjunction with emerging technologies will make a significant impact on the future of healthcare.

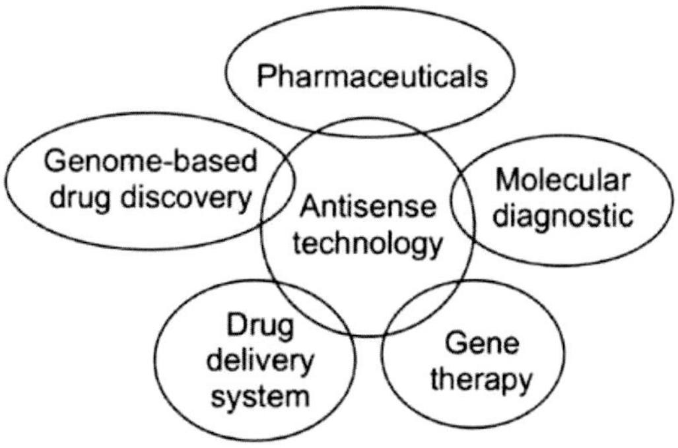

Fig. (1). Antisense technology and biopharma industry.

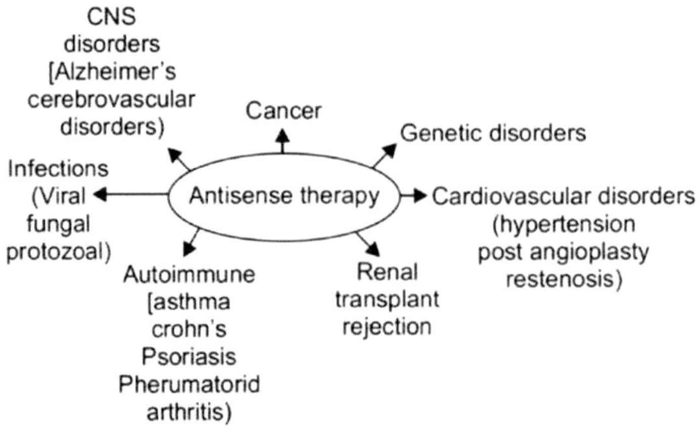

Fig. (2). Potential clinical applications of antisense therapy.

Theoretically, all infections and diseases due to genetic overexpression should be amenable to antisense approaches.

Antisense therapy interferes with the expression of disease-causing proteins, thus offering a direct and selective intervention in the disease process. Other key antisense technologies that have an impact on drug discovery and molecular diagnostics are antisense gene therapy ribozymes, triple helix-forming oligonucleotides and peptide nucleic acids (PNA).

Antisense approaches are compatible with emerging trends in drug development, genomic-based therapeutics, and the integration of diagnostics with therapeutics Fig. (**3**).

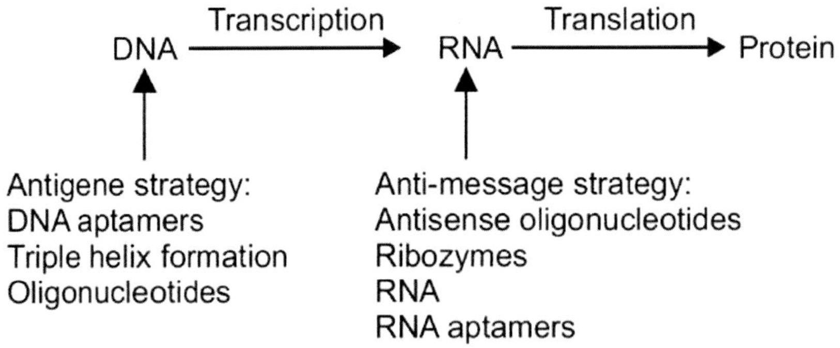

Fig. (3). Antisense strategies.

The main advantage of the antisense approach is that the antisense compounds target a disease at its genetic origin whereas conventional pharmaceuticals merely counteract the manifestations of diseases by inhibiting gene products (proteins) (Table **1**).

Table 1. Antisense technology as gene therapy approaches.

• Antisense RNA using vectors.
• Single strand (SS) DNA oligonucleotide mediated antisense.
• Insertion of a gene that will produce specific antisense nuclei in cells
• Chimeric RNA/DNA antisense oligonucleotides delivered by viral vectors.
• Decoy oligonucleotides delivered by ex vivo pressure transfection
• Ribozymes
• Triple helix forming oligonucleotides delivered by viral vectors
• Vector-mediated antisense RNA approach

GENE SILENCING

RNAi (RNA Interference)

For years, RNAs have been thought to carry out just two broad functions in cells, namely, gene expression (mRNA) and protein synthesis (rRNA, tRNA). With the discovery of RNA interference (RNAi) in 1998 by Andrew Fire, Craig Mello and colleagues—the silencing of gene expression was done by double stranded DNA molecules—in nematode worms. It is an evolutionary ancient method of genome defect in many organisms, predating the evolutionary divergence of plants and worms Fig. (**4**).

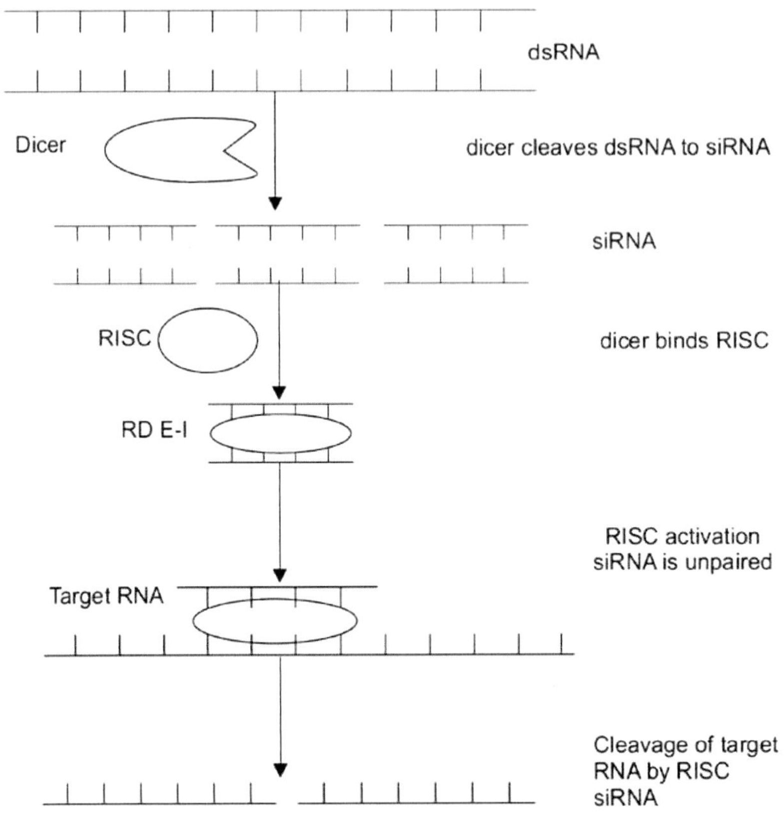

Fig. (4). Mechanism of RNAi.

Mechanism of Gene Silencing

RNAi is a mechanism for gene silencing that is induced by double-stranded RNA (dsRNA). ds RNA is normally destroyed by living cells of all organisms and RNAi destroys mRNA that has same sequence as double-stranded RNA detected in the cell. Long dsRNA is processed by the action of dsRNA-specific endo nuclease known as Dicer to short interfering RNA (siRNAs) [21–24 nucleotide in length]. siRNA are bound by nuclease complex known as RISC (RNA-induced silencing complex). A helicase in RISC unwinds the duplex siRNA and base-pairs to mRNA having sequence complimentary to siRNA. Then, RNAase *"Slicer"* within RISC proceeds to degrade the target RNA.

The complementarity between the antisense strand of the unwound siRNA and the target RNA governs the sequence-specificity of gene silencing.

RNAi probably served as an ancient defence mechanism against mobile genetic elements such as RNA viruses and transposons. Also, RNAi has a role in gene regulation and formation of heterochromatin. RNAi is harnessed as an experimental tool to explore gene function, is revolutionizing our ability to perform large-scale genetic screens, and shows therapeutic potential.

siRNA

siRNA may have a general role in silencing of transposable elements (jumping genes), repetitive genes (including transgenes) and viruses. About half of the sequences in human genome were generated. by duplication and insertion of transposons. Silencing of these mobile elements is crucial for the stability of genome and RNAi-related processes involving the generation of short RNAs are essential to this silencing processing in many organisms.

MRNA SURVEILLANCE

Micro RNA

They are abundant, single-stranded RNA (few thousand to 40,000 molecules per cell), sharing properties in common with siRNA. They do not produce protein, rather regulate the gene expression by blocking translation of mRNA. They do not promote degradation of mRNA, but block translation by binding to mRNA in 3′-untranslated region.

They are found in worms, insects, mammals and plants. The first mRNA detected in C. elegans were termed as small temporal RNA (stRNA) because they regulate the timing of worm development during conversion of larva into the adult.

Genes encoding miRNA seem to make up 0.5–1% of the predicted genes in all multicellular organisms and so far, some 175 of these human miRNA genes have been confirmed and little is known about their function.

Tiny Nonencoding RNA (tncRNA)

A newly discovered class of short, 20–22 nucleotide RNA encoded by genome of C. elegans. tncRNA don't have highly complementary sequences nearby in the genome, and so may not be processed from hairpins. They are not evolutionarily conserved. Their function is still not known.

Small Modulatory RNA (smRNA)

A short dsRNA, non-protein-coding, 20-nucleotide dsRNA, isolated from neural stem cells in the hippocampus of adult mice. It is evolutionarily conserved in vertebrates and is bound by regulatory protein.

RNAi into the Lab and Clinic

RNAi promises to be one of the most useful lab tools yet. Silencing genes with RNAi makes it possible to analyze many gene networks in mammals.

Target gene has been silenced experimentally in C. elegans by injecting dsRNA and soaking them in a solution of dsRNA or feeding bacteria expressing dsRNA. About 19,000 genes in worms and libraries of 12,000 different dsRNA have been used to screen this animal for genes involved in complex phenomena such as obesity, ageing. In fruit flies, purified long dsRNA has been used to define the role of specific genes in cholesterol metabolism and heart formation.

In human cells in vitro, chemically synthesized siRNAs have been used to define gene functions and short RNA might even be used to treat diseases such as cancer. In humans, major obstacle therapeutic gene silencing is 'delivery problem' – the necessity of introducing short dsRNAs into specific organs.

Therapeutic Applications

Many disorders have been targeted by RNAi in in vitro and in vivo model systems, namely, oncogenesis, infectious diseases, viral hepatitis.

Oncogenesis

siRNAs specific for BCR-ABL transcript in myelogenous leukaemia have been shown to silence the oncogenic fusion transcripts without affecting expression levels of normal C-ABL ad C-BCR transcripts.

In pancreatic and colon carcinomas, RAS genes are often mutated (point-mutation). Introduction of RNAi specific for oncogenic variant of K-RAS (called K-RAS V12) reduces levels of K-RAS V12 transcripts and loss of anchorage independent growth and tumorigenicity.

siRNA have been used to decrease drug resistance of cells in vitro by inhibiting expression of MDR1 (multidrug transporter).

Viral Hepatitis

siRNA targeted to FasRNA and delivered by high-pressure infection into tails of mice have been demonstrated to reach the liver and inhibit Fas expression and protect mice from hepatitis.

Infectious Disease

RNAi have the most application in treatment of infectious diseases since RNA targets are exogenous and can be inhibited without affecting cellular functions.

In HIV, incoming viral RNA can be targeted by RNAi in some studies while others indicate that it is resistant to RNAi (shielded from RNAi by a nucleocapsid). Also, it may be added here that RNA silencing is an antiviral defence and viruses have evolved to counteract it. Silencing effect of RNAi is highly specific and potent and requires that sequence of the target RNA be known.

RNA-based therapeutic strategies like antisense RNA and ribozymes suffer from limitations. No ribozyme has been approved for clinical use and only one (DNA) antisense agent: Fomivisen has been approved by FDA for treatment of cytomegalovirus retinitis in HIV.

For Genetic Diseases

SNPs in mutant allele transcript can be used as selective targets for RNAi in genetic diseases such as Huntington's disease.

Obstacles to Therapy

The single biggest obstacle to development of RNAi-based therapeutic agents is delivery.

Target RNAs can be expressed from vectors or delivered as artificial siRNAs. A variety of strategies or delivered as artificial siRNA with use of plasmid and virus vector-based cassettes have been explored. The well-documented hazards of inserting foreign vector sequences into chromosomal DNA include insertional activation and inactivation of cellular genes. Silencing effect of siRNA is short-lived because siRNAs eventually decay within the cells, and it is not clear whether there are selective tissue sites for uptake of siRNAs. In nutshell, RNAi is attractive as a therapeutic approach owing and RNAi-based therapeutic agents are not-too distant future.

Antisense Therapy

It is based on assumption any sequence longer than a minimum number of nucleotides (~20 ntd) occurs only once within the human genome. It involves delivery of oligonucleotide that are complementary to mRNA or viral RNA of interest into cells, which are then able to seek out and bind to RNA target. (Fig. **5**). This leads to suppression of expression of protein either by sterically blocking critical steps of the translation process or through expression of protein.

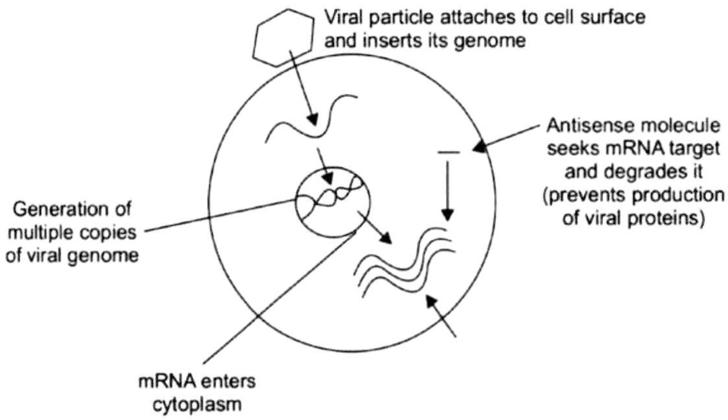

Fig. (5). Inhibition of gene expression with antisense technology in case of viral infection

The original antisense technology developed in 1978 used antisense oligonucleotides complementary to sequence within their target mRNAs to inhibit gene expression. Oligonucleotides (DNA, RNA) of 18–25 nucleotides have been used in antisense studies with first step in mechanism of gene knock down in common.

Various Antisense Technologies are shown in Figs. (**1** and **2**).

1. Antisense oligonucleotide hybridizes to target mRNA, which is then degraded by intracellular enzyme RNase H that cleaves RNA strand of RNA/DNA duplex.

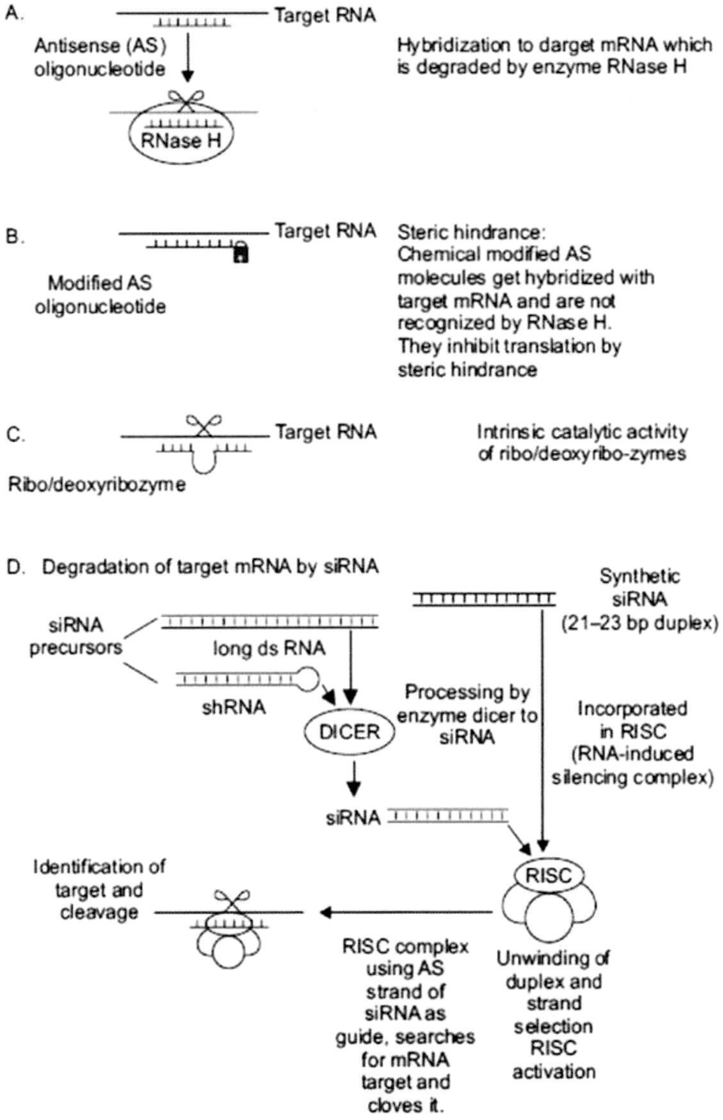

Fig. (6). Mechanism of indignation of gene expression through various "antisense" technologies.

2. AS molecules translation by steric hindrance
3. *e.g.*, modified nucleic acid derivatives such as morpholinos, 2′-0-methyls, 2′-0-allyls, locked nucleic acids, peptide nucleic acids.
4. Intrinsic catalytic activity of ribozymes and deoxy ribozymes

5. Ribozyme bind to RNA *via* Watson-Crick base pairing and cleavage of phosphodiester backbone of RNA target by transesterification.
6. Degradation of target mRNA is siRNA

When long double-stranded RNA molecules are introduced into these organisms, they are processed by endonuclease Dicer into 21-to-23-nt small interfering RNAs (siRNAs). siRNAs are then incorporated into multicomponent RNA-induced silencing complex (RISC), which unwinds the duplex and Fig. (**6**) uses the AS strand as a guide to seek and degrade homologous mRNAs.

Synthetic short siRNAs (20–25 bp) that can be either delivered exogenously or expressed endogenously from RNA polymerase II or III promoters, resulting in a powerful tool for down regulation of target mRNAs.

siRNA Therapeutics

After choosing target gene for down regulation, there are several hurdles in identification of candidate therapeutics for clinical trials.

Challenges for AS-Based Approaches for Gene Knock Down

1. Identification of effective sequence.
2. Identification of sequence that provides most potent knock down at lowest possible concentration (dose) of agent.
3. Accessibility of target site because of local, internal secondary structure and steric occlusion.
4. Identification, analysis of target sequence in terms of greatest probability of success for a given mRNA.
5. High specificity, off-target and other toxic effects in cell culture experiments.
6. Sense strand may be selected by RISC complex rather than AS strand resulting in inhibition of unintended genes.
7. Delivery of AS molecules to desired cell types, tissues or organ. Since RNAs do not readily cross the cell membrane on their own owing to their large molecular mass and high negative charge.
8. siRNA expressed from viral vectors with opposing promoters result in inefficient hybridization and poor silencing activity.

9. shRNA is more difficult to synthesize chemically because of its >50 nt size. But has advantage over siRNA in case of viral delivery as it is expressed as a single molecule resulting in high level of activity.
10. siRNA have very short-half life in blood (less than minutes), they should be chemically modified to make them resistant to serum RNases.
11. Obstacles in gene-therapy vectors: insertional mutagenesis, malignant transformation, immune response to proteins expressed from viral vectors.
12. Effects of long-term expression of siRNA is not known.
13. Points to ponder: While designing siRNA therapeutics

- Choose effective target site on mRNA or viral RNA that does not cause off-target effects on gene expression.
- Decide:

a. whether to use:

- siRNA
- or shRNA

b. whether or not it should be chemically synthesized or expressed in vivo (from a range of vectors)

- Synthetic siRNA are useful where long-term silencing is not required, e.g., in treatment of acute viral infection)
- Encapsulation of siRNAs in lipid complexes, attachment to fusogenic peptides, antibodies or cell surface receptors allow further improvement of potential drug candidates.

Delivery Strategies for RNA

1. Use of chemically synthesized RNAs that have been modified for improved pharmacokinetic properties.
2. Use of viral or non-viral vectors to express RNA within the cells.

Potential RNAi-Based Therapies

Inhibition of viral replication by RNA interference has been demonstrated in vivo for a variety of RNA viruses such as HIV, influenza virus, hepatitis C & D, rota virus, respiratory syncytial virus (RSV) and dengue virus; and DNA viruses such as human papilloma virus, hepatitis B, herpes simplex virus. Viral infections, neurodegenerative diseases, septic shock, macular degeneration and caner are candidate diseases for siRNA-based therapies.

Systemic route of delivery is the ultimate goal in developing siRNA drugs. Development of new siRNA-based drugs is feasible but it will take at least several more years (Table **2**).

Table 2. Studies of RNAi therapeutic efficiency in products.

Tissue	Disease	Target	RNAi formulation	Route
Eye	Neovascularization	VEGF VEGF	siRNA siRNA	Intracellular Intravitreal
CMV	Retinal Neovascularization Age-related macular degeneration (AMD)	CMVIE2 VEGF	siRNA drug* (orm versen) anti VEGF** (and 5 siRNA)	Intravitreal
Respiratory system	Influenza RSV	Viral genes NS 1	siRNa siRNA (Alnylan)*	Intranasal

*Phase I trial.

*Phase II trial.

RNA Interference Analysis

A key experimental approach to elucidate the function of a gene in vivo is the selective depression of its activity or expression followed by phenotypic analysis compared to controls. A variety of techniques are available, namely, gene disruption approaches that include conventional genetic screens and knockout technology; use of antisense oligonucleotide and antibody microinjection.

The RNAi analysis has become a popular approach for loss-of-function experiments. Also, RNAi technology in post genomic era is considered a strong method in genome-wide high throughput analysis of gene function.

dsRNA/siRNA/shRNA libraries for systemic RNAi screens of most predicted genes have been established for studies using *C. elegans*, Drosophila cultured cells and several mammalian cell-lines. With the help of these libraries, large-scale functional RNAi experiments resulted in dissection of genetic pathways and systematic analysis of the genome.

Also, RNAi can be harnessed to silence disease-causing genes and holds great promise for development of RNAi therapeutics. siRNAs have been reported to have clinical potential in treatment of viral infections, cancers, several disorders, and neurodegenerative diseases.

Since several diseases involve over-expression of a particular gene, much effort has gone towards finding drugs that can down regulate gene expression on the DNA, RNA or protein level: RNAi therapeutics.

mRNA SURVEILLANCE

In eukaryotes, an elaborate set of mechanisms have evolved so that multistep process of gene expression is a accurately executed and adapted to cellular needs.

In RNA surveillance works by assessing the quality of mRNAs to ensure that they are suitable for translation. mRNA surveillance facilitates detection and destruction of mRNAs containing premature termination codons (by nonsense-mediated decay NMD), thereby preventing synthesis of truncated and aberrant proteins can have deleterious effects.

Thirty per cent of human inherited genetic disorders result from premature termination codon mutations (PTC) and NMD underlie the recessive nature of many of these diseases. e.g., β thalassemia (recessive-trait) results from PTC mutation occurring in first or second exon of β-globin gene and individual is healthy since NMD destroys the resultant mRNA. However, if PTC is present in third and final exam it escapes detection by decay machinery causing the disease.

Also, NMD is critical during normal cellular development, e.g., immunoglobulin and T-cell receptor genes in mammalian lymphocytes undergo rearrangements resulting in upto 60% of frame-stuffed genes with PTCs NMDs down regulate PTC-containing mRNAs in lymphocytes by 90–99% preventing synthesis of defective proteins.

Thus, mRNA surveillance function to maintain proper levels of normal transcripts and to deplete aberrant transcripts from the cell.

Role of Translation

The requirement for ongoing translation to detect mRNAs having PTCs is well-documented both NMD and nonstop decay depend on translation by different mechanisms. NMD in mammals could be an entirely nuclear process for some transcripts.

Evolution

mRNA surveillance pathway is conserved across eukaryotes from yeast to humans. It is speculated that it is evolved to mitigate the potentially harmful gain-of-function and other dominant-negative effects of truncated proteins. mRNA surveillance may serve as a safeguard to allow organism to accumulate a reservoir of mutations while masking otherwise deleterious phenotypic consequences.

USING BIOTECHNOLOGY AGAINST BIOWEAPONS

Bioterrorism

It is use of biological materials as weapons to harm humans and even plants and animals. Aim of biotechnology is to improve quality of life for humans and other organisms, but bioterrorism represents a most extreme abuse of living organisms.

Tracking down the history, in 14th century bubonic plague was spread, using bodies of victims during wars in Russia and other countries (Back Death Plague of Europe). Measles smallpox and influenza were spread to native Americans by early European settlers. After September 11, 2001, anthrax (dried powder spores of Bacillus anthracis) scare was noticed.

Microbes as Bioweapons

Everyday all around the world, new strains of infectious and potentially deadly pathogens are evolving.

These microorganisms may be used as bioweapons of mass destruction in future (Table **3**).

Table 3. Potential Microbial Bioweapons.

Agent	**Disease threat**
Brucella	Fever, lethargy
Bacillus anthracis	Cutaneous lesion, flu, pneumonia
Clostridium botulinum	food poisoning, respiratory paralysis and cardiac arrest
Ebola virus	Haemorrhagic fever, joint pain
Influenza virus	Flu
Rickettsia	Typhus, fever
Variola virus	Smallpox
Yersinia pestis	Plague

Also, there is possibility that unknown organisms could be used as bioweapons since they would probably be difficult to detect and neutralize.

Variola virus that causes smallpox is a possible bioweapon of concern since its vaccination has been stopped over 20 years ago and WHO declared the disease to be eradicated the throughout the world. Recent monkey smallpox outbreaks may revive smallpox as a concern. After 2001 anthrax events, with possible threat for use of smallpox as bioweapon, in USA smallpox vaccines are produced and stocked by biotechnology firms.

In addition to direct threat to humans, there is recent concern over possible bioweapon attacks that could cause severe damage to crops, food animals and other food supplies. This could cripple agricultural economy and cause scarcity of food (Table **4**).

Table 4. Bioweapon targets on food sources.

Agent	Target	Disease
African swine fever virus	Pigs	African swine fever
Foot and mouth virus	Livestock	Foot and mouth disease
Puccinia	Wheat, barley, oat	Stem rust
Phytophthora infestans	Potato	Potato blight
Brucella melitensis	Livestock	Brucellosis
Japanese encephalitis virus	Mosquito	Japanese encephalitis
Bacillus anthracis	Livestock	Anthrax

Using Biotechnology against Bioweapons

After 2001 anthrax incidents numerous agencies have worked to develop legislations for minimizing dangers of bioterrorism and responding to possible strikes/attacks.

US government has initiated Project Bioshield to combat biological and chemical terrorism by developing and purchasing substantial amounts of vaccines and drugs to treat or protect people from bioweapons.

However, no measures can guarantee that bioterrorism will never occur or that one can detect as well as protect, against illnesses from such attacks, if they occur. There is, hence, urgent need of worldwide efforts to prevent bioterrorism.

How Biotechnology can help to Detect an Attack

Field tests are essential for detection of an attack. Many tests involve antibody-based tests, *e.g.*, Elisa for determination of pathogen or specific molecules from pathogens present in a water or air sample. However, these instruments are not very sensitive and there is need for development of more sensitive biosensors.

Hand-held protein-based immunoassays and protein microarrays have been developed to detect airborne spores of anthrax and smallpox virus.

Some field based micro-assays can detect whole pathogens or their proteins or spores.

Recent approach is to extract nucleic acid from environmental samples such as soil, water, air, body fluids and tissue samples. PCR is performed with help of broad-based sets of primers specific for different pathogens. PCR can serve as an important tool for tracking the source of a bioterrorism sample of bacteria by comparing similarities and differences in its DNA sequence of over 12 different strains of B. anthracis, genome of one strain has already been sequenced and plans are underway for others.

Battling bioterrorism will require coordinated efforts of scientists, physicians, politicians, and emergency response teams and clean up personnel. Also, countries must build up a stockpile of drugs and vaccines. However, vaccines must be administrated before exposure to bioweapons. If a bioterrorist attack involves organisms that have been engineered against most conventional treatments or if an unknown organism is used as bioweapon. A greater awareness of bioterrorism and implementation of strategies to prevent and defuse bioweapon attacks is need of the hour.

MOLECULAR CYTOGENETICS

Mutations can occur in germline, somatic cells and can be induced or spontaneous in occurrence chromosomal aberrations are major cause of congenital anomalies mental retardation and infertility in humans and chromosomal analysis is the gold standard for the diagnosis and prognosis of these disorders. Also, in tumour genetics conventional single cell and metaphase cytogenetics is essential for monitoring of disease, staging and research purposes for identification of chromosomal regions harbouring tumour suppressor and proto-oncogenes.

Multiple molecular cytogenetic strategies and applications are used to design diagnostic approaches to detect and characterize genetic changes ever the base pair levels.

Conventional Techniques

Karyotyping

Staining of chromosomes at metaphase and detection of numerical and structural chromosomal abnormalities.

Banding techniques to detect chromosomal aberrations.

Detectable chromosomal aberrations

Numerical:

Aneusomies of whole chromosomes:

Trisomy 21, 18, Chromosome constitution 45, X.

Structural:

Inter-chromosomal:	Detection Duplication Inversion
Inter-chromosomal:	
	Balanced and unbalanced Translocation Insertions

Marker Chromosomes

They are structural abnormal chromosomes of which the origin of euchromatic content cannot be determined by conventional cytogenetic analysis alone.

FISH (Fluorescence in Siter Hybridization)

In situ hybridization (ISH) on metaphase spreads or interphase nucleus can analyze genetic changes at single cell level. Molecular cytogenetics is based on fluorescence in situ hybridization skip (FISH). It is a sensitive and specific method (Fig. 7).

Targets for FISH

Routine diagnostics:

Interphase nuclei

Metaphase chromosomes of:

peripheral blood (T-lymphocytes)

primary fibroblasts

bone marrow cells

Prenatal diagnostics:

Amniocytes

Chorionic villi cells.

Non-dividing or archived cells:

Fresh frozen

Paraffin embedded tissue slices

Touch preparations of pathological tissues

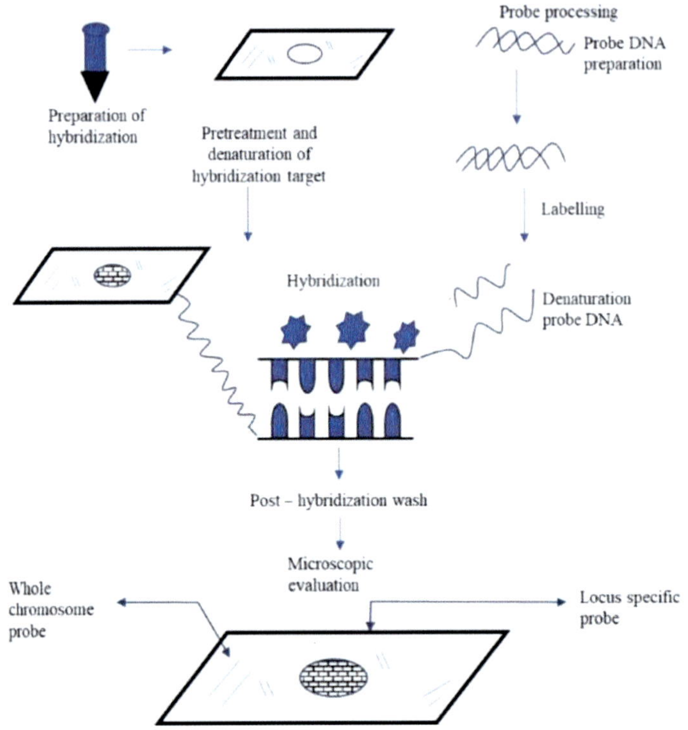

Fig. (7). FISH standard steps.

Preparation of DNA Probes for FISH

Prepared by:

1. Locus-specific PCR amplifying single genes.
2. Cloning of large human DNA fragments by:

Chromosome microdissection

Flow sorting of whole chromosome

3. Also, DNA probes are commercially available.

4. Region or band-specific chromosomal DNA can be cloned in vectors of various sizes (cosmid, plasmid, PI-derived artificial chromosomes PACs bacterial artificial chromosomes BACs or yeast artificial chromosomes YACs

Labelling of Probe

Fluorochrome: conjugated nucleotides:

Fluorescein isothiocyanate

FITC-dUTP

Reporter molecules:

Biotin-dUTP

Digoxygenin (DIG-dUTP)

Labelling Strategies

Based on: Enzymatic in corporation of label—conjugated nucleotides in a newly synthesized strand e.g., amplification degenerated oligonucleotide primer (DOP)

Nick translation

Random priming by hexamer primers

Terminal fluorochrome-labelling reactions for small oligonucleotides (Table **5**).

Table 5. Types of FISH Probes.

Type	**Target**
PCR amplified micro-dissected or chromosomal bands (Micro-FISH)	: chromosome part
PCR products *in situ* (PRINS)	: telomere repeats
PCR primer for specific chromosomal loci, gene	: microdeletions single genes
Locus specific probes* (microdeletion and microduplication)	: sub-microscopic chromosomal loci
Centromere specific α satellite probes*	: centromere
Whole chromosome Probes (WCP)	: whole chromosome

(Table 5) cont.....

Tumour probes*	: Chromosomal loci (Translocation break points) gene amplification
Telomere probes (Q-FISH) *	: telomere repeats

*are commercially available.

Whole Chromosome Painting (WCP) Probes or Painting Probes

These probes are DNA libraries representing a cocktail of DNA fragments or single chromosome (Tables **6**, **7**).

They allow, labelling of individual chromosome in metaphase spreads and their subsequent identification and characterization.

Table 6. Special Probes

Special Probes
Primed in situ labelling PRINS: Centromeric satellite DNA Single-copy FISH probes (SC-FISH): microdeletion and sub-microscopic deletions

Immunotyping of Cells and FISH have been combined to generate MACISH and FICTION approaches

MACISH-Morphology, antibody, chromosomes, in situ hybridization

FICTION: Fluorescence immunophenotyping and interphase cytogenetics

These approaches allow examination of numerical and structural chromosome abnormalities of immunologically classified cells.

Table 7. Multicolour FISH Assays.

Assay	Target	Detect
Cen M-FISH and CM-FISH	Centromere (metaphase)	numerical aberrations
TM-FISH, M-Tel FISH, S-COBRA	Sub-telomeres	cryptic terminal detection, duplication, and translocation
SKY/M-FISH	Whole Chromosome	Inter-chromosomal translocation
Chromosomal bar codes	whole chromosome	Inter- and intra-chromosomal translocation, deletion duplication, inversion
Multicolour banding (MCB)	Whole chromosome	Inter- and intra-chromosomal translocation, deletion duplication, inversion
CGH comparative genomic hybridization	Whole chromosome	Inter- and intra-chromosomal imbalances, gene amplification, marker chromosomes
Matrix-CGH/Array CGH	Spotted defined DNA probes	Inter- and intra-chromosomal imbalances, gene amplification, marker chromosomes

Molecular Karyotyping—Array CGH

It is based on the combination of molecular genetics and cytogenetic techniques to detect complementary nucleic acid sequences in situ on metaphase chromosomes or in the cell nuclei. Automated analysis of genetic imbalances such as small deletions or gene amplifications are available as matrix based CGH array commercially.

Convention and molecular cytogenetic techniques are important for medical diagnostics. Recently whole genome array technology is offering opportunity to investigate whole genome with high resolution in one experiment.

ALLELE- SPECIFIC MUTATION DETECTION

To detect known nucleotide variations in DNA, three PCR-based approaches are used:

1. Amplification refractory mutation system, PCR-ARMs

2. Allele-specific oligonucleotide probes hybridization, PCR-ASO

3. Competitive oligo-priming

PCR-ARMS

PCR-based approach for analysing known point-mutations in DNA and distinguishing between normal hetero- and homozygous mutant genotypes.

It is also referred to as PASA (PCR amplification of specific alleles) and ASPCR (allele-specific PCR). This approach has been applied to analyze known disease mutations associated with α1- antitrypsin deficiency, amyloidotic polyneuropathy, phenylketonuria sickle cell disease. Also, this strategy is applicable to analysis of any known point mutation or SNP.

Principle:

A mismatch between 3′ nucleotide of a PCR primer and the template reduces or prevents primer extension by Taq polymerase.

Taq DNA polymerase lacks 3′ to 5′ exonuclease activity and cannot correct mismatches at 3′terminus of primer. Complementary base pairing at 3′ and of primer is required for efficient amplification by Taq polymerase. Normal allele will be amplified and mutant being having a mismatch with 3′ residue is not amplified. Conversely, mutant will be amplified of 3′ residue of primer is complementary to mutant allele and not normal allele. This specificity of 3′ terminal can be further enhanced by incorporating an additional mismatch near 3′ end (Fig. **8**).

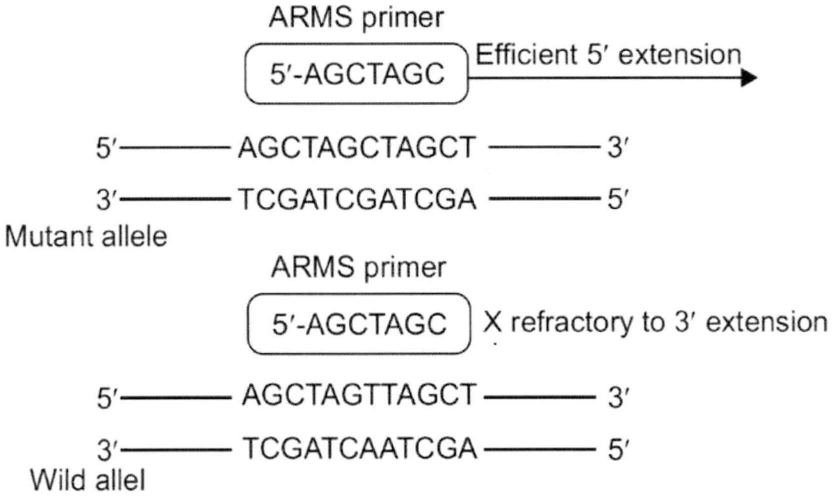

Fig. (8). PCR-ARMS.

Application of PCR-ARMS

1. PCR-ARMS is applied commonly for detection of individual point mutation.
2. To determine genotypes for individual mutations or SNPs.

To establish haplotypes of individuals in absence of samples from relatives.

Types of PCR-ARMS

1. Single—detects single mutation.

2. Multiplex—can detect upto 4 to 6 different mutations in single-tube detection, e.g., Senith- Lemli-Opitz syndrome has—DHCRT gene mutations.

Advantage of PCR-ARMS Assays

- PCR-ARMS assays are ideally suited for molecular diagnostic applications requiring detection of small numbers of mutations.
- Easy to develop validate and implement multiplex assays.
- Non-radioactive
- Does not require expensive and sophisticated detection system.

Limitation of PCR-ARMS Assays

- Can be used to detect only point mutations and polymorphism.
- Impractical to apply it other diagnostic strategies such as sequencing.

PCR-ASO

(ASO: Allele-specific oligonucleotide probes). It is based on the principle that even single nucleotide mismatches between a probe and its target destabilizes the hybrid. ASO probes are used to detect any known mutation or SNP within amplified DNA fragment.

ASO Primer Selection

- Involve considerable amount of trial- and error testing of candidate probes.

- Several versions of a given probe are synthesized to attain allele specificity under the assay conditions

ASO Probe

- Short nucleotide (–15 to 17-mers).

- Have 30–50% G + C content.

- Designed with discriminating nucleotide located near the middle probe.

Types of ASO Formats

1. Forward
2. Reverse

Forward ASO Format

PCR-amplified DNA fragments are immobilized onto a nylon membrane which is then hybridized specific, complementary to a labelled oligonucleotide probe. On wishing, imperfect matches to target are washed off. Then, oligonucleotide probes (phosphorylated at 5′ end with γ–32 P) or biotinylated at 5′ end) are subjected to detection of probe-target hybrids (X-ray or streptavidin) conjugated with horse radish peroxidase, HRP (detected spectrophotometrically with tetramethyl benzidine and hydrogen peroxide or Chemiluminescence)].

Draw Back

Cumbersome because it requires separate labelled probes and hybridization cycles for each allele.

Reverse ASO Format

It has immobilised array of ASO probes to a membrane strip and its hybridization to PCR-amplified DNA. In earlier version, poly (dT)tails were added to 3′ termini and immobilized on nylon membrane. Nowadays, 5′ amino linkers are covalently bound to ASO probes. Reverse ASO formats are widely used tools for routine screening of numerous mutant alleles and kits for mutant screening of several genetic diseases, namely, thalassemia (both α, β), cystic fibrosis and genotyping SNPs for foremost identity testing.

Advantage PCR ASO (Reverse)

Simple approach

Non-radioactive

Does not require specialization treatments.

Drawback PCR-ASO (Reverse)

Costly and time-consuming to identify and develop panel of oligonucleotide probes.

Competitive Oligo-Priming Assay (COP)

COP is used to detect known sequence variations, based on allele-specific amplification using ASO (Table **8**).

Table 8. COMPARISON.

Allele-specific amplification	**Vs.**	**COP**
• Mismatching between primer and template DNA prevents extension of DNA synthesis		• Mismatching prevents primer annealing
		• Uses three primers
• Uses two primer		• It is system of allele-specific amplification through differential primer annealing.

Three primers of DNA synthesis in one PCR are used for differential primer annealing in COP:

Forward primer: a pair of competitive oligonucleotides-carry mutant or normal configuration at mutation site in the middle of their sequence

Third primer: common reverse primer for respective PCR

Mismatches can be formed within forward primmer, usually in the middle and at 3′ end of forward primer in some cases.

Use of Forward Primer

To detect DNA sequence alterations in COP

Stages of COP

1. Ist stage: DNA amplification by COP

2. Second stage: Detection of genetic identity—mutant versus normal—of the amplified material

Advantage COP

- Easy
- No need of heavy equipment or complex procedure

- Cost-effective: most labels are commercially available in routine
- Mutation detection system can be used almost anywhere
- Possibility of multiplexing: primer competition for correct annealing to DNA is possible and detection of several mutations in one tube or one PCR run.

Disadvantage COP

- Difficulty in differentiating equal size DNA molecules produced in one PCR.
- Long and laborious optimization procedure is required to specific exact conditions for each mutation, namely, elimination of misprinting, improper differential detection of PCR products that may interfere with interpretation of results.
- Allele-specific mutation detection is feasible using PCR-ARMS, PCR-ASO and COP assays that have high degree of accuracy and specificity. Potential of COP has not been fully exploited.

MUTATION DATABASE

Advances in technology have led to identification of numerous mutations in genes ranging from point mutations to large rearrangements.

Genetic or Mutation Databases

Genetic or Mutation Databases are online repositories of mutation data, described for single (locus specific) or more (general) genes or for a specific population or ethnic groups (national/ethnic).

Applications of Mutation Database

- To facilitate diagnosis at DNA level
- To define optimal strategy for mutation detection
- To provide information about mutation specific phenotypic patterns
- To correlate locus-specific variant information with genome-wide features: repetitive elements, gene structure, interspecies conservation, mutation hot spots, recombinant frequency, *etc.*

Mutation Resource on Net

OMIM

Online Mendelian Inheritance in Man is a database of mutations that is updated on daily basis. Hugo-MDI

Human Genome Organization-Mutation Database Initiative

HGMD

Human Gene Mutation Database

(a general mutation database (MD))

www.hgmd.ord

HbVar Database

Haemoglobin variants and thalassemia mutations database

(a locus-specific database, (LSDB))

www.hgmd.org, www.hgvs.org

NEMDB databases

National/Ethnic Mutation Database

Other DNA Variation Databases

dbSNP www.ncbi_nlm.nih.gov/projects/SNP

HAPMAP Data Coordination Center www.hapmap.org

Human Genome Variation Database HGVD www.hgvbase.org

NEMDBs

NEMDBs record extensive information of an ethnic group or population.

National Genetic Database and National Mutation Frequency databases are available that give comprehensive information of inherited disorders whose disease-causing mutation spectrum is defined.

FINDbase: Frequency of Inherited Disorders database records frequencies of causative mutations and pharmacogenetic markers worldwide NEMDBs can be helpful in molecular diagnostic testing by providing reference information for development of customized genetic tests for various populations/ethnic groups.

GEN2PHEN *(www.gen2phen.org)*

It is proposed integrating project of 19 academic and corporate entities to unify human genetic variation databases to genotype-to phenotype (G2P) data and link it to other biomedical knowledge sources *via* genome browser.

To conclude, biomedical community must first appreciate overwhelming need for improved genetic/mutation database systems and solutions will then presumably follow!

ANALYSIS OF HUMAN SPLICING DEFECTS

Identification of DNA variations that cause aberrant splicing is not as simple. Variations in splicing regulatory elements in coding and non-coding regions may result in unexpected deleterious effect on pre-mRNA splicing. Thus, differentiation between benign and disease-causing sequence substitutions and identification of nature of regulatory elements of splicing are challenging for medical geneticists.

Splicing Process

Pre-mRNA splicing is a fundamental process is gene expression and generation of proteome diversity. In nucleus, splicing process acts on precursor (pre-)mRNA, recognizes protein coding exonic sequences and joins them together to form nature mRNA. The nature mRNA gets transported Fig. (**9**) to cytoplasm and translated into protein.

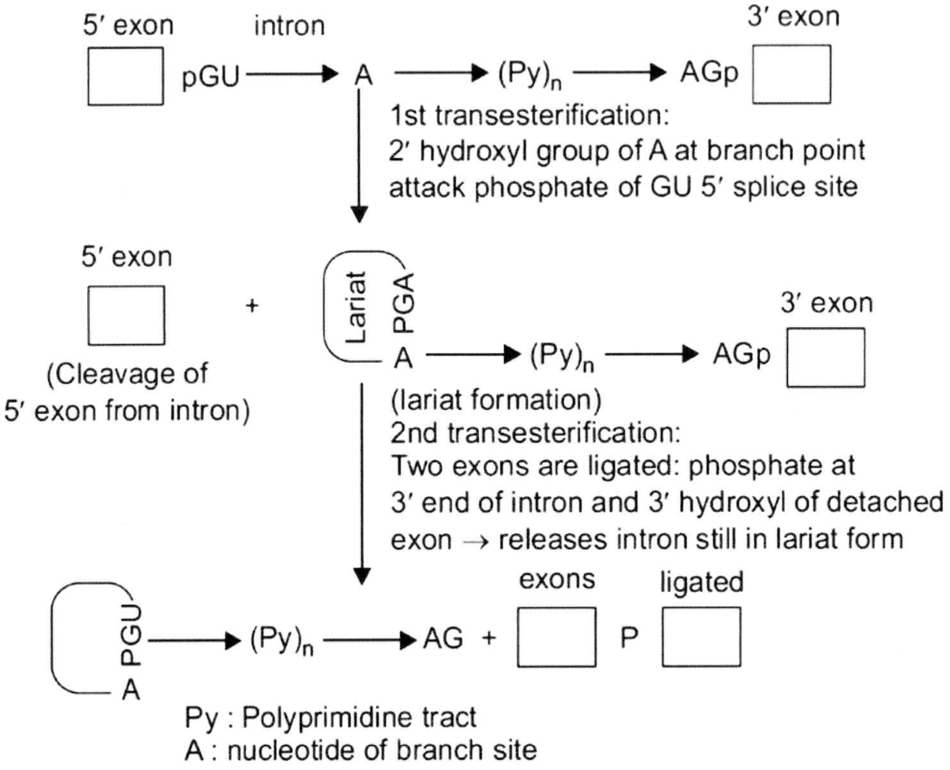

Fig. (9). Splicing process.

5′ splice site marks the exon/intron junction at 5′ end on intron and hallmark is GU dinucleotide. 3′ exon end of splice site region has 3 conserved elements: branch site, the polypyrimidine tracts, terminal AG. The process of splicing consists of two transesterification steps.

Alternative Usage of Different Splice Sites

- It is a common event in human cells.
- Majority of exons are constitutive, *i.e.*, they are always included in final mRNA
- It may occur in different manners:

a. usage of alternative splice sites

b. mutually exclusive exons

c. exon skipping/inclusion

d. intron retention

- It results in production of multiple isoforms from same transcription units
- It is responsible for complexity of proteome 59% of human genes generate multiple mRNA that is responsible for law unexpected number of genes found in human genome
- Alternative spliced transcript has a restricted developmental and/or cell-type regulations
- They respond to a variety of external stimuli.

Elements Regulating Splicing

Correct splice site needs to be differentiated from abundant pseudo-splice site. Also, cis-acting elements (enhancers or silencers) on pre-RNA (assist splicesome in selection of splice sites) are required for fine-tuning regulation of alternative splicing process.

Enhances and silencers can be located either directly in exons (ESE and ESS) and they overlap with selection of amino acid sequence and codon usage. In introns, enhancers and silencers (ISE and ISS) are located at a very long distance from splice site.

Splicing can be constitutive or alternative and lack a well-defined consensus sequence. Enhancers and silencers are involved in both types of splicing are not equivocally defined and their functions may overlap.

Trans-acting splicing factors can interact with enhancers and silencers. They belong to two groups: numbers of serine/arginine-rich (SR) proteins and heterogenous nuclear ribonucleoproteins (hnRNPs). SR protein bind at ESE and facilitate exon recognition and hnRNP are inhibitory. RNA binding proteins have one or more RNA-binding domains are involved in protein-protein interactions.

Human Gene Defects Due to PRE-mRNA Splicing

Distinguishing between benign polymorphisms and disease-causing variations is a difficult task. Identification of disease-causing mutations is based primarily on linkage of the mutation with disease phenotype and effect of mutation on gene expression Fig. (**10**).

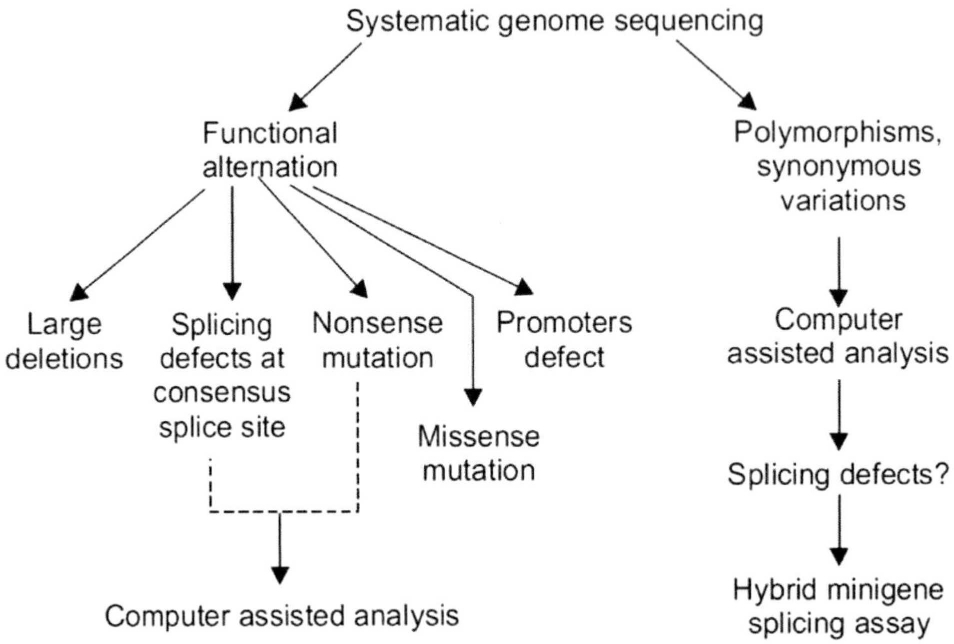

Fig. (10). Strategies to detect mRNA splicing alterations.

Prediction of Sequence Variations

Easy to Predict.

- Large deletions
- Nucleotide changes at consensus GU/AG splice sites
- Exonic variations that produce: stop codons, radical amino acid changes
- Promoters variations

Difficult to Predict

- Variation in nucleotides flanking GU/AG dinucleotides
- *Computer-based approaches: Fact file*

- Can identify:
- Splicing regulatory elements on consensus sequences
- SNP disrupt
- Cannot identify: degenerated splicing regulatory elements

The best way to establish which DNA substitution affects splicing is by direct analysis of processed transcript. However, sample is not available for some tissue-specific expressed gene, e.g., brain- or heart-specific genes, then hybrid minigene assay is of help.

Minigene Assay

Any genomic region of interest suspected of causing a splicing defect can be amplified from normal and affected individuals and cloned into minigene which on transfection followed by transcription and post mRNA processing result in mature mRNA Fig. (**11**).

Interpretation of Gel

WT multigene shows correct inclusion of exon

Mut 1 shows an aberrant spliced form

Mut 2 causes significant exon skipping:

- Co-transfection with positive regulatory splicing factor
- siRNA mediated inhibition of negative splicing factor induces exon inclusion restoring normal splicing.

The mRNA splicing pattern is analyzed by RT-PCR with primers for processed minigene transcripts.

siRNA—mediated silencing of splicing factor is a powerful approach for identification of transacting splicing factor. In vitro splicing assay using labelled preformed RNA molecules incubated in nuclear extracts to produce spliced product (lariat) that can be evaluated.

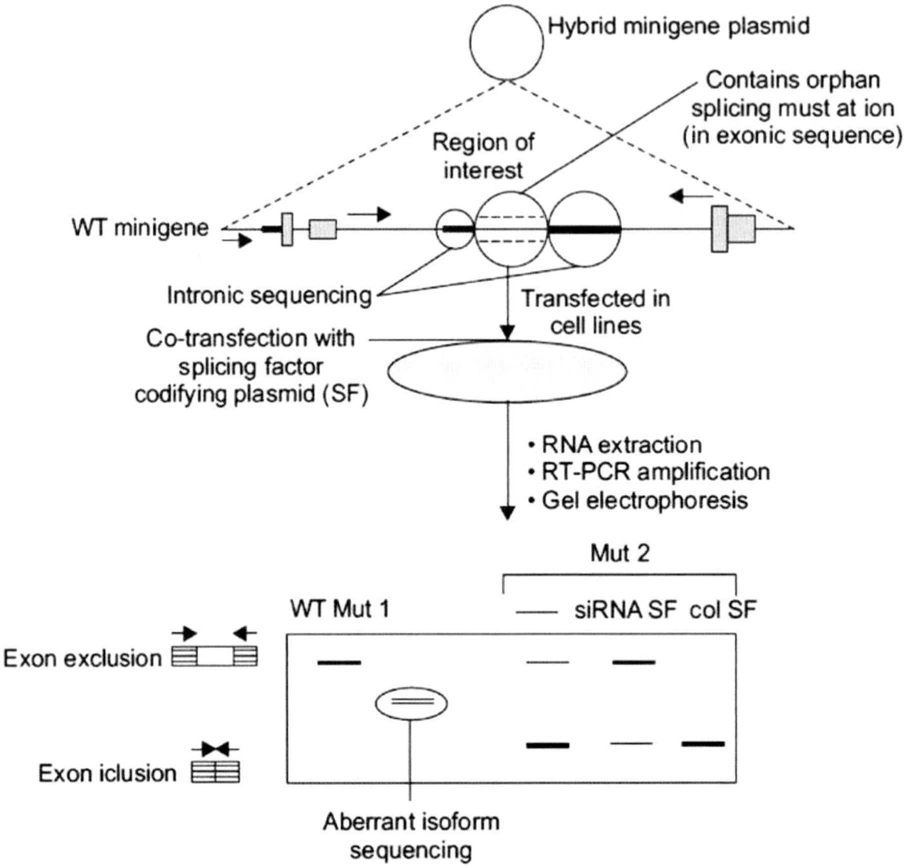

Fig. (11). Hybrid minigene splicing assay.

Applications Hybrid Minigene Assay

1. 3′ splice site variations: cystic fibrosis (Box **1**): CFTR: aberrant exon 9 skipping
2. Nucleotide substitution in exonic regulatory elements involving splicing: missense and silent mutation:

(i) CF: exon 12 skipping: D5656 and G576A missense mutations. Nonsense mutation: introduction of stop codon in

(ii) Neurofibromatosis type 1 (NF1): exon 37,

(iii) SMN2 (spinal muscular atrophy): survival motor neuron 1(SMN1) gene is duplicated, and its homologous copy is

3. Variations at 5′ splice site:

- Variation near AG/GU are not easy to evaluate
- NF1: exon 3 + 5 G > C substitution causing aberrant skipping of exon 3

4. Deep intronic mutations:

Ataxia telangiectasia (ATM) gene: intron splicing processing element defect (15 PE) infecting intronic element: Box **1**,-**3**.

Box 1: CFTR intron 8/exon 9 junction:
• Contain variable number of UG repeats (9–13) followed by U repeat (U5, U7, U9) in normal population
• US allele associated with alternative splicing of CFTR exon 9
• Exon 9 encodes part of functionally important first nucleotide binding domain and its skipping produces a man-functional CFTR protein
• UG 13 U_3 allele found in classical CF.

Box 2: NF1
• NF1 autosomal dominant single gene disorder 17 Q 11.2 chromosome NF1 gene is tumor suppress or gene contain 60 exons.
• NF1 gene transcribes several mRNAs (11–13 kb).
• Neurofibromin (2818 amino acid is most common transcript and 50% of mutations result in aberrant splicing stop codon introduced in exon 37

Box 3: SMN
• SMN2 differ from SMN1 by five nucleotides which can be intronic or exonic and are translationally silent.
• Silent C > T substitution in exon 7 causes in ability to compensate for SMN1 defect in the patients.

Mapping Intronic Splicing Regulatory Elements

Identification of a particular disease gene involving gene splicing regulatory elements and evolution of their contribution in aberrant splicing events can be done by hybrid minigenes along with insertion of ribozymes to break off nascent transcript.

In diagnostic field, hybrid minigene assay can be used to distinguish between benign polymorphisms from disease-associated splicing mutations.

DETECTION OF GENOMIC DUPLICATIONS AND DELETIONS

Gene and chromosome duplications being the fundamental evolutionary mechanisms, are associated with a direct change in gene dosage.

Pathological Consequences

Supernumerary chromosomes:

- Turner
- Trisomy 21 (Down syndrome)
- Trisomy X
- Klinefelter syndrome (XXY)
- *Microdeletions:*
- Di George syndrome
- Criduchat syndrome
- *Subtelomeric deletions:*
- Mental retardation
- *Gene deletions or duplications:*
- cancers
- Duchnne-muscular dystrophy
- Spinal muscular atrophy
- Chariot-Marie-Tooth disease
- Fanconi anaemia
- Congenital adrenal hyperplasia

Diagnostic Techniques

For identifying supernumerary chromosomes and large deletions, classical cytogenetic techniques are used. FISH, single copy probes allow detection of microdeletions (Table **9**).

Table 9. Diagnostic Techniques.

Technique	**Detected**
Southern Blot	Deletion, Duplication
Microsatellites	Supernumerary chromosome large deletion or duplication
Multiplex quantitative fluorescent PCR (QFPCR)	Trinucleotide repeat markers in aneuploidy
SNP array	Allele imbalance or loss of heterozygosity of SNPs caused by deletions in tumour cells
PCR	Measurement of gene dosage • large gene and chromosome rearrangements
MAPH (Multiple amplifiable probe hybridization)	Copy number measurement
MLPA (multiplex ligatable probe (amplification)	Detection of aneuploidy, unbalanced cryptic translocations whole or partial gene duplications or deletions.
Long range PCR	Full characterization of duplication or deletion
Array-based CGH	Gene duplications and deletions

Human Genome Variation Society has taken responsibility of establishing a standard mutation nomenclature that includes:

- deletions and
- duplications

(www.hgvs.org)

Gene Dosage Applications in Tumour Profiling

Loss of heterozygosity LOH (due to partial chromosomal loses) occur in a large number of tumour types. LOH analysis of polymorphic microsatellite markers are sued for detection differential diagnosis and typing of tumours.

MLPA: Detection of DNA/mRNA copy number of methylation changes

MLPA (multiplex ligation dependent probe amplification is a PCR-based technique to detect copy number changes in DNA or RNA. MLPA can amplify upto 50 nucleic acid sequences in one cycle with a resolution down to single nucleotide level. MLPA is now routinely used in molecular cytogenetics and often replaces FISH. Since it can detect upto 50–70 mt.

Aberrations disrupting single genes are too small to be detected by FISH. MLPA is cheaper and technically simple as compared to CGH Box **5**, **6**.

Box 5. Routine MLPA
Routine MLPA
Her 2-neu (ERBB2) testing in breast tumor

Box 6. Methylation of MLPA
Methylation specific MLPA analyzes aberrant methylation of CPG is London tumour samples.

Use of MLPA

- Analysis of complicate genomic areas:

CYP21A2/CAH region SMN1/S MN2 genes

- Detection of copy-number changes in well-microdeletion syndromes of Subtelomeric regions, centromeric region in one reaction.

- Tumour diagnostic
- Pharmacogenetics
- Detection and subtyping of microorganisms

MS-MLPA

Methylation specific MLPA detects changes in cytosine methylation in specific genomic areas. It can detect aberrant methylation of imprinting regions, CpG islands near tumour suppression genes. It can quantify copy number and methylation upto 50 different sequence per reaction, however, its sensitivity is low Fig. (**12**).

Detection Methods for MLPA

Capillary electrophoresis

Microfluidics

Bead arrays

Microarrays

MOLECULAR TECHNIQUES FOR DNA METHYLATION STUDIES

DNA methylation is the best studied epigenetic biomarker and has a great potential as diagnostic and predictive tool therapeutic target.

DNA Methylation and Disease

DNA methylation and chromatin structure are strikingly altered in many pathological situations such as cancer and a number of genetic variations associated with disease susceptibility have been identified. Aberrant methylation patterns have been identified in neuro developmental disorders, autoimmune disease. In cancers a global loss of DNA methylation of genome occurs that can initiate and propagate oncogenesis *via* chromosomal instabilities and transcriptional activation of oncogenes and metastatic gene. Hypermethylation of CpG is binds occurs in promotor region of tumor suppressor or cancer related. gene is associated with transcriptional silencing of associated gene. Also, genes of pathways involved in single transduction, DNA repair, detoxification cell cycle regulation, differentiation, angiogenesis, apoptosis, are inactivated by DNA methylation.

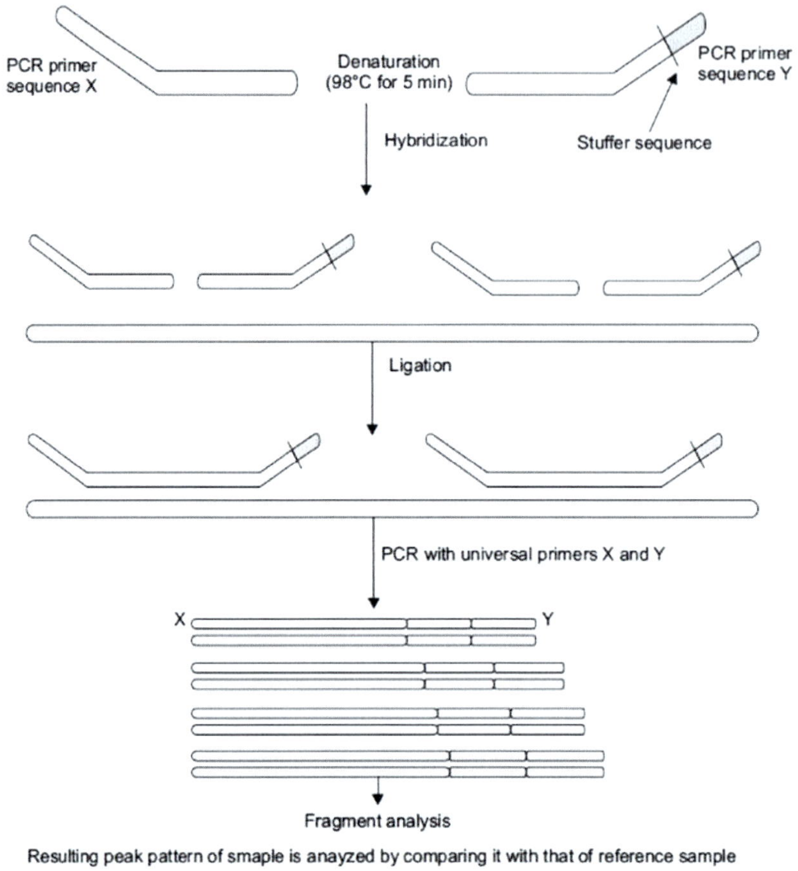

Fig. (12). Outline of MLPA technique.

Both hypo- and hypermethylation are found in the same tumour, but the mechanism is not known.

Methods for DNA Methylation Analysis

- Digestion/hydrolysis to mono nucleoside
- Chemical derivatization
- Methyl transferase assay
- Solid-phase primer extension
- Cytosine extension assay

- Luminometric methylation assay
- Immunological detection
- Self-primed-in-situ labelling (SPRINS)

DNA methylation analysis will play a key role in diagnosis, prognosis and treatment of various diseases. Predictive epigenetic biomarkers will allow a personalized treatment of disease based on the individual methylation profile.

PHARMACOGENETICS, PHARMACOGENOMICS, AND NUTRIGENOMICS

Pharmacogenetics

This term was coined by Vogel in 1959 to describe inheritance of an aberrant drug metabolism.

Pharmacogenetics has been defined as variation in drug response as it relates to an individual's genetic makeup.

Pharmacogenomics

It refers to a broader use of genome-wide association, studies (GWAS) and potential complex interactions as well as alteration in gene expression that correlates to drug response.

Analytical Methods in Pharmacogenetics

1. Candidate gene approach: SNPs are correlated to phenotype Fig. (**13**)
2. Candidate pathway-based studies: Several genes are investigated with respect to pharmacology of a specific drug, disease, or biological pathway for variations that may contribute to phenotypic differences
3. GWAS: Thousands of SNPs are spaced throughout the genome.

Candidate gene approach narrows focus to a few important genes/SNPs and therefore has higher power (Table **10**).

Pharmacokinetic Effect are due to

Interindividual differences in absorption distribution, metabolism, or excretion of drug. Pharmacokinetic genes are targets for pharmacogenetic research.

Pharmacodynamic effects my lead to interindividual difference in a drug's effect despite the presence of appropriate concentration of active drug at site of action (Table **11**).

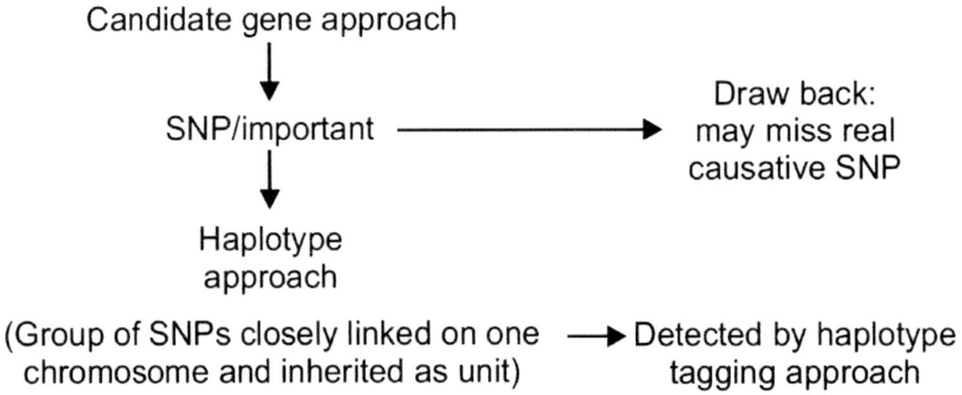

Fig. (13). Candidate gene approach.

Table 10. Enzymes of pharmacogenetic relevance to drug therapy:

Enzyme	Drug
(a) Phase 1 Enzymes:	
Aldehyde dehydrogenase	Acetaldehyde
Alcohol dehydrogenase	Ethanol
CYP1A2	Caffeine
CYP2A6	Nicotine Coumarin

(Table 10) cont.....

Cyp2C9	Phenytoin Glipizide Fluvastatin Tolbutamide Warfarin
CYP2C19	Amitriptyline Imipramine Mephenytoin Omeprazole
CYP2D6	Clomiphene Tamoxifen
CYP2E1	Caffeine
CYP3A4	Erythromycin
CYP3A5	Tacrolimus
Cholinesterase	Benzoylcholine Butyrylcholine
Paraoxonase	Paraoxon
(b) Phase II enzymes	
Acetyltransferase	INH Dapsone Procainamide

(Table 10) cont.....

	Sulfamethazine
Dihydropyrimidine dehydrogenase	Uraols
Thiomethyl transferase	2-mercapto ethanol captopril
UDP-glucuronsyl transferase	Bilirubin

Table 11. Pharmacodynamic genes that effect drug response.

Gene	**Drug/disease**
ApoE2	LDL-C
ACE	ACE inhibitors (hypertension)
β-adrenergic receptor	Beta blockers (hypertension)
CRH	Antidepressant
Dopamine receptor	Depression (inhibit serotonin uptake)
EGFR	Gefitinib Cetuximab Cancer
ER-α	Bone mineral density
FCGR3A	Infliximab (Crohn's disease)
HMG CoA reductase	Statins
5-Lipoxygenase	Monteleukast (asthma)
NEF3	Response to antipsychotics

(Table 11) cont.....

Serotonin receptor	Depression (inhibit serotonin uptake)
TNF	Anti-TNF (Crohn's, rheumatoid arthritis)
VK0RC1	Warfarin (anticoagulant)

Ethical Implications

Most important ethical issues are privacy and confidentiality of genetic information of patient. For routine clinical decision-making, most pharmacogenetic tests are used, *e.g.*, CYP2D6 SNP testing), genetic tests to predict disease susceptibility may have an impact on patient's life, family or third-party interests. GINA (Genetic Information Non-discrimination Act) is bill regarding discrimination and genetic testing to prohibit discrimination on basis of genetic information with respect to health insurance and employment.

Issue of secondary information garnered as a consequence of pharmacogenetic testing is also a matter of concern.

Nutrigenomics

(Sometimes called nutritional genomics)

Nutrigenomics is interactions between foods or dietary supplements and an individual's genome and consequent downstream effects on their phenotype.

Analytical Techniques for Nutrigenomics

SNP genotyping	:	RFLP, Sequencing, arrays
Copy-number variants	:	CGH array, PCR-based methods, MLPA

Human Clinical Trials

Clinical trials are ultimate proof that a nutritional Fig. (**14**) intervention is beneficial to health utilizing genomically based diagnostic techniques.

Study Population

↓

Stratify by genotype

↓

Randomize to control or experiment diet

↓

Monitor biomarkers

↓

Clinical expression of disease

Fig. (14). Study design for human trial of foods.

For nutrigenomic studies, data management, biostatistics and bioinformatics need to be developed accordingly so that microarray and proteomics data on gene expression and identified affected genes are extrapolated to giving information on human health or disease.

PREIMPLANTATION GENETIC DIAGNOSIS AND PRENATAL DIAGNOSIS

Preimplantation Genetic Diagnosis (PGD)

Preimplantation embryos are obtained in vitro and genetically analyzed for genetic defect if any before transferring.

Indications for PGD

- To detect

(i) Monogenic diseases:

- Cystic fibrosis

- Spinal muscular atrophy
- Sickle cell disease
- β-thalassemia
- Huntington's disease
- Marfan's disease
- Duchenne's muscular dystrophy
- Hemophilia A and B
- Retinitis pigmentosa

(ii) Chromosomal aberrations:

- Reciprocal translocation and
- Robertsonian translocation:
- Mental retardation
- Recurrent miscarriage
- Infertility

(iii) Aneuploidy:

- Monosomy
- Trisomy
- Triploidy

Techniques for PGD:

i. *ART* (Assisted reproduction technology)

- By controlled ovarian hyperstimulation, a large cohort of mature oocytes are obtained in regular IVF.
- Intracytoplasmic sperm injection (ICSI) is preferred over IVF. After 16 hours in culture, normal fertilization can be observed if two pronuclei and two polar bodies are present.

ii. *Biopsy*

- *Polar body biopsy:* FISH analysis for translocations (1st polar body extruded at metaphase II and second polar body extruded after normal fertilization, thus can be retrieved for analysis).
- *Cleavage stage biopsy:* FISH analysis PCR amplification (one or two blastomeres are biopsied on day 3 at 8-cell stage through ZP, zona pellucida).
- *Blastocyst biopsy:* Trophectoderm (TE) biopsy on emerging approach. (opening in ZP by laser on day 3 or 4 opposite ICM to allow TE to herniate TE cells are aspirated by biopsy papilla)

PGD for Monogenic Disease Techniques

Single cell PCR

Allele drop-out (ADO) and preferential amplification

Whole genome amplification

Single cell cytogenetics: FISH

CGH

PGD is still labour intensive and time-consuming, and introduction of newer technologies has made it safer and more reliable (Table **12**).

Prenatal Diagnosis

Table 12. Standard techniques.

Technique	**Disorder**
Non-invasive	
Maternal serum screening	

(Table 12) cont.....

α-fetoprotein (αFB)	Neural tube defect
Triple test	Down syndrome
Ultrasound	Structural abnormality
Invasive	
Amniocentesis	
Fluid	
Cells	Neural tube defects chromosomal abnormalities molecular defects metabolic disorders
Chorionic villus sample	Chromosomal abnormality metabolic disorders molecular or defects
Teratoscopy blood	Chromosomal abnormality haematological disorders congenital infection
Liver	Metabolic disorder
Skin	Hereditary skin disorders.

Indications for Prenatal Diagnosis

- Advanced maternal age
- Previous child with chromosomal abnormality
- Family history of chromosomal abnormality
- Family history of a single gene disorder, neural tube defect, other congenital abnormalities.

- Abnormalities identified during pregnancy
- Other high risk factors: parental consanguinity, history of unexplained three or more miscarriages maternal illness.
- Poorly controlled diabetes, evaporate medication

Assisted Conception and Implications for Genetic Disease

IVF

Due to defective genetic imprinting, dysmorphic syndromes: Beckwith Wiedemann syndrome can occur.

ICSI

Intracytoplasmic sperm injection can result in chromosomal abnormalities or rearrangements, heritable chromosomal abnormalities from men.

Donor insemination (DI)

There is risk of transmitting chromosome disorders from donors and increasing risk of new germline mutations.

Assisted Conception that Require Licencing

In vitro fertilization

Intracytoplasmic sperm injection

Sperm donation

Preimplantation genetic diagnosis

Egg donation

Embryo donation

Surrogacy

Fetal Cells in Maternal Circulation

Non-invasive means of prenatal diagnosis for chromosome and DNA abnormalities are also available antibodies specific to fetal trophoblast, use of PCR to detect paternally derived DNA marks in maternal blood can be analyzed. Prediction of rhesus status, nucleated RBCs of fetal origin can be analyzed for prenatal diagnosis

Prenatal Treatment

Prenatal diagnosis and screening for abnormalities during pregnancy has led to the possibility of treatment in vitro. In congenital adrenal hyperplasic (CAH) a possible mode for successful model for prenatal treatment after diagnosing by giving dexamethasone.

Also, gene therapy is promising treatment.

NEXT GENERATION DNA SEQUENCING TECHNIQUES

Starting from Sanger enzymatic sequencing and Maxam and Gilbert chemical degradation, fascinating opportunities are available for next-generation DNA sequencing!

Techniques Developed for Sequencing Human Genome in HGP

Capillary array DNA sequencer (Japan) Automated sequencing by Venter (ABI and Amersham, USA)

Next-Generation DNA Sequencing Platforms

They provide high sequencing speed and throughput (Table **13**), and sequence data can be determined from amplified single DNA fragment. Also, they offer novel and rapid ways for genome-wide characterization (upto 1 Gb/run) and analysis of profiles of mRNAs, small RNAs, transcription factor binding sites, genetic variations, chromatin structure and DNA methylation patterns, microbiology, and metagenomics

Table 13. Next-Generation DNA Sequencing Platforms.

Platform	Principle
Illumina-Solexa genome analyzer	Sequencing-by-synthesis chemistry with fluorescent dye labelled reversible terminator nucleotide 1.5 Gb data/run, 750 Mb/day
ABI Solid system (Sequencing by Oligo ligation and detection)	Unique sequencing chemistry based on ligation and catalysed by DNA ligase 3–10 Gb/run
Gs454 Life Science	Sequencing by-synthesis in open wells of a fibreoptic slide using pyrosequencing protocol. (1.6 million wells).
Helicos single-molecule sequencing device: Helioscope	Single molecule-chemistry: DNA sequencing without PCR (or amplification) from a single DNA molecule by hybridizing to primers anchored on solid surface (of glass coverslip) in a flow cell and polymerase enzyme is added. Next base incorporated in synthesized DNA detected by photon detection systems.

Techniques under Development

Single-molecule DNA sequence determination of sequencing without need for cloning is a very promising approach. It uses “Realtime sensor” DNA polymerase with acceptor fluorescent dye and four donor fluorescent dyes for four nucleotides close to active site. When correct nucleotide is found, selected and entered in active site of enzyme, donor dye label in polymerase comes into very close proximity with acceptor dye label on nucleotides for integration in growing DNA chain during synthesis) energy is transferred from donor to acceptor dye to generate FRET (fluorescent Resonance Energy Transfer) light signal.

Use of real-time single-molecule nano-sequencing technology will enable researchers to sequence entire human genome in less than a day for under $1000 by 2011 (VISI Gen Biotechnologies) with speed of 50 to Mb/second.

Pacific Bioscience is working on next-generation DNA sequencing instrument at speed of 100 Gb/hour or diploid human genome in 4 minutes.

Single-molecule real-time (SMRT) technology of Roche, Illumina, Applied Biosystems will be based on zero mode wave guides (ZMWs) of nanoscale holes in 100 nanometre metal film.

Use of artificial nanopores for rapid DNA sequencing, lithographically fabricated nanogap for DNA molecule translocation are also under process for faster and cheaper platforms for sequencing.

Bionanomatrix and complete Genomics are developing technology to sequence human genome in eight hours for $100 by using sequencing chemistry and nanofluidic technology

1,000- Genomes Project

Researchers are preparing a concrete plan for a project to sequence 1,000 human genomes, that will allow creation of a reference standard for analysis of human genomic variations. Illumina, Roche 454 Life Sciences and Applied Biosystems decided to help with the project. This project will identify variants present at a frequency of 1% over most of the genomes and as low as 0.5% within genes. Similar genome wide analysis is planned for stem-cell-lines.

RNA Sequencing

Next generation sequencing may be applied to characteristics of mRNA, methylated DNA, DNA, or RNA regions bound by certain proteins and other DA or RNA regions taking part in gene expression and regulation.

Sage: Serial analysis of gene expression technique concept is used by next-generation technology to analyze RNA transcripts in a biological system by obtaining short sequence tags 20–35 bp long from each transcript in the sample. Using computer informatics sequence tags allow location of each of them to be determined and mapped in reference genome.

This technique has been applied by Cloonam on transcriptome profiling in stem cells.

RNA-SEQ Technique

It provides insights into alternative splicing patterns of human genome by sequencing CDNA derived from RNA to map and compare transcriptomes in two different human cell types.

CHIP-SEQ

Sequencing of chromatin immuno precipitated fragments to identify and localize DNA sites with which DNA binding proteins can interact and bind. There is also a microarray-based method termed ChIP-on-Chip technique.

Future DNA Sequencing Techniques and Medicine

The availability of ultra-deep sequencing of human genomic DNA will transform the medical field in future in terms of diagnosis and drug development.

Also, this technology will be useful in microbial genomics.

Human Microbiome Project

(also termed Second Human Genome Project)

This has been proposed to study collections of microbomes in and on the human body that will be one of the factors in understanding human health and disease. Changes in microbial communities in body have been link to immune system, obesity and cancer. Human body contains ten times as many bacterial cells as human cells (*i.e.*, 1,000 bacterial gene for every human gene). Understanding of human microbiome antibiotics may lead to development of pro- and pre-biotic approaches for maintaining human health. Each person's microbiome will become his/her medical biometric in future!

To conclude, efforts to find a cost-effective and rapid technique for whole genome sequencing along with miniaturization are going on.

SINGLE CELL BIOPSY

Single-Cell Analysis

Single-cell analysis has entered the multiomics age (single-cell multiomics field) with evolution of rapidly growing collection of software tools.

Single-cell analysis is study of genomics, transcriptomics, proteomics, metabolomics and cell–cell interactions at the level of single cell. Using fluorescence-activated cell sorting (FACS) for precise isolation of selected single cells from complex samples, and high throughput single cell partitioning technologies, analysis of genome and transcriptome of single cells and quantification of their proteome and metabolome is possible. For proteomic and metabolomic analysis of single cells, Mass spectrometry techniques are used.

With transformative new methods to profile genetic, epigenetic, spatial, proteomic and lineage information in individual cells, along with single-cell RNA sequencing *technologies, Integrative single-cell analysis has become feasible.*

Single-Cell Isolation

Dielectrophoretic digital sorting, enzymatic digestion, FACS, hydrodynamic traps, laser capture microdissection, manual picking, microfluidics, micromanipulation, serial dilution, and Raman tweezers are used for this.

Microfluidics allows for the isolation of individual cells for further analyses.

SINGLE CELL MANIPULATION TECHNIQUES

They have long been studied and is currently a critical method in the fields of biosensing, biorobotics, single cell screening and analysis as well as cell-level therapies

Single Cell Sequencing

Single cell sequencing uses optimized next-generation sequencing (NGS) technologies to examine sequence information from individual cancer cells for example to provide a higher resolution of cellular differences and a better understanding of the function of an individual cell in the context of its microenvironment.

Applications

Cancer sequencing, Microbiomes (microbial genome sequences without cultivation),

Single-cell DNA methylome sequencing, Single cell transposase-accessible chromatin sequencing. Using machine learning methods, data of gene expression profiles and other applications can be sorted and analyzed in terms of to study gene dynamics, RNA splicing, and cell typing in a better way to determine the identity of cells that don't have known genetic markers.

Approach of Automated Organelle Biopsy on Single Small Cells is Feasible

Newer method through 3D printing and micro- and nanofluidic equipment is making it easy to perform single-cell biopsies and robot-aided single-cell surgery system using microfluidic chips, micropipette mounted onto a 3-DOF micromanipulator and a computer operated high-precision XY stage are being developed to perform high-precision and high-throughput single-cell biopsy and under experimental trials.

Automated extraction of mitochondria and nucleus from human acute promyelocytic leukemia cells and human fibroblast cells and single cell surgery such as manipulation or removal of subcellular components or/and organelles from single cells are increasingly explored used for the study of diseases and their causes in precision medicine. Also, Preimplantation genetic diagnosis a procedure within ART (Assisted reproductive technologies) using robotic micromanipulators, computer vision and automation algorithms are in experimental phase and presents a step towards fully automated ART.

Affordable future applications in high throughput single live cell analysis on a lab-on-a-chip platform and potentially minimally-to-non-invasive surgery are in trial phases and would be a reality.

From Single Gene Analysis to Single Cell Profiling: A New Era for Precision Medicine

Molecular profiling of DNA and RNA provides a valuable new insight into the genetic basis of non-malignant and malignant disorders, and has increased the understanding of basic mechanisms regulating the human development and disease.

Recent technological advances enabling the analyses of alterations in gene-based structure or function in a comprehensive, high-throughput fashion have shown that each tumor type typically exhibits distinct constellations of genetic alterations targeting one or more key cellular pathways that regulate cell growth and proliferation, evasion of the immune system, and other aspects of cancer behavior.

Single Cell Profiling: From Bench to Bedside

Advancing technologies for single-cell analysis have been developed the past years that are making it possible to monitor dynamic changes in tumor heterogeneity at genomic, transcriptomic, proteomic, and functional levels. scRNA-seq technique to enable the detection of rare cell types and finer distinctions among different cell subtypes and disease subphenotyping paving way be advanced robotics single cell biopsy and surgeries.

CRISPR, GENE EDITING

Genome Editing Tools before CRISPR

The initial genome editing techniques emerged following discovery of restriction enzymes and meganucleases *e.g.*, Zn-finger nucleases (zFN). ZFN editing technology was expensive and time- consuming with limitation of one genome can be edited at a time. This was followed by TALENs (transcription activator- like effector nucleases) utilizing engineered enzymes containing a DNA- binding domain and a separate DNA- cleaving domain. TALENs have advantage over ZFNs owing to their flexibility and feasibility to target a wider range of sequences. Techniques using restriction enzymes and rAAVs (recombinant adenovirus-associated viruses) have limitation to accommodate a small amount of genetic material.

CRISPR technology has changed the face of genetic engineering and relies on interactions between DNA and RNA that were challenging to design and manipulate prior to its inception.

What is CRISPR

CRISPR are **Clustered Regularly Interspaced Short Palindromic Repeats** are repeated segments of genetic material. Bacteria, archaea use CRISPR- Cas9 system for protection against bacteriophages. Following phage infection, bacteria employs cas-9 (CRISPR- associated nuclease) to create double- stranded break (DSB) and snip off viral DNA from its target loci and retains memory for future infections and has been used to manipulate genes in different ways (Box 7).

Box 7. Components of CRISPR.

DNA endonuclease targeted CRISPR trans reporter

Combines in a single reaction:

Cas12a

guide RNA

Fluorescent reporter molecule

Recombinase polymerase amplification.

Applications of CRISPR

CRISPR technology are a set of DNA sequences involved in immune system of prokaryotes adapted for genome engineering.

CRISPR Based Diagnostics Available

CRISPR- based diagnostics are currently in development. Its ability to detect and rewrite the underlying cause of genetic disease with CRISPR has huge medical potential.

Medical Potential

CRISPR has huge medical potential and has been used to manipulate genes in different ways. CRISPR is enabling advances in scientific fields especially in Human diagnostics & therapeutics.

Several advantages of CRISPR-based diagnostics compared to traditional PCR-based methods for detection. These include high specificity due to enzymatic recognition of the target and they have fast turnaround times due to signal amplification.

TRANSFORMATIVE ADVANCES IN REGENERATIVE MEDICINE

There is need of development and introduction of newer, efficient therapies to improve patient care and latest advances in 3D printing or bio printing would be of great value in therapeutics in future (bio printing has already been diseased).

Regulatory issues are causing barrier in 3D printing and policies are yet to evolve. Even, FDA has not issued any regulations on bio printing since 3D printed organs do not fit clearly into any category may be medical devices or biological product under law.

3D printing may be used for medical research in vivo drug testing and in vivo transplantation using comparable 3D scaffolds, printed cells & tissues. Since living cells and biomaterials are involved in 3D printing processes raise ethical, policy and regulatory issues, issue of disposal of 3D printing materials, their intended use and long term effects in vivo.

Also, regulatory guidelines are required for safety and quality of bio printed materials in animal and human trials and there are regulatory gaps in this regards that are required to be identified and addressed.

Biomimetic Medical Material

They mimic natural material, structure and architecture and are useful in tissue regeneration, development of material for drug testing. With development of innovative technologies such as nano biotechnology, bio sensors, tissue engineering and regenerative medicine and 3D printing, development of new biomaterials is getting feasible that mimic biomolecules, peptide sequences, chemical and physical structures and morphology. Also, formulation of new bioinks, 4D bio printing with smart hydrogels and technology to fabricate human-scale tissues require regulatory polices to address social, ethical, and regulatory issues concerned with bio printing. Certain policy makers propose 3D printed organs to be regulated as biological products or analogous products applicable to treatment, cure or prevention of diseases in human being.

Advancing transformative technologies and therapeutics in regenerative medicine includes advanced stem cell therapeutics (cellular and molecular based therapeutics, fertility preservation and precision medicine); development of *disease- in- a- dish model* and organism systems (to study disease etiology, advance diagnostics, prevention and/ or treatment), biomechanics and tissue regeneration, precision medicine therapies (for restoration of health life and fertility), wound healing and tissue regeneration, engineering of muscle skeletal tissues (for reconstruction of complex defects due to trauma, congenital defects, tumor resection).

ENCODE, EXOMIC STUDIES, ANCESTRY STUDIES

Encyclopedia of DNA Elements (ENCODE)

ENCODE is a public research consortium that can be accessed through the project's freely accessible database portal for identifying all functional elements of human and mouse genomes. ENCODE was started in 2003and contains a massive data-collection to catalogue the 'functional' DNA sequences and learn when and where they are active in cells and how they affect the process of genome packaging, regulation and reading. It has already revealed some of the genome's dark corners of genome and has facilitated the understanding of how genetic variations can affect human traits and diseases.

In *ENCODE "Encyclopedia" data is organized at two levels of annotations:*

1) *Integrative- level annotations*, including a registry of candidate cis-regulatory elements

2) *Ground- level annotations* derived directly from experimental data.

The fourth phase of ENCODE (ENCODE 4) in February 2017 to continue and a new component, functional element characterization, has been added to expand understanding of the human and mouse genomes and expand the catalogue of candidate regulatory elements in their genomes (Box **8**).

Box 8. Components of ENCODE 4

Functional Element Mapping Centers

To map biochemical activities to identify candidate functional elements in the human and mouse genomes.

Functional Element Characterization Centres

To characterize the role of candidate functional elements in specific biological contexts.

cont.....

Computational Analysis Groups
Pilot new applications of ENCODE data
Data Coordination Center (DCC)
It processes and shares ENCODE metadata and data, and provides a portal for the community to visualize and download data.
Data Analysis Center (DAC)
Specifies data processing pipelines and quality metrics for major data types, design and perform *integrative analysis* of ENCODE data

Exome is the sequence encompassing all the exons of protein coding genes in genome and they cover between 1 and 2% of genome. It can be extended to target functional nonprotein coding elements (*e.g.*, micro-RNA, long intergenic noncoding RNA, *etc.*) and specific candidate loci.

Two Main Categories of Exome Capture Technology: Solution-Based and Array-Based.

Exome Sequencing

Whole exome sequencing (WES) is a new and powerful technique where genomic DNA binds to a predefined target of known exons is sequenced using next-generation technology, to capture the protein-coding portion of the genome.

Exome sequencing technology allows exploration of the most well-understood portions of the genome: protein-coding sequence and functional elements.

Also.it allows identification of genetic variants that affect heritable phenotypes, including important disease-causing mutations and natural variation.

ANCESTRY STUDIES

Genetic ancestry testing, or genetic genealogy, is a way for knowing the family history (genealogy) by examination of DNA variations that can provide clues regarding where their ancestors might have come from and about relationships between families.

Certain patterns of genetic variation are often shared among people of backgrounds. The more closely related two individuals, families, or populations are, the more patterns of variation they typically share.

Three types of genetic ancestry testing are commonly used for genealogy.

Y chromosome testing

Mitochondrial DNA testing

Single nucleotide polymorphism testing

Limitations

Genetic ancestry testing has a number of limitations. Test providers compare individuals' test results to different databases of previous tests. Thus, ethnicity estimates may not be consistent. Since most human populations have migrated many times throughout their history and mixed with nearby groups, ethnicity estimates based on genetic testing may differ.

In ethnic groups with a smaller range of genetic variation, most members share many SNPs, and it may be difficult to distinguish people who have a relatively recent common ancestor, such as fourth cousins, from the group as a whole.

Applications

Genetic ancestry plays a central role in population pharmacogenomics.

Ancestry-informative markers are enriched in pharmacogenetic loci located in both protein-coding and non-protein-coding regions, and trans-ancestry differentiation in population pharmacogenetics studies must be carefully considered.

Whole-genome analysis is necessary for an unbiased examination over pharmacogenetic loci.

Genome-wide association studies (GWAS) a5re done to identify where genetic variants responsible for causing disease and searching for gene variants that confer risk of disease.

Encode, Exomic studies, ancestry studies.

CONCLUSION

Antisense RNA approach is designed to specifically interfere with virus replication. A complementary DNA strand of a gene can be inserted in reverse orientation (3′ → 5′) and is termed antisense gene. Antisense therapy refers to inhibition of translation by using a single stranded nucleotide. Also, it is possible to inhibit both transcription and translation. Antisense approaches are compatible with emerging trends in drug development, genomic-based therapeutics, and the integration of diagnostics with therapeutics. Everyday all around the world, new strains of infectious and potentially deadly pathogens are evolving. These microorganisms may be used as bioweapons of mass destruction in future. A greater awareness of bioterrorism and implementation of strategies to prevent and defuse bioweapon attacks is need of the hour. Multiple molecular cytogenetic strategies and applications are used to design diagnostic approaches to detect and characterize genetic changes even the base pair levels. DNA methylation is the best studied epigenetic biomarker and has a great potential as diagnostic and predictive tool therapeutic target. Pharmacogenetics has been defined as variation in drug response as it relates to an individual's genetic makeup. It refers to a broader use of genome-wide association, studies (GWAS) and potential complex interactions as well as alteration in gene expression that correlates to drug response. Nutrigenomics is interactions between foods or dietary supplements and an individual's genome and consequent downstream effects on their phenotype. Preimplantation embryos are obtained in vitro and genetically analyzed for genetic defect if any before transferring. PGD is still labour intensive and time-consuming, and introduction of newer technologies has made it safer and more reliable.

CONFLICT OF INTEREST

No potential conflict of interest is declared by the author. It is also declared the complete work is an individual effort by the author and there was no financial/ administrative/academic support availed from any individual/ institution /organization.

EXERCISE

1. What is antisense RNA technology

2. Discuss Gene silencing

3. How to do mRNA Surveillance

4. How biotechnology can be used against bioweapons

5. Discuss molecular cytogenetics

6. Describe allele specific mutation detection. What are mutation databases.

7. Techniques for analysis of human splicing defects

8. How detection of genomic duplications and deletion done by molecular techniques for DNA methylation studies

Short notes:

i. Pharmacogenetics

ii. Pharmacogenomics and nutrigenomics

iii. Preimplantation genetic diagnosis and prenatal diagnosis

Next- generation DNA sequencing techniques (NGS)

Single cell biopsy

CRISPR and gene editing

Transformative advances in regenerative medicine

BIBLOGRAPHY

[1] Wilson K, Hofmann A, Walker JM, Clokie S, editors. Wilson and Walker's principles and techniques of biochemistry and molecular biology. Cambridge university press; 2018 Apr 19.

[2] Karp G. Cell and Molecular Biology. John Wiley & Sons Incorporated; 2007.

[3] Hartl DL, Jones EW, Hartl DL, Jones EW. Genetics: principles and analysis. 1998.

[4] Creager AN. Recipes for recombining DNA: a history of molecular cloning: a laboratory manual. BJHS Themes. 2020;5:225-43.

[5] Primrose SB, Twyman R. Principles of gene manipulation and genomics. John Wiley & Sons; 2006 Feb 10.

[6] Glick BR, Patten CL. Molecular biotechnology: principles and applications of recombinant DNA. John Wiley & Sons; 2022 Mar 15.

CHAPTER 11

Ethics in Science & Technology

"History of the world civilizations shows that societies have risen to a higher level not through mechanical or technological efficiencies but by practising sound moral and ethical values".

— Swami Bodhinanda (Gita & Management)

LEARNING OBJECTIVES

This chapter gives an overview of ethics, values, and morals concerning research; Indian research at a glance and violation of ethical issues in India and worldwide; Virtual embryo – virtual life, artificial bacteria -ethical issues; ethics in the era of covid19 and challenges in precision medicine. Also, the ethical responsibilities of scientists, technologists, institutions, firms, policy-makers, governments, international organizations and citizens are discussed.

Abstract: This chapter discusses conceptual issues in arguing for the ethics of science and technology. Since we live in a world where scientific knowledge and new technologies are continuously challenging our values, and we have to live our daily lives and make decisions based on the fundamental values of human dignity in our civilisation, scientists are no exception. Governments and private sectors have recognized the importance of ethics required to reconcile the human imperatives of development and sustainability. It is necessary to conduct both in-depth research on ethics and strengthen ethics education in science and technology to solve the problems brought about by rapid developments in the field. Stem cell research, genetic testing, and cloning are giving human beings new power to improve health and control development processes of all living species. Concerns about the social, cultural, legal and ethical implications of such progress are the most significant debates of the past century and a new word has been coined to encompass these concerns, *i.e.* bioethics.

Keywords: Ethics, Plagiarism, Ecological issues, Policy issues, Global ethics experiences, Society for Scientific Values.

ETHICS VALUES MORALS

Ethics are a set of principles and a sense of purpose which are fundamental to a civilized society. It is said that science is ethics–neutral but scientist is not! Ethics can be universal or functional and profession dependent which cannot be taught but must be cultured and nurtured through experience, analysis, introspection, and a sense of responsibility.

Simmi Kharb, Akshat Singh, Abhyuday Singh & Deepa Kharb (Eds.)

Ethics can be exercised at the level of individuals, communities, professions, and countries. At a philosophical level, ethics include abortion, genetic testing, organ transplant, gene therapy, etc. At the professional level, ethics include research integrity and scientific values. At the regulatory level: biosafety, bioethics, EIA, clinical trials, and field trials are the main concerns. The fields of biotechnology and bioethics have coevolved and impacted each other.

Professional Ethics: Issues

Plagiarism

Duplicate publication

Author credit and accountability

Research supervision

Data: quality and integrity

Special Facilities: Sharing and use of peer review.

IPR

Development, acquisition and commercialisation of technology

Ecological issues

Professional Ethics: Secondary Issues

Policy issues

Interaction with the public and media

Science vs Society

Science vs market forces

Regional, communal and caste factors

Political interventions

Recruitment and assessment

Corruption and kickbacks

Issues Regarding Scientific Values and Research Integrity in India

Favouritism and victimization in:

Recruitments and promotions

Grants, awards, peer reviews

Caste, region, religion

Feudal work culture

The bureaucratic, non-transparent system, poor accountability

Corruption

Plagiarism, false data/claims, authorships, conflict of interest

Public Protests Against Biotechnology

Since biotech is one of the battlefronts in the fight against globalization, liberalization, capitalism and privatization. However, biotech needs to be democratized and negotiable.

INDIAN RESEARCH AT A GLANCE

In India about one lakh scientists, engineers and technologists are working in various S & T Institutions, producing around 20,000 research papers/articles. Also, 3,000 PhDs are produced every year, most of which flock to the west.

Science and technology Institutions in India

>250 universities

> 100 deemed to be universities

8 IITs

4 IIITs

19 NITs

40 DRDO Labs

40 ICMR Labs

40+100 CDIR Labs & Centres

49 ICAR Institutions

20 MIT

19 Autonomous research institutions

Indian researchers are preferred in most countries and many Indian scientific institutions have active links with western labs and participate in several bilateral and multilateral S & T programs. India has become a research superpower third in the world and globally Indian names galore in research publications and patents.

VIOLATION OF ETHICAL ISSUES IN INDIA

- "Silent" supervisors claim co-authorships of research papers.
- People publish (in national journals) re-hash materials published elsewhere.
- Purchase of degree and honours
- Ghostwriters for PhD thesis
- Plagiarism
- Political, and regional factors in appointments, honours and national awards.
- Corruption and kickbacks in S & T funding agencies
- Grooming deemed-to-be universities without minimal faculty and infrastructure for teaching and R & D

It should be remembered that S & T is another dimension of patriotism and IP is the wealth of a nation. For improving the S & T knowledge, the following points need to be implemented:

1. Global protection of IPR
2. Globally competitive S&T
3. International research, collaboration and global networking.

4. International law and watchdogs to protect IPRs

Fields where S & T ethics are Important

Medical sciences and technology

Bioengineering and biotechnology

Molecular/Nano-scale life sciences: genetic modifications

Agro-biotechnologies—GM

IT

Global biosphere and ecology

UN Declaration on Bioethics and Human Rights: Principles

Human dignity and human rights

Benefit and harm

Autonomy and individual responsibility

Consent: prior, free and informed

Special protection to those who lack the capacity for consent

Respect for human vulnerability and personal integrity.

Privacy and confidentiality

Equality, justice and equity

Non-discrimination and non-stigmatization

Respect for cultural diversity and pluralism

Solidarity and cooperation

Social responsibility and health

Sharing of benefits

Protecting future generations

Protection of environment, biosphere, biodiversity

(Adopted by Declaration on 19th October 2005 by 23rd session of General Conference of UNESCO)

UNESCO has a division of ethics of S & T and Global Ethics Observatory. Also, there exists International *Bioethics Committee* and Division for mapping global Ethics Experiences. Various data banks concerned with Ethics exist, namely, Who's who in Ethics. Ethics, Institutions and Ethics Training Programmes are patronised by UNESCO.

In India also, societies promoting integrity, objectivity and ethical values in S & T exist namely, Society for Scientific Values *(SSV)*. *S & T* institutions should introduce formal/informal studies/discussions on ethical conduct to sensitize people concerned about ethical practices and issues of national and global importance.

VIRTUAL EMBRYO – VIRTUAL LIFE, ARTIFICIAL BACTERIA - ETHICAL ISSUES

Ethical Issues

Artificial Life and Ethics

Reports of the successful creation of artificial life have worried the philosophers. Advances in synthetic biology in future will make the distinction between artificial and natural life a difficult and fluid one.

A major stream of Artificial Life research aimed at building synthetic life forms is operating in virtual worlds, implemented as computer programs. A clear long-term target for such research is the evolution of digital life forms with a complexity of structure and behaviour analogous to biological life forms, potentially exhibiting intelligence and self-awareness.

The creation of intelligent, self-aware digital life forms will have clear ethical implications, but there is no current research into how these ethical issues might be addressed and such ethical research and building up of a solid philosophical foundation for the consideration of these ethical issues. are required.

Bioethicists have reacted with caution to the announcement that scientists in the US have created the first synthetic living cell. Dr Craig Venter's team announced their landmark discovery in Science magazine. They have succeeded in transplanting synthetic DNA for a bacterium into a host cell and what the ethicists called "playing God", and what that means is the capacity to be a creator. There will be very important ethical issues since this work had proceeded without any real regulation at all. Since the bad guys are out there and weaponizing all sorts of things will be much, much easier. These scientists can be their own worst enemy since they are using words like "clone" or "synthetic life, lest thing doesn't become a national or international threat because more safeguards haven't been made.

The moral significance of the creation of artificial life has failed, because the creation of artificial life is morally problematic in a way that the derivation of organisms from existing life forms is not. Decisive moral consideration is not how life is created but what non-genealogical properties it possesses.

Ethics of Realism in Virtual Life and Reality

The golden rule of reciprocity ("treat others as you would have them treat you") of most philosophical traditions and religions is a fundamental human moral imperative. The first and most positive aspect of virtual reality (VR) is that VR can place people virtually in the body of another, such that a member can temporarily occupy the body and position of another member of different skin colour or age or height.

Superrealism

Also, very high-quality visual and behavioural realism of virtual humans will become likely and available shortly. For example, Facebook has been carrying out research and development in this area. The benefits of superrealism are clear and realistic virtual scenarios can make the applications more efficacious. For example, aviators can be better trained in the virtual simulation; in exposure therapy in which a patient is presented with a realistic virtual version of the agent they are afraid of and this may be more efficient if the agent seems real. As occurs with most things in the world, with benefits come potential misuse, abuse or neglect, all of which bring about ethical concerns. The challenge now is for researchers, content creators, and distributors of these systems to determine what should be within this code of conduct.

Emerging ethical dilemmas and policy issues in science and technology
Personalized genetic tests/personalized medicine
3-D printing
Adaptation to climate change
Low-quality and counterfeit pharmaceuticals
Autonomous systems: human-controlled, to automated, to autonomous, with the ability to act on their own without human input
Human-animal hybrids (chimaeras)
Data collection and privacy: genetic data, medical treatment
Human enhancements: Pharmaceutical, surgical, mechanical and neurological enhancements.

ETHICS IN ERA OF COVID19

The coronavirus disease 2019 (COVID-19) pandemic has placed an extraordinary demand on health systems and healthcare providers throughout the world and has presented a number of unprecedented challenging ethical issues. COVID-19 pandemic raised unique ethical dilemmas, but the key issue has been the need to ration scarce critical care resources. Difficult life and death decisions have to be made in emergency rooms and intensive care units and other ethical issues have arisen related to conducting clinical trials during the pandemic, vaccines and the increase in domestic violence during the quarantine period.

Arrival of vaccine has raised many ethical issues. Many researchers would prefer to test the efficacy of other vaccines, for the same virus, in clinical trials involving human subjects. Question arises if it is ethical to conduct a trial on another vaccine and to deprive subjects in the trial from the benefit of an effective vaccine already in hand? In medical ethics, a robust principle is that no effective treatment or vaccine would be withheld from the patients, if their survival may rely on it. It is feared that if such studies are carried out in less-resourced healthcare systems, then a major concern would be that withholding an efficient safe vaccine in any trial would probably affect the vulnerable populations. On the contrary, this is argued that whether it is justifiable to conduct a trial with another vaccine that has clear advantage over the existing product. Thus all measures should be taken to protect the vulnerable research subjects by pharmaceutical companies and researchers who are conducting the vaccine trials and provide appropriate compensation to trial participants, and further share the financial rewards of the successful vaccine with the involved people. Also, informed consent should be obtained in culturally and linguistically appropriate way.

WHO Working Group on Ethics and COVID-19

WHO has established an international Working Group on Ethics and COVID-19 in order to develop advice on key ethical questions that Member States need to address.

The expert group also advises WHO's technical units regarding ethical aspects of their COVID-related work. Since its formation in February 2020, the group has been engaged in the following activities:

- Advice on ethical considerations in COVID-19 research
- Practical guidance on the application of ethical values central to COVID-19 research published in the journal "Public Health Ethics"
- A policy brief on resource allocation and priority setting in COVID-19 care
- Providing ethics input into the WHO's Clinical Management Guidelines and training
- Feedback provided on the Solidarity Trial protocol
- Development of emergency standard operating procedures for human research committees to facilitate rapid review of protocols during the COVID-19 pandemic
- Advice on the criteria that must be satisfied for SARS-CoV-2 challenge studies to be ethically acceptable
- Considering other areas: Immunity certificates, MEURI (i.e., monitored emergency use of unregistered and experimental interventions) and the fair global allocation of vaccines, therapeutics, and diagnostics.

CHALLENGES IN PRECISION MEDICINE

With medical and technical advancements in genomics, proteomics, data analysis and other fields, there are gradual development of laser-focused drugs and ability to predict personal risk factors of a person for particular diseases and how individual responses to various treatments might differ. However, despite the many advantages of personalized medicine, there are numerous issues would arise, including ethical, legal and social problems.

In the era of social diffusion of information, any material can reach a large number of people in less than a minute. Digital tools are able to connect the patient and healthy subject to medical information and this expanding phenomenon along with patient empowerment by a specialist is essential and required to be discussed in a medical environment in order to block any uninformed and unsafe influence. Thus, now emphasis is to focus on how ethics review boards or research ethics committees work, organs responsible for monitoring compliance with transparency, informed consent process and patient empowerment. The innovating medical process should also be performed by ethics education and training of healthcare professions.

Thus, transition from a conception of reactive to a pro-active medicine, associated with the innovation and the ethical issues that is inextricably linked to it, must be considered as a primary goal in the health system and scientific community. Intellectual property rights ensure that the individual who first has an idea has the exclusive right to develop it, this includes copyrights, patents and trademarks. However, with the development of genetic technology, these rights will have to be reassessed. For example, some argue that patenting DNA sequences may have a negative influence upon research and slow down the overall development process.

Regulatory frameworks are required to ensure that the standard of genetic testing and research is maintained at a high and reliable standard, however the current frameworks cannot be applied to personalized medicine. Also, ethical and social issues that arise regarding confidentiality and privacy of patients and another major issue within the field of personalized medicine is the ethics surrounding patient information.

There are many ethical concerns relating to incidental disease discovery, occurrence of false-positives can lead to a plethora of both ethical and medical issues. Whilst a patient is being screened for one disease, the presence of another life-changing disease may be identified. This is particularly an issue if there are no available treatment options, as the prognosis of the patient is not improved during this process. Discovering that one has a disease can also have a very serious psychological impact on patients, leading to further ethical issues and sometimes issues of stigmatization of individuals with certain diseases can arise. If patient's genetic data was leaked, many issues may be presented. For example, inappropriate use of this information by insurance companies, who may not offer policies to certain individuals with genetic diseases. Additionally, this information may also be used by employers, who may not employ someone based upon their genetic disease. This therefore highlights the importance of the security and confidentiality of genetic information.

EXERCISE

1. What is meant by ethical question in science?

2. Can ethics be applied in science and technology?

3. What are the emerging issues in ethics?

4. Why is ethics important in science and technology?

5. Discuss ethical issues of virtual life and artificial life.

6. What are ethical issues in covid 19 research and technology development.

7. Discuss ethical issues of precision medicine.

CONCLUSION

Ethics are a set of principles and a sense of purpose which are fundamental to a civilized society. Ethics can be at the level of individuals, communities, professions, countries. At professional level, ethics include research integrity and scientific values. At regulatory level: biosafety, bioethics, EIA, clinical trials, field trials are the main concerns. The fields of biotechnology and bioethics have coevolved and impacted each other. In India also, societies for promoting integrity, objectivity and ethical values in S & T exist namely, Society for Scientific Values (SSV). S & T institutions should introduce formal/informal studies/discussions on ethical conduct to sensitize people concerned on ethical practices and issues of national and global importance.

BIBLOGRAPHY

[1] Wilson K, Hofmann A, Walker JM, Clokie S, editors. Wilson and Walker's principles and techniques of biochemistry and molecular biology. Cambridge university press; 2018 Apr 19.
[2] Karp G. Cell and Molecular Biology. John Wiley & Sons Incorporated; 2007.
[3] Hartl DL, Jones EW, Hartl DL, Jones EW. Genetics: principles and analysis. 1998.
[4] Molecular Cloning: A Laboratory Manual : Joseph Sambrook And David Russell.
[5] Primrose SB. Principles of gene manipulation and genomics by Sandy B Primrose and Richard Twyman.
[6] Glick BR, Patten CL. Molecular biotechnology: principles and applications of recombinant DNA. John Wiley & Sons; 2022 Mar 15.

CHAPTER 12

Medical Biotechnology

LEARNING OBJECTIVES

After completing this chapter, you should be able to:

- Provide examples of current applications of biotechnology in medical sciences
- Understand the purpose of gene therapy, regenerative medicine, pharmacogenomics

Abstract: Medical biotechnology incorporates many of the topics that have already been discussed in this book. Right from developing new drugs to prospects of stem cell use and cloning, the possibilities are enormous.

Keywords: Homologs, Personalize medicine, nanodevices, Nanoparticles, Regenerative medicine, Xenotransplantation, Biocapsules, Stem cells.

DETECTION AND DIAGNOSIS OF HUMAN DISEASES BY MOLECULAR BIOLOGY

Molecular biology offers powerful tools for diagnosing and combating human diseases. Mice, rats, worms, and flies have played critical roles in helping scientists study human diseases.

Various model organisms are used for the identification of disease genes and testing of gene therapy and drug-based therapeutic approaches.

Homologs

Many important genes are conserved from species to species and genes identified in model species have been related to human genes termed as homologs.

The human genome project and comparative genomics studies have demonstrated that human beings share a large number of genes with other organisms *e.g.*, humans share 50% of genes with fruit flies and about 61% of genes mutated in 289 human disease conditions are found in fruit flies. This group includes genes involved in leukemia, cystic fibrosis, pancreatic cancer, prostatic cancer and other human genetic disorders. Heart disease, and HIV model organisms are used by scientists to study disease processes and test therapies to combat the disease. Molecular biology offers possible biomarkers for the detection of diseases at an early stage,

Simmi Kharb, Akshat Singh, Abhyuday Singh & Deepa Kharb (Eds.)

e.g., in the case of cancer, early detection is critical for treatment and improving patient survival.

Biomarkers are proteins produced by diseased tissues or their production is increased when the tissue is diseased. They are released into body fluids such as blood, urine, and body cavity fluids. Also, the detection of genes or gene expression patterns also provides important biomarkers for early detection and diagnosis and monitoring of diseases and microarray offers promising results in this regard.

GENETIC DISEASES

Many different genetic diseases have been detected by molecular biology techniques. Until recently, fetal genetic testing was done more for fetal sex detection than the detection of genetic diseases. Amniocentesis and chorionic villus sampling are used for the detection of genetic diseases. Karyotyping, FISH (fluorescence in situ hybridization) and spectral karyotyping are useful in identifying missing or extra chromosomes. A number of diseases due to chromosomal abnormalities occur when a portion of a chromosome is deleted or swapped from one chromosome to another, *e.g.*, chronic myelogenous leukaemia where DNA is exchanged from chromosome 9 to 22 and vice versa and this exchange can be detected by FISH.

Mutations in specific genes also result in many genetic diseases and require more sophisticated techniques for their detection in both fetuses and adults.

RFLP (restriction fragment length polymorphism) pronounced "*riflips*" analysis can detect genetic diseases in embryos and adults from amniotic fluid and blood respectively. Also, RFLPs are used for DNA fingerprinting. Another approach is allele-specific oligonucleotide (ASO) analysis that allows the detection of a single nucleotide change in the gene. In the ASO technique, DNA is isolated from cells and amplified by PCR using primers flanking genes of interest. This technique can be used to screen gene defects from single cells from 8 to 32 cell-stage embryos created by in vitro fertilization, termed as *Preimplantation Genetic Testing*.

SINGLE NUCLEOTIDE POLYMORPHISMS (SNPS), EXOME SEQUENCING

SNPs, single nucleotide changes in DNA sequences, (pronounced "*snips*") are the most common genetic variations in humans. SNPs occur in approximately every 1,000 to 3,000 base pairs (bp) in the human genome and over 1.4 SNPs have been identified. Most SNPs occur in introns (non-protein coding regions) and have no effect on a cell. But, when an SNP occurs in a gene sequence, it may cause a change in the protein structure that produces diseases or influences traits in a variety of ways, including conferring susceptibility for some types of diseases. Since SNPs occur frequently throughout the genome, they serve as a valuable genetic marker for identifying disease-related genes.

HapMap

Hap is an abbreviation for haplotype and Hap Map is an international effort to identify and catalogue chromosomal locations (loci) of >1.4 million SNPs present in 3 billion bp of the human genome. Many SNPs on the same chromosomes are clustered in groups called haplotypes and this may have a role in diagnosis and treatment.

Microarray analysis using DNA microarrays, and protein microarrays will also play an important role in the detection of genetic and other diseases.

Applications of Biotechnology

Major areas of medical biotechnology are the identification of novel drugs and developing new ways for the treatment of diseases. Different proteins, *e.g.*, insulin, human GH have been produced using recombinant DNA technology and are used to treat human diseases. Also, therapeutic proteins such as monoclonal antibodies, blood products and enzymes produced by living systems can be thought of as biotech drugs (Table **1**).

Biotechnology proteins have revolutionized the healthcare and pharmaceutical industries. Newer strategies for treating different types of cancer are promising and oncogenes and tumor suppressor genes are getting attention.

Work is going on to identify proteins made by these genes are targets. For inhibition and activation to fight the disease.

Table 1. Recombinant therapeutics.

Protein	*Application*
Monoclonal antibodies	Therapeutics: cancer, Rheumatoid arthritic Diagnostic

(Table 1) cont.....

Interferons	Cancer Asthma, allergy Arthritis Infections
Interleukins	Cancer HIV Radiation- or drug-induced bone marrow suppression
Coagulation factors	Hemophilia Blood clotting disorders
Erythropoietin	Anaemia
Human growth factor	Growth deficiency
Insulin	Diabetes mellitus
Insulin growth factor	Diabetes mellitus

(Table 1) cont.....

Vaccines	Hepatitis Herpes Malaria

Genome Editing

Already discussed in chapter 10.

Personalized Medicine & Targeted Cancer Therapy

PERSONALIZED MEDICINE

SNPs discovery is responsible for a newly emerging field of Pharmacogenomics: customized medicine. Small molecule drugs are designed based on genetic profile of a patient to personalize medicine and improve drug delivery. Pharmacogenomics is based on different response of different individuals to same drug in terms of degree of effectiveness and adverse effects due to genetic polymorphisms (**Fig. 1**).

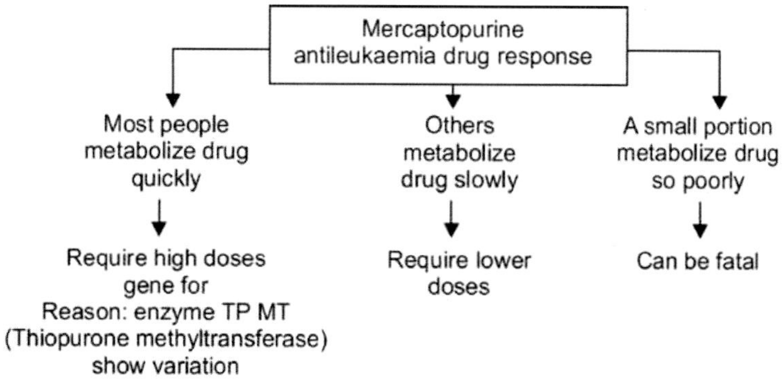

Fig. (1). Pharmacogenomics after blood test, indivisuals can be give dosage tailored to their genetic profile.

Cancer chemotherapy requires so-called magic-bullet drugs that destroys only cancer cells and not normal body cells.

An example of pharmacogenomics in action is breast cancer therapy: women with defective BRCA1 or 2 gene copy are at increased risk of breast cancer, as compared to those cases that do not exhibit clear mode of inheritance. Extraction of DNA from cancerous breast tissue for SNP and microarray analysis could be used to determine genes which are involved and to design drug treatment strategy that is specific and most effective against particular type of cancer. Similarly, for women with HER-2 positive breast tumours. Herceptin, a type of monoclonal antibody, has proven to be effective in some women.

Another example is Gleevec used to treat chronic myelogenous leukaemia (CML) and it targets a protein BCR-ABL fusion protein produced by the swapping of DNA that occurs in CML.

DNA Microarray analysis of gene expression will be used to diagnose patients based on gene they express to provide them with a pharmacogenomic treatment based on those genes.

Apart from drug designing, improvement for drug delivering also required to maximize their effectiveness. Microspheres sprayed into airways have been successful in asthma, lung cancer, emphysema, tuberculosis. Implanting of microspheres with anticancer drugs in body adjacent to growing tumours are also under research.

PERSONALIZED MEDICINE & TARGETED CANCER THERAPY

Personalized Medicine

Personalized medicine is having impact in patient care and clinical research pouring way for more technological advances. It is the tailoring of individualized medical treatment of each patient based on their unique molecular and genetic profiles that makes them susceptible to certain disease. This approach can help physician to select a molecular profile– based individualized therapy or treatment protocol that will have minimum side effects and successful outcome. This involves risk assessment by genetic testing for predisposition to a disease to institute preventive measures for preventing a disease lifestyle dietary/ behavioral/ treatment intervention. Also, early detection of disease at molecular level, molecular diagnostics for individualized treatment strategy and management of disease for successful outcome of disease.

Personalized medicine is helping in patient care in various condition such as breast cancer (*e.g.*, HER 2 protein), melanoma (BRAF protein inhibitor, cardiovascular disease (gene expression profiling and tailored immunosuppressive drug regimens) and disease signature in other disease are also available such as T2DM, prostate cancer, Parkinson's disease, age related macular degeneration etc.

CAR, TREGS CELL THERAPY

Chimeric Antigen Receptor Technology (CARs)

CARs are made up of two major domains the ectodomain and end domain. Ectodomain sits on outside of cells, interacts with environment and endodomain lies inside the cell, relays signals from outside of cell to inside.

Chimeric antigen receptors (CARs) are (artificial) surface receptors introduced into somatic cells by genetic engineering, acts as recognition molecules in similar way as antibodies or T cell receptors.. Chimeric antigen receptors combine antigen specificity of antibody with biological properties of T- lymphocytes linked together to form variable regions of a monoclonal antibodies linked together to form a single antibody.

Gene transfer of CARs generates antitumor responses in cancer patients and produces remarkable clinical response in these patients. In clinical applications for inserting CARs in T- lymphocytes, retrovirus lentiviruses are used to integrate into host genome and produce robust expression of the gene in human T cells and their progeny Adaptive transfer of T cells collected from autologous peripheral blood engineered to express chimeric antigen receptors (CARs) has produced impressive clinical responses in patients with malignancies and solid tumors.

Progress in the development of chimeric antigen receptors and in genome editing (including the application of CRISPR-Cas9) over the past two decades has facilitated the genetic optimization of primary T cell therapy for cancer.

Treg Therapy

(Treg = Regularity cells)

Treg are a small subject of immune cells that curb excessive immune activation. They are specialized CD4+ subpopulation of lymphocytes with regulatory functions, maintain immune homoeostasis and self-tolerance. Tregs maintain are immune balance *via* suppression of immune responses.

Polyclonal Tregs are promising in cell therapy in transplantation & auto immunity as evident preclinical models & clinical trials. CD4+Tregs can be developed as central Tregs with thymus or in various tissues after thymus development in presence of factors such as TGF-B & 1L-2. Treg adoptive cell therapy can be non-engineered or engineered. Adoptive non engineered Tregs have used in preclinical trials in auto immune diseases, T1 DM using polyclonal antibodies. Genetically engineered Tregs using antigen targeted namely, TCR- transgenic Tregs have been used in preclinical trials in diabetes, autoimmune diseases, multiple sclerosis models and have been shown to be beneficial. Engineered T cells immunotherapy is rapidly expanding and includes therapeutic Tregs.

Tregs therapy are promising in suppressing immune responses in organ transplant, immune suppression in avoiding or minimum use of immune suppressive drugs. Tregs. may be useful to improve transplant tolerance and control immune response in transplantation in future.

Tolerogenic Vaccines

They represent technology design based on knowledge of Treg niche namely, antigenic, cytokine and APC niches that are preferential Treg microenvironments. They are autoantigen specific; interventions preserve host defense and avoid opportunistic infections associated with broad spectrum immunosuppression.

In contrast to conventional vaccines, tolerogenic vaccine are preventive & provide humoral immunity and they have therapeutic action and potential to reverse pre-established auto immune disease and they act *via* in activation of pre-existing pathogenic effectors or memory T-cells directly along with induction and even expansion of suppressive Tregs for producing long- lasting immune tolerance. They include peptide based vaccines, nucleic acid based vaccines with genetic or viral vectors, nano particle embedded with auto antigens and immunomodulatory drugs such as rapamycin, cyclosporine, cell based passive vaccines with polyclonal Tregs or tolerogenic dendritic cells (DCs). At present no tolerogenic vaccines have been approved for clinical interventions though early phase clinical trial is going on.

Oral Antigen Based Oral Immuno Therapy (OIT)

OIT can be used for alleviating allergies and autoimmune diseases. They take the advantage of regulatory mechanism that are utilized by GIT to promote unresponsiveness against food antigens and non-viral commensals of GIT and are shown to be useful in food allergy and autoimmune diseases. They are used as replacement in genetic diseases to prevent anti-drug antibody response.

ART ASSISTED REPRODUCTIVE TECHNOLOGY

Assisted Reproductive Technology

Centers for Disease Control and Prevention (CDC) defines ART as "any treatment where oocytes and sperm are handled outside the body for the purpose of establishing a pregnancy." It consists of controlled ovarian stimulation (COS), oocyte retrieval, IVF, and transfer of the embryo or embryos into the uterus.

Ovulation induction is the stimulation of ovulation by using fertility medications. It can treat oligoovulation or anovulation and also helps in development of ovarian follicles.

Transvaginal oocyte retrieval (TVOR) or oocyte retrieval (OCR) is the removal of *oocytes from the ovary of a woman to perform fertilization outside the body.*

In vitro Fertilization (IVF)

In vitro fertilization (IVF) with or without in vitro maturation (IVM) involves retrieval of oocytes from ovarian follicles, fertilized in vitro and then subsequently the resulting embryo is transferred into the uterus.

Nowadays single embryo transfers (SET) is usually performed as multifetal gestation can increase the risk of both maternal and fetal morbidity and mortality as it increases risk of preterm birth, preeclampsia and other pregnancy related complications.

• *Intra cytoplasmic sperm injection (ICSI)*- It is an in vitro procedure in which a single spermatozoon is injected into the oocyte cytoplasm.

• *Assisted hatching (AH)*- It is also an in vitro procedure in which the zona pellucida of an embryo is perforated or thinned out by using mechanical, chemical methods or *via* laser to cause the separation of the blastocyst. The embryo reaches the blastocyst stage in 5–6 days following fertilization.

• *Gamete intrafallopian transfer (GIFT)* is an in vitro procedure in which both gametes *i.e* sperm and oocyte are transferred into the fallopian tube.

• *Zygote intrafallopian transfer (ZIFT)* is an in vitro procedure in which the zygote is *transferred into the fallopian tube.*

INTRAUTERINE INSEMINATION (IUI)

Intrauterine insemination (IUI) is a procedure in which the motile sperms which are processed and concentrated are placed directly into the uterine cavity. This procedure is mainly used when the cause of infertility is related to the male partner.

Risks Associated with ART:

Multifetal gestations

Prematurity

Low birth weight

Small for gestational age

Perinatal mortality

Placenta previa

Abruptio placentae

Preeclampsia

Birth defects

OHSS (Ovarian Hyper Stimulation Syndrome)

Ectopic pregnancy

Ovarian torsion

NANOTECHNOLOGY & NANOMEDICINE

Nanotechnology and Nanomedicine

Application of nanotechnology for improving human health is nanomedicine and it is of particular interest in medical biotechnology. Nanodevice sensors, nanoparticle devices that unclog block arteries and detect and eliminate cancer cells are also in pipeline. Many nanotechnology-based drugs are available in market nowadays. Even smart drug using viruses, tiny nanoparticles, *e.g.*, gold particles have been developed to deliver drugs to treat (tumour seeking) or destroy (tumour killing) cancer cells with few side effects.

Nature Nanomachines

Within all living organisms are the engines of life *i.e.*, large, highly structured proteins are nanomachines that are highly structured, active assemblies to do all the work in the cell and ATP synthase is "the-nanomachine-that-synthesises-the-ATP-molecule." Even all diseases involve malfunctioning protein nanomachines. The nanomachines of nature regulate the great global cycles.

Drug Delivery Systems – Nano Cubes, Nanotubes

In nanomedicine and nano delivery systems materials in the nanoscale range are used to serve as diagnostic tools or to deliver therapeutic agents to specific targeted sites in a controlled manner.

Nanotechnology offers multiple benefits in treatment of chronic human diseases by specific, and target-oriented delivery of precise medicines and a number of applications of nanomedicine include chemotherapeutic agents, biological agents, immunotherapeutic agents etc. for treatment of various diseases.

NANOBOTS & DIAGNOSTICS

Nanobot

Nanobot is study of manipulation of matter on atomic and molecular scale based on nanotechnology. Nanobots are of the size of 1 to 100 nm and have a role in medicine targeted interventions for drug delivery. Self-propelled nanobot-biodegradable nano devices (of bio nano components) for preclinical trials are available that can transport programmed delivery of molecular preboards for cancer treatment. They can be programmed to perform specific biological functions.

Nanobots and Diagnostics

Nanobots in Healthcare

1. *Blood content monitoring bots* using special sensor nanobots that can be inserted in blood. Various blood contents can be measured *via e.g.*, microbiology haematology, toxicology.

2. *Motorized self-propulsive nanobot* for drug delivery based on enzyme- based on propulsion.

cont.....

3. Nanobots for oncology diagnostics and therapeutics.
4. Futuristic: DNA nanobots, CRISPR bots.

Nanobots have the advantage of speed causing minimal or no trauma, requiring less recovery time (rapid response a change), longevity, specificity, accuracy, and they disassemble and get excreted after completion of task. Ease of programmed from remote sensing/ compt. However, they are expensive and complicated to design. Also, nanobots can even be used as bioweapons or misused by terrorists and can be a threat to society if they enter into wrong hands. Their biodegradability is another issue and if nanobots self- replicate then they can challenge human immune system.

Nano Robotics

They can be used in targeted cancer therapy, body surveillance (continuous monitoring of vitals and wireless transmission of this data and sound an alert for example if blood sugar levels are suddenly high in a case of a diabetic.

Multi-Functional Bots

They can convert themselves into stents for example to remove/open up blockage of blood vessel, as tool to sense and repair anomalies in the body for example removing blockages in circulatory system. Using swarm intelligence (to share information available and take collective action), intrabody nanobots can create a single, strong shield against pathogens and toxins.

Advanced Microsurgery

Microsurgery of eye, retina can be performed using nanobots and even fetal surgery can be possible. Nanobots can be used in endoscopy even nanobot mouthwashes are being used.

They can be used as cochlear implants in ear, stem cell delivery in regenerative medicine and nanobotics have a wider scope in the field of medicine in vaccine delivery and development.

Nanobots in Vaccines

They are one of the best methods for vaccination because of precise, accurate, target specificity and rapid acting features. Nano size delivery systems are still under developmental stages nanobots can be programmed robots to dispense vaccine in host, increase speed of vaccine development, precise and accurate vaccine delivery.

Nanobots Debris

It is much harmful since it is non soluble, can block blood vessels of any organ causing organ failure. Nanobot are programmed to release digital signature and could be hacked and if more than one type of nanobots are present in the body then they can be theoretically trend into a network to communicate and do their bidding and exploiting for ransom wire threat by hacker!

FUTURE OF DNA BIOENGINEERING: AI, SUPERCOMPUTERS, ORIGAMI, DESIGNER DRUG

Future of DNA Bioengineering

With development of newer approaches in biotechnology, in future there will be shift from the current system of generalized medicine based on population averages to precision medicine based on each patient's individual biology to predictive medicine based on AI-generated estimations of a person's future health state. This shift in the healthcare would ensure that the genomes of millions and billions of people will be sequenced to form a foundation of their personalized treatment. Big data analytics will then be used to compare their genotypes with their phenotypes (how those genes are expressed over the course of their lives). The healthcare applications of the genetics revolution are immense and realistic since Artificial intelligence has become the pet anxiety of luminaries like Elon Musk, Bill Gates, and Stephen Hawking. In the coming decades, advanced pharmaceuticals, bioelectronics, rejuvenation technologies and genetic interventions will boost human physical and people will live longer, healthier lives and even bioenhancement in near-future society in space!

With breakthrough in gene editing technology, CRISPR researchers were able to tinker with embryos to repair DNA and help fend off disease-causing mutations. Beyond the whole concept of designer babies and epigenetics, even resistance to cancer could be engineered into DNA at the time of conception.

However, these evolving technologies would raise ethical and political issues since this would cause emergence of “biologically bifurcated humankind” with broader inequality between enhanced citizens of affluent nations and unenhanced citizens of poor nations and impending psychological impact on society & potential of human genomics to create new ‘sociogenetic’ classes.

Human genomics are converging with computing technologies such as blockchain, cloud computing and machine learning. Artificial intelligence and machine learning have enabled deep analysis of thousands of molecules with potential to become future drugs and human genomic data. Also, deep learning is being used molecular structure to predict the efficacy of antibiotic candidates. There is an advancing trend towards the development and approval of personalised therapeutics, cell therapies where medical treatments would be tailored towards individuals that would account for their likely response based on genomic and epigenetic data. However, these treatment modalities are costlier owing to their sophistication and lower demand.

The misuse of technology by state or non-state actors are the ongoing concerns around. Examples included various bioweapons and the misuse of DNA databases. In developed countries most powerful supercomputer have been developed and installed in premiere centres that will enable top scientists and healthcare experts to use the powerful combination of AI and simulation to accelerate the digital biology revolution and bolster the world-leading life sciences industry.

GENE THERAPY

Gene therapy is transfer of therapeutic genes into the human body for correcting defects in faulty gene(s) that cause diseases. Two strategies of gene therapy include: ex vivo gene therapy and in vivo gene therapy.. In ex vivo therapy, cells with faulty genes of a person with disease are removed, manipulated in the lab for their reintroduction for the treatment of the patient. It is more effective than in vivo approach. In in vivo gene therapy, corrected genes are introduced directly in the intended tissues and organs of the body without removing body cells. Here, viruses, liposomes artificial chromosome are used as vectors for gene therapy.

BIOMIMICRY

Term biomimicry and biomimetics come from the *Greek* words *bios*, meaning life, and mimesis, meaning to imitate. Other terms often used are bionics, bio-inspiration, and biognosis.

Biomimicry or biomimetics is examination of nature, processes to take inspiration from to solve human problems. With the emergence of smart materials and structures, this has become feasible to make smart sensors and actuators capable of mimicking biological transducers, bio-inspired signal-processing techniques, modelling and control of manipulators resembling biological limbs, and the shape control of flexible systems. These are the primary areas where recent technological advances have taken place.

Some key applications of these technological developments in the design of morphing airfoils, modelling and control of anthropomorphic manipulators and muscle activation modelling, and control for human limb prosthetic and orthotic applications are discussed. Also discussed, with some typical examples, are the related developments in the application of nonlinear optimal control and estimation, which are fundamental to the success of biomimetic robotics.

Nature also makes extensive use of fibres, from nanoscale collagen fibres in tendons to microscale wood fibres, terminal hairy fibres in gecko feet pads to high-tenacity spider silk. Understanding this structure– function relationships is key in developing textile products for example, adaptive, thermoresistant, superhydrophobic, or self-healing.

Lotus plant wards off water drops and while it rolls off to collect all the dirt along with it. Keeping clothes and other textile materials self-cleaning and water repelling for use in outdoor clothing, carpets, and architectural fabrics became feasible on this knowledge. Similarly, development of a textile fabric adopted from functionality of duck feathers product is developed on cotton and polyester fabrics, layering it with chitosan for surface roughness and coating it with silicon. The application of the fibre optic transmitters' act like photonic crystals in textiles can be used to make thermal insulated fabrics. Mimicking microstructure of butterfly wings can be applied to produce structural colors in textiles. Biomimicry in textiles can translate into designing solutions that are sustainable and developed in a way that cause the least environmental impact.

Biomimetic Sensors

Biomimetic sensors can be potentiometric, voltametric or impedance spectrum sensors modified by specifically designated biomimetic materials. Using nanotechnology and microfluidics and enzyme as sensing elements, various biosensors and chips based on sensory cells such as gustatory cells, nerves cells have been developed. Biomimetic sensors have many applications in biomedical field such as early diagnosis, monitoring, & therapy; for food quality control; in the field of forensics and for environmental analyses.

EXAMPLES FOR BIOMIMETIC SENSORS

Acoustic sensors:

Cochlear amplifier and speech recognition system

Sonar receiver based on Dolphin

Chemical sensors:

Artificial chemical recognition sites

Artificial human tongue

Artificial human nose: based on Conducting polymer, Piezoelectronics, or Chemo-fluorescence

Electric sensors for:

Electrolocation

Vision: Fly based vision system based on:

Hexagonal oriented vision

Non- camera motion detection

Primate or human eye-based vision

Posture monitoring

Artificial organs/tissues:

Muscle : Artificial muscle monitoring

Skin: Artificial electronic skin

Mechanical cells/ tissues:

Artificial muscle spindle

Artificial blood corpuscles

Artificial crustacean antenna

Thermal sensors:

cont.....

Photo-mechanical sensors
IR Sensor
Sensing skin: Thermal Skin

EVOLUTION BIOTECH SOLUTION, TRACKING ANCESTRY

Already discussed in chapter 10.

ANTISENSE RNA TECHNOLOGY & RNAI FOR GENE THERAPY

Antisense RNA technology blocks translation of mRNA molecules to silence gene expression. Antisense RNAs is a promising way to turn off disease genes as a gene therapy approach. RNAi has reinvigorated gene therapy approaches by gene silencing. Double-stranded RNA molecules are delivered into cells where dicer enzyme chops them into 21 nt-long pieces: siRNAs (small interfering RNAs) that join with enzyme complex known as RNA-induced silencing complex (RISC). RISC shuttles siRNAs to their target mRNA, siRNA binds by complementary base pairing. RISC complex then degrades siRNA-bound mRNAs so that they cannot be transformed into proteins.

In vivo delivery of antisense RNA, dsRNA or siRNA is challenging because they degrade quickly in the body and are difficult to penetrate cells and target right tissue. Plasmid vector, liposome, lentivirus, attachment of siRNA to cholesterol and fatty acids are used to deliver silencing RNAs. In macular degeneration, VEGF gene is targeted for gene silencing. Other target diseases for siRNAs are different cancers, influenza, diabetes, multiple sclerosis, neuro degenerative diseases.

Gene therapy in SCID (severe combined immunodeficiency) with defect in adenosine deaminase gene(ADA), cystic fibrosis (CFTR gene defect) has been tried successfully. Over 500 gene therapy clinical trials have been carried out and over 600 are ongoing. There are still many hurdle in making gene therapy a safer and reliable therapeutic approach.

BIO-PRINTING, 3-D & 4-D PRINTING

3D Printing

In this technique, individualized materials are being developed with the aim to customize the architecture and produce customized functional products. They would serve as a powerful tool for the production of bioengineered manufacturing implants based individual-specific anatomy, and can be used as phantoms that can be used in education , planning surgery and production of disease models.

Wound Healing

Anatomically adaptable dressings; poly(ethylene glycol) (PEG)- homogenized pericardium matrix based - 3D-printed hybrid scaffolds have already been developed by scientific community for promoting wound healing of vascular grafts for supporting surgical reconstruction of injured vessel wound; and congenital heart defect reconstruction by developing vascular grafts.

Implants and Prostheses

3 D printed implants and prostheses can be fabricated for personalized therapy. Also, preparation of individualized, 3D printed products can cater to individualized needs based on patient- specific anatomy and pathology. These customized prosthetics, and devices would enable restoration of mobility and functions of organ(s) and would restore the normal appearance that was lost by various types of deformations or traumas.

Applications: 3 D Printing of

Ovarian, fallopian tube, ureter (*e.g.*, CA uterus: ureter is compromised by tumor invasion) prosthesis: 3D printed using stem cell.

Stem Cell Generation of Ovaries in Infertility

Models for Surgical Planning and Training, Phantoms: education and surgical planning.

The production of 3D printed models would enable better evaluation and assessment of pathological changes in organ(s), better & accurate diagnosis, and further visualization of individual -specific anatomy of organ)s). This would help in providing significant amount of information and better preoperative planning and thus reducing incidence of complications and patient loss. 3D printing of realistic models of organs for surgical training can ease and shorten duration of operation and it would further decrease intra-operative complications.

Bioprinting and Organs-on-Chip

Regenerative medicine is one of the most challenging and most promising technology and it involves fabrication of multilayer object from various soft biological matter namely, living cells. The futuristic personalized/ individualized patient- centric medicine involves development of biological constructs for restoration of architecture and functions of tissue(s), along with additive fabrication for preparing various tissue/organ constructs *e.g.*, blood vessels, cartilages, bones, kidneys, liver, or heart tissue. using Bioinks with alginate and nanocellulose.

3D printing can be used in creating drug delivery systems and multidrug devices and preparation of personalized drug formulations having accelerated release characteristics to ensure desired therapeutic results with minimum or nil adverse effects! They are helpful to prioritize the development of pediatric and geriatric dosage forms in personalized dosing and dimension-specific drug formulations to ensure desired therapeutic effect.

Risk of rejection of 3D-printed constructs can be minimized by using autologous source of cell derived from biopsies or their differential bio harvesting.

4th Dimension of Printing

It involves production of self- evolving materials having shape memory & structures and they may serve as actuators for developing biorobotics, biomedical devices, and drug delivery systems and in tissue bioengineering.

Biomimetic ink with hydrogel matrix with embedded cellulose fibrils following immersion in water, exhibit localized anisotropy and they have been used in production of shape-morphing systems to be used serially for production of smart textiles and biomedical devices.

These additive biomanufacturing of dynamic, reconfigurable, functional materials would pave way for newer avenues for creation of designer architectures with shape- mobility to be used in tissue bioengineering, production of biomedical devices, soft robotics and even more.

MICROFLUIDICS

Already discussed.

VIRTUAL CELL, IN-SILICO MODELLING

Already discussed.

REGENERATIVE MEDICINE AND ORGAN TRANSPLANTATION, TISSUE AND ORGAN ON CHIP

Another hot area of medical biotechnology is Regenerative Medicine. Treatment of human illnesses by doctors include various approaches namely, surgery, radiation therapy or drugs. But, none of these approaches provide the complete answer for curing human disease since they neither produce tissue regeneration, nor restore the functions of damaged organs *e.g.*, the tissue damage after heart attack or stroke cannot restored back to original, normal state prior to illness. It is highly unlikely that drug(s) could be used to stimulate several hundred charges in gene expression with proper timing for tissue regeneration and restore organ function. Regenerative medicine , being an exciting new field of biotechnology, seems promising for growing various cells and tissues to replace or repair the cells, defective tissues and organs, and this will radically change the practice of medicine and health care delivery.

Organ transplantation, though not a new idea, is relatively new aspect of medical biotechnology research.

Fetal tissues grafts have been of long proposed to treat Parkinson disease and other neurological conditions. Bridge implants from fetal neural tissue in damaged area of severed spinal cord have shown promise in dogs and rats.

ORGAN TRANSPLANTATION

Autografts

Autografts are transplantation of one's own tissue from one part of the body to another, *e.g.*, coronary artery bypass from vein of leg, skin grafts.

Heart or liver transplants are carried out after histocompatibility matching (MHC). Most transplant recipients require immunosuppressive drugs for rest of their lives to minimize organ/graft rejection and there are chances of opportunistic infections in these subjects. Scarcity of donors and rejection directed scientists to look at other ways of providing donor organs. One such approach is *Xenotransplantation:* transfer of organ from different species and baboons and pigs were considered. Owing to threat of transmission of viruses from pigs to humans and other health problems, transplant scientists are combining molecular techniques and transplantation technology to produce cloned pigs to overcome organ rejection and viral disease transmission.

Xenotransplantation does not always have to involve the transfer of a whole organ and efforts are going on to develop ways to deliver small clusters of cells for cell and tissue transplantation raising a new term Cellular Therapeutics. This involves use of living cells encapsulated in tiny beads or tubes: Biocapsules or Microcapsules.

Biocapsules may contain therapeutic molecules or cells, *e.g.*, insulin producing (beta cells) from pancreas can be implanted in type I diabetes patients. These Biocapsules protect cells from being attacked by recipient immune cells since immune cells and antibodies cannot enter the capsule and these capsules are only permeable to nutrient exchange and allow molecules produced by the encapsulated cells to escape and enter bloodstream. This approach would likely to require change of Biocapsules every few months.

Tissue engineering is emerging science and may someday provide bioengineered, healthy tissues and organs for replacing diseased or damaged tissues. At present, bioengineered human skin sheets are beneficial in treatment of burn patients. Also, bioengineered bone(s) for healing the bone fractures have been shown to serve their purpose and scaffolding to engineered teeth has shown promise. Field of tissue engineering is in its infancy and engineered organs will be a reality in future.

STEM CELL TECHNOLOGIES, POTENTIAL APPLICATIONS AND CLONING

Stem Cell Technologies

There is tremendous promise and controversy surrounding stem cells in future, stem cell research may affect lives of millions of people throughout the world.

Potential Applications of Stem Cells

Stem cell technology has been used to grow healthy tissues, genetic manipulations for treating birth defects & other disorders, gene delivery for gene therapy, tissue bioengineering to create functional tissues, scientists are hoping to develop stem cell treatments for diseases such as stroke, heart disease, Parkinson's disease, diabetes and other conditions.

Promising examples of uses of stem cell are use of stem cells to make WBCs in leukaemia, umbilical cord stem cells to provide RBCs for sickle cell patients and patients with other blood deficiencies. Repairing of heart tissue by stem cell technology has shown strong potential. Another promising treatment is used of IP cells to correct sickle cell anaemia.

Promising Stem Cell-Based Therapies

Autoimmune disease

Cardiovascular disease

Cancers

Degenerative retinal disease

Diabetes

Neuro degenerative diseases

Osteoporosis

Phenylketonuria

Severe combined immuno deficiency (SCID)

Sickle cell disease

Cloning

Cloning refers to making a copy of a gene, a cell or an entire organism. With announcement of cloning of Dolly (sheep) in February, 1997, prospect of human closing also opened up.

Human Cloning Application: Implications

Two approaches to cloning are:

- Reproductive cloning
- Therapeutic cloning

Reproductive cloning is intended to create a baby and Dolly was produced by reproductive cloning.

Therapeutic cloning provides stem cells that are a genetic match to a patient requiring a transplant. Chromosomes from patient's somatic cells (*e.g.*, its skin) are injected into an enucleated egg (egg with its nucleus removed) that is stimulated in culture to create an embryo till blastocyst stage. It is then used to harvest stem cells that can be introduced into the donor and there is no chance of immune rejection. Term somatic cell nuclear transfer is preferred over therapeutic cloning.

Human Genome Project (HGP)

HGP has revealed disease genes and scientists have been developing "maps" showing location of normal and disease genes on all human chromosomes. HGP has to of development of many projects, *e.g.*, Cancer Genome Atlas Project (TCGA) to identify genomic changes involved in a variety of different cancers. HGP has provided us with unprecedented knowledge about human chromosomes and the genes they contain. However, much work lies ahead to determine functions of genes, then complex proteins coded by them that play roles in normal cell activity and diseased conditions.

Astro-Biotechnology – Space Biotechnology

Astrobiotechnology is a molecular step towards the boundaries of space exploration. Astrobiotechnology being a relatively new branch has found an important place in space research and exploration missions(SRE). Biotechnology techniques such as PCR, gene expression, or proteomics can be of help to identify and monitor potential extra-terrestrial biological contaminants from any mission involved in search for life-forms. It is not only important for the planetary protection, but also for further astrobiology research, and for studying the limits of life-forms in space, and possible evolution of life forms in the other environments!

Research Applications of Astrobiotechnology

Modern molecular biology and biotechnology includes various high-throughput "omics" technologies for analyzing various biological samples. The omics technology spans across the genomics, transcriptomics, proteomics, and metabolomics techniques. These techniques allow in-situ measurements and analysis , real-time monitoring of the biological environment and sampled data more accurately.

Various biological experiments involving micro-organisms, cell(s), tissue(s), cell cultures, smaller plants & invertebrates; *in-situ* detection of various microbial contaminations; and pathogen detection in samples taken from air, surface, and water in spacecraft or samples from outer space during space walk or using probes can be done. Amplification and *in situ* detection of bacterial and fungal contaminants that are based on real-time nucleic acid sequence-based amplification and molecular beacon detection technology are now possible.

Potential of Astrobiotechnology

Astrobiotechnology applies modern biology tools to advance space exploration that are focused on identification of the technology gaps in longer missions and to applying various transition methodologies & experience derived from experiments based on Earth to other planets. Future long-term missions in the space would require a generation of a significant amount of food, water, and oxygen on-board for the crew's necessities, since this huge quantity of mass can neither be supported by the available launch systems nor would be cost effective. Thus, final goal of Astrobiotechnology is to make space missions completely independent without relying on any supplies from Earth, and biotechnology along with 3D printing would be meeting the needs of long-term, and even extra- milky way space missions in future.

Research and development of space biotechnology is highly expensive and newer technologies such as 3D-printing would enable the astronauts/ space-crew to produce a wide variety of tools, food and even bioengineer biological materials such as autologous human tissues on board on- demand. Pharmaceutical and biotechnology companies are conducting experiments regarding various protein crystallization techniques for developing immunotherapeutics & drugs and testing newer technologies cellular function assessment so as to improve drug effectiveness and safety. It is expected that fundamental progress in space medicine would protect astronauts from diseases and their treatment. This would help to mitigate effects of space-related stressors; advances in these fields could be useful also on Earth in long run.

Thus, field of space bioprocessing or biotechnology has three major areas namely, separation and purification of biological materials for therapeutic or diagnostic applications; enhanced protein crystallization for use in pharmaceutical research; and research into the effects of weightlessness on basic biological processes.

Bioterrorism, Medical Terrorism

The world has recently witnessed the devastating effects of disease outbreaks of Ebola and the Zika virus and covid- 19 virus, even omicron – and they seemed to be natural in origin. The malicious use of biotechnology could lead to medical bioterrorism meaning that future outbreaks would be started on certain purpose. The perpetrator would be a state actor or a terrorist group who can be responsible for development and release of a bioweapon, *e.g.*, a new designer poison or infectious disease that could be hard to detect and even harder to stop. Unlike a bullet or a bomb, these self- replicating and mutating deadly cells or poisons could continue to spread long after their deployment. The governments around the world have to take this threat very seriously, and the threat of bioweapons to the environment should not be taken lightly either.

Even assembly of an arsenal containing “anthrax, botulism, hemorrhagic fever, plague, smallpox, typhoid, and yellow fever,” ready in case of attack could be kept by terrorists. And the newer gene editing technologies are adding nails to these the odds and the fact that a hypothetical bioweapon targeted at a certain ethnicity, or even a single individual like a world leader might be a reality!

As the attacks using traditional weapons require much less expertise, dangers of futuristic bioweapons should not be ignored. At present, it might seem convincing that bioweapons cannot be made without plenty of these expensive materials and confidential scientific knowledge. However, with the invent of do-it- yourself technology and easy online procurement system with restrains, and with the recent advances in biotechnology, the production of bioweapons outside a specialized research lab might even be easier. The falling cost to chemically manufacture strands of DNA implies that affordable to ‘print’ deadly proteins or cells at home would a reality soon. With openness and easy-access of scientific knowledge online, can freely Google the details of chemical structure and manufacturing of deadly neurotoxins. And the most controversial aspect of biohacking is another challenging aspect in era of gene-editing.

SMART USE OF GENOMIC DATA IN RESEARCH, CONSERVATION OF SPECIES, SAFER GMOS, IN INDUSTRY, MEDICAL DIAGNOSIS TREATMENT

Already discussed.

Creating New Life and Implication

Venter lab in 2010 announced creation of the first bacterium with an entirely synthetic genome wherein Mycoplasma mycoides genome was stitched together from simple chemical building blocks and then inserted into a bacterium from a different Mycoplasma species whose genetic contents had been removed. It was a giant step for synthetic biology.

This was reported to be the first instance of 'artificial life.' This prompted a meeting of the U.S. Presidential Commission for the Study of Bioethical Issues and an ensuing ethical report (2010), it was widely assumed that the creation of artificial life is itself morally significant.

The worries philosophers have about artificial life do not, for the most part, depend on the artificiality of a given organism. Advances in synthetic biology will make the distinction between artificial and natural life a difficult and fluid one.

DNA Biohacking, CRISPR, Ethical Issues, Designer Babies

Today, not only can you genetically modify food and animals, but you can even modify DNA. Deoxyribonucleic acid (DNA) is the carrier of genetic information, present in living organisms. DNA in the wrong hands can have serious ramifications. Genetic hacking' is a risk of online genealogy and growth of home DNA testing has opened up an opportunity for genetic hacking, research finds. A growing number of amateurs join the do-it-yourself molecular biology movement outside academic laboratories. (More details are discussed under specific sections).

Extra-Terrestrial Life, Disease

Extraterrestrial life is life that may exist and originate outside the planet Earth. Earth being the only place in the universe currently known by humans to support life. Existence of extraterrestrial life seems to be hypothetical since no evidence of any planets that can support life, or shown to have actual presence of any life form. Most scientists hold that evolution of life could have occurred independently in different places in the universe. Alternatively, it could be that life in the universe might have stemmed from a smaller number of points of origin, and then spread across the universe, from habitable planet to habitable planet.

At present there are no evidence that what will happen if alien life form reaches Earth or if it can cause any disease. Following covid-19 pandemic, an awareness has grown amongst Astro scientific community that due precautions have to be taken regarding any microbe being transferred to Earth along with various rock, soil samples or the rocket returning back carrying any contaminants!

NASA is poised to launch a new rover to Mars to look for microbial life and collect some rock and soil samples to be brought back to Earth which might potentially be containing that microbial life—on a later mission, since there is a risk that Martian microbes find us hospitable hosts. NASA has a long history of working to protect the Earth from biohazards from other planets and to protect other planets from biohazards from Earth.

The Office of Safety and Mission Assurance (OSMA) division of Space agency has a mission is to "carefully control forward contamination of other worlds by organisms and organic materials carried by spacecraft" and to "rigorously preclude backward contamination of Earth by extraterrestrial life."

ISSUES IN GENETICS SAFEGUARDS FOR SAFETY BY DESIGN FOR RISK MANAGEMENT IN SYNTHETIC BIOLOGY

Genetic Safeguards for: Safety-By-Design

Synthetic Biology

This is new interdisciplinary area of engineering and science that redesigns and creates novel artificial biological pathways or synthetic biomolecules.

Convention on Biological Diversity defines synthetic biology as technological applications using the biological systems, living organisms, or derivatives and making or modifying new products or processes for specific use.

The potential of genetic engineering has been extended by synthetic biology by inspiring researchers to bioengineer biological systems for performing specific tasks in area of therapeutics, diagnostics, bioenergy, bioremediation and biomanufacturing of high-value biomolecules through biological pathway design and optimization.

Comparison between Synthetic Biology And Genome Editing

Synthetic biology in some ways is similar to genome editing, since both involve changing genetic code of an organism. In synthetic biology, long stretches of DNA are stitched together that can be genes or novel stretches which are then inserted into genome of an organism. In genome editing, tools are used to make smaller changes in the organism's own DNA. Also, genome editing tools can delete or add small stretches of DNA in the genome.

Both these technologies have ethical and social implications that would be discussed in relevant sections.

Risk in Synthetic Biology

Synthetic biology is a new technology that provides innovative biotechnological solutions to address various environmental and health challenges. Various risks in the field of synthetic biology can be technical risks, *e.g.*, accidental release of artificial organisms in environment or dangers due to evolving do-it-yourself (DIY) biology and easy online availability of materials that can be misused in bioterrorism.

Therefore the concept of responsible research and innovation should be the strategy so that both technological concerns as well as societal concerns can be handled. Scientists should be encouraged to anticipate, discuss, reflect and act upon the impending risks in this field in an open, transparent way, right from the beginning of a research project till their entry in the market.

Also, there can be issues of non-technical risks, such as institutional demands having an impact on the career, health and social relationships, and even economic pressures and there may be a risk of laboratory accident or inadvertent release.

Possible risks to human, animal end environmental health result from the products that emerge from methods and tools. Risk assessment only makes sense at the level of the biological system, not for parts in isolation. Since Misuse of these technologies and a failure to account for unintended consequences could cause irreversible environmental damage.

The potential far-reaching impacts of synthetic biology demand governance methods and research guidelines that promote its ethical and responsible use. Under the precautionary principle, stringent risk assessment and the inclusion of diverse stakeholder perspectives should be applied in the development and handling of innovative synthetic biology applications and products. The precautionary principle states that when human activities may lead to unacceptable harm that is scientifically plausible but uncertain, action should be taken to avoid or diminish that harm. Another emerging development is Do-It-Yourself Biology, also known as "DIY Bio". It's a movement of "citizen scientists" interested in synthetic biology experiments that has become an international phenomenon over the last decade. Often with little prior knowledge of the field, enthusiasts meet in makeshift labs to take crash courses in biotechnology and conduct hands-on experiments. Simple protocols found online and specialized kits costing US$150–US$1,600 have driven the movement's rapid expansion. DIY Bio labs can be found in most major cities, and by 2017 there were about 168 groups worldwide.

Regulating the use of easily accessible and low-cost technologies like CRISPR will likely be a challenge for authorities. There is also growing concern that the technology could be misused by extremist groups.

Risk assessment could be carried out building upon commonly applied principles which are established in Annexes of the Directives 2001/18/EC and 2009/41/EC, which examine the magnitude of potential hazards or adverse effects of genetic engineering on human health and on the environment and the likelihood of the events leading to that hazard (exposure chain).

GENETIC BIOSENSOR DESIGNING – GENE CHIP, SURVEILLANCE, EPIDEMIOLOGY

Genetic Biosensor Designing

Genetic biosensors are powerful tools for real- time monitoring of natural product biosynthesis in microbial cell factories. Coupled design of genetic biosensors with high-throughput analytics in biofoundries can accelerate the process for selecting genetic parts, metabolic pathways, and producer strains. Combining transcription factors and riboswitches to complement one another's functions has emerged to improve natural product biosynthesis.

Biosensors are enabling major advances in the field of analytics that are both facilitating and being facilitated by advances in synthetic biology. The ability of biosensors to rapidly and specifically detect a wide range of molecules makes them highly relevant to a range of industrial, medical, ecological, and scientific applications. Approaches to biosensor design are as diverse as their applications, with major biosensor classes including nucleic acids, proteins, and transcription factors. Each of these biosensor types has advantages and limitations based on the intended application, and the parameters that are required for optimal performance. Specifically, the choice of biosensor design must consider factors such as the ligand specificity, sensitivity, dynamic range, functional range, mode of output, time of activation, ease of use, and ease of engineering.

SINGLE-CELL DIAGNOSTICS:

Metabolic Engineering, and Synthetic Biology Applications

As producing, purifying, and transforming whole biosensor components into individual cells is costly and time consuming, the majority of single-cell biosensing is focused on biosensors that can be genetically encoded. While this is difficult for single-stranded DNA aptamers, it has been achieved for single stranded RNA aptamers [78, 87]. These RNA aptamers rely on a fluorescent output, which can then be visualized on a single cell basis *e.g.*, fluorescence-assisted cell sorting. Moreover, riboswitches have been employed successfully as genetically encoded in vivo biosensors. Their ability to be encoded within messenger RNA (mRNA) transcripts, effecting downstream gene expression, allows riboswitches to trigger cell survival phenotypes and function as parts of gene regulatory circuits.

By using engineered microbial cell, overproduction of small-molecule chemicals is possible which helps in reducing the cost of production and promotes environmental protection. Rapid and sensitive evaluation of *in vivo* levels of products of interest can facilitate optimization of cell factories. *In vivo* biosensors of small molecules can easily detect them using fluorescence, absorbance, and cell growth parameters and they can aid high-throughput screening of small-molecule products. These biosensors can be protein-based biosensors and RNA-based biosensors.

Genetically encoded small molecule biosensors, which provide the means to couple metabolite concentration to measurable or actionable outputs, are highly promising solutions to the bottleneck. Here we review recent advances in the design, optimization and application of small molecule biosensor in metabolic engineering, with particular focus on optimization strategies for transcription factor (TF) based biosensors.

Prediction, Surveillance and Follow up of Endemics, Epidemics and Pandemics and Epidemiology of Diseases : Future Prospective – Wearable Biosensors/ Non-Invasive Tech, Urine, Skin Patches to Predict, and at Level of Community Waste Storage, Possible Role in Bioterrorism.

Already discussed.

Microbial Cell Factories

Microbial cell factory is an approach to bioengineering which considers microbial cells as a production facility in which the optimization process largely depends on metabolic engineering. Microbial cell factories are used for many applications in industrial microbiology.

Low yield and low titre of natural products are common issues in natural product biosynthesis through microbial cell factories. One effective way to resolve such bottlenecks is to design genetic biosensors to monitor and regulate the biosynthesis of target natural products. In this review, we evaluate the most recent advances in the design of genetic biosensors for natural product biosynthesis in microorganisms. In particular, strategies for selection of genetic parts and construction principles for the design and evaluation of genetic biosensors are already being discussed.

Microbial cell factories (MCFs) are gaining much scientific attention owing to their potential to synthesize a range of compounds to fulfil current demands of commodities in a sustainable manner. MCF is a production facility of organisms that aims at achieving a high yield of both native and non-native metabolites by rewiring and optimizing the production process with the help of metabolic engineering and synthetic biology. In the past few decades, several natural microorganisms have been identified and used for the production and optimization of value-added biomolecules for therapeutic, biotechnological, and industrial applications.

Microbial cell factories: applications

Production of microbial products: recombinant therapeutic proteins

Therapeutic proteins and enzymes:

Antibiotics, antitumor agents, immunosuppressants, antivirals, anthelmintics, nutraceuticals, polymers, enzyme inhibitors

cont.....

Vaccines, hormones, interferons, growth factors
Agricultural and industrial products:
Surfactants, bioherbicides, biopesticides
Industrial proteins: recombinant production of protein-based polymers & enzymes: used in food, feed, detergent, textile, and waste treatment processes
Futuristic:
Antibody mimetics:
Promising biotherapeutics: future alternatives to mAbs
Small antibody-based formats: Single-chain variable fragments (scFvs), fragmented antigen-binding (Fabs)
Non-antibodies:
Interferons (*e.g.*, IFNα-2b), cytokines [*e.g.*, granulocyte colony stimulating factor (G-CSF) and tumor necrosis factors (TNFs)], hormones [*e.g.*, insulin glargine and human growth hormone (hGH)], and interleukins (IL-2 and IL-11)
Production of new or improved microbial strains for biotechnological applications.

Future of in- House Production of Medicines: Drugs and Complex Biologicals

There are several unusual characteristics of pharmaceutical industry in terms of the structure and nature of their business operations. Little is known about them outside the industry, however these issues can affect the process of bringing new pharmaceuticals to the patient materially. Since development of a new pharmaceutical product is extremely costly , very time consuming, and have a high risk of failure and a very little chance of having a successful outcome!

Need of the hour is development of a greener pharmacy with likely future commercial and technical developments in business.

A vast majority of existing pharmaceutical products consist of small molecules that being produced *via* chemical synthesis. However, recent advances in the understanding of genomics and proteomics, coupled with latest technological capabilities in manufacturing very large molecules are getting preference for being used as biologicals as compared to conventional chemical- based therapies.

The fastest growth biologics are monoclonal antibodies and they are considered to be the perfect human medicines by some. They have major therapeutic advantages int terms of their exquisite specificity, high potency i,e., patient dosage can be small and are required to produced only on small-scale manufacturing platform. They can be targeted to human receptor sub-types implicated in pathology/disease process and have least potential for side effects.

Second therapeutic revolution though in infancy is also stemming from advancing field of genomics, and this is termed as "*personalised medicine*". the recent rapid advances in the mapping of the human genome and subsequent development of the scientific disciplines of genomics, proteomics and metabolomics is leading us to a better understanding of the molecular signals of many diseases. The expectation is that molecular screens combined with clinical data will point to more precise treatment options for each patient sub-group. This should enable much more precise and effective prescribing to occur which will, in turn, mean less overall drug use, since every prescribed dose will be effective first time. The next generation of human pharmaceuticals will certainly leave smaller residues in the environment as compared to those resulting from the usage of current medicines.

Biologics

Biologics are one of the fastest growing classes of therapeutic compounds, rapidly outpacing the growth of small-molecule drugs. By 2020, analysts are expecting biologics to make up over a quarter of the entire pharmaceutical market. This drive towards biologics is due to their ability to reach targets considered 'undruggable' using small-molecule therapies, and because of the benefits, or rather the reduced side-effects, offered to patients through better-targeted therapies. Biologics will continue to show robust growth for decades to come. The field of biologics is representative of a wider shift in focus away from 'one size fits all' treatments and towards more targeted medications to treat specific groups of patients.

Biologic Treatments

Biologic treatments, as the name suggests, are derived from biological processes – for example, copying an individual's ability to grow or develop antibodies. Instead of being chemically synthesised, biologic pharmaceuticals are manufactured and harvested directly from the cell's biological processes.

Biologic treatments can excel in targeting receptors and proteins that cannot be achieved using small molecule therapies and potentially achieving more potent interactions with the drug target, or with less potential for off-site interactions.

Antibody–drug conjugates (ADCs) are a class of drugs produced by combining biologics with molecular chemistry. ADCs are one of the most advanced oncology treatments to have been developed in recent years, and they were conceived as targeted cancer treatments. All ADCs are constructed from three individual components: an antibody scaffold; a chemical linker; and a highly cytotoxic molecular payload. By using the ability of antibodies to couple specifically to certain proteins known as antigens, a triggered release of the cytotoxic molecule within the desired cell can be achieved, mitigating off-site cytotoxicity that may lead to unwanted side-effects, and they show promise as more active cancer treatments and overcome many of the safety concerns.

Battlefield Medicine: Role of Biotechnology – Do-It-Yourself Approach

Modern biotechnology has played an important role in treatment of war injuries, prevention and diagnosis of diseases, and protection against biochemical toxic agents; it will show its advantages in strengthening the power to fight, resist fatigue, sense and monitor the battlefield, and develop military biomaterials.

Biotechnological weapons can cause destruction that is both more powerful and more civilized than that caused by conventional killing methods like gunpowder or nuclear weapons.

Biotechnology plays a critical role in treating war injuries, preventing, and diagnosing disease, and protecting the force against exposure to harmful agents. While effective in its ability to provide medical intervention, biotechnology's non-medical side reveals opportunity to create a "superhuman" soldier who is more effective in combat and equipped to survive the rigors of war. Scientists in the field have proposed ideas on how to neurologically and physically enhance soldiers at the genetic level. These developments may help build soldier resistance to battle fatigue, increase endurance, and enhance intelligence making soldiers more decisive on the battlefield. Creating soldier that are stronger, faster, and able to counter unpredictable enemy tactics will increase the military's ability to adapt to changing battlefield conditions and conduct major operations using a smaller force. This thesis examines performance and cognitive enhancement of the soldier *via* genetic engineering and its potential ability to arm the military with the capabilities to maintain rapid deployment cycles despite the reduction in force and fight wars using sophisticated techniques to reduce casualty rates. Understanding the ends and means of soldier enhancement and the novel ethical issues associated with genetic modification is critical to its future in military application.

Do-it-yourself battlefield medicine saves lives. Quick care on the battlefield, sometimes by a wounded soldier himself, led to a 92 percent survival rate for one Army regiment over more than seven years, a study found. With advances in 3D or bioprinting, it is expected that bioprinted skin, medicines and equipments and tools will be of great help in helping the injured soldier.

Introduction: Time Line, Types of Biotechnology – Colours

Biotechnology is responsible for the manipulation of living organisms or their components to produce products that are of benefit to humankind. Due to the wide range of applications, colors have been used to differentiate the main areas of research, such as white (industrial), green (agricultural) and blue (marine and fresh water), among others. Thus, this review outlines the impacts of these areas of biotechnology, emphasizing their impact and potential to replace carbon-based technologies with more sustainable technologies.

Biotechnology is responsible for the manipulation of living organisms or their components for the production of products that are of benefit to humankind. Due to the wide range of applications, colors have been used to differentiate the main areas of research, such as white (industrial), green (agricultural), and blue (marine and fresh- water), among others.

Color Code Classification of Biotechnology

Due to the vast application of Biotechnology in various fields like medical, agriculture, dairy, textile, food, and many more industries, Biotechnology can be classified using a color code.

Based on the application field, the colourful types of biotechnology are Green, Red, White, Gold, Grey, Blue, Yellow, Violet, Brown, and Dark.

S. No	Color Code	Biotechnology Branch/ Field
1	Green	Agriculture Biotechnology
2	Red	Medical Biotechnology

cont.....

3	White	Industrial Biotechnology
4	Gold	Bioinformatics
5	Grey	Environment Protection Biotechnology
6	Blue	Marine (Aquatic) Biotechnology
7	Yellow	Food Nutritional Biotechnology
8	Violet	IPR, Ethics and Biosafety
9	Brown	Arid & Desert Biotechnology

Medical "Red" Biotechnology

Medical biotechnology is all about human health and medicine. So, medical biotechnology will involve producing new pharmaceutical drugs, antibodies, vaccines, and more.

Industrial "White" Biotechnology

Largest branch of biotechnology! Its focus is on using technology to create new processes with the use of fewer natural resources and energy as compared to conventional methods.

Environmental and Agricultural "Green" Biotechnology

Green biotechnology concentrates on technologies related to agriculture,

Marine "Blue" Biotechnology

It refers to the study of marine organisms with a focus on using these organisms for various human purposes, such as creating new medicines or food supplements to enhance human health.

Animal Models to be Replaced

Animal models are still indispensable in some research areas. They provide the only way of modelling the effects of a new medicine on an entire organism, with all its organs and the complex interactions that take place in the body. Long-term effects can often only be demonstrated in animal models, and that is also why authorities responsible for licencing drugs still insist on them as part of the approval process.

On the other hand, it is known that animal models are not always transferable to humans. Drugs may cause effects in humans that are not seen in animal models, just as some effects in animals may not be relevant to humans. To reduce animal testing and improve translatability of results to humans, we are intensively researching various alternative methods.

Organs on a Chip

One of these methods is to model human physiology outside the living organism, for example on a chip, or to use computer models to test the behaviour of a medicine in the body. *Organs on a chip* is among the latest developments and flexible synthetic chips about the size of a USB stick serve as carriers for various human organ cell structures and can be used to screen drug candidates for efficacy and safety at a very early stage. The technology provides a sneak preview of a newly-discovered molecule and its potential effects on humans many years before it is used in a real human.

Tissue Bioprinting

3D printing has revolutionized the tech world for its potential to produce complex machine parts from a digital file. The same is starting to be done using bioinks that carry cells to make living tissues. Few companies in the world use bioprinted tissues in the drug discovery process.

Organoids

While cell cultures are tried and tested methods for screening drugs, how human cells behave in a dish is not necessarily how they behave in the body. One alternative could be miniature organs, called organoids. These 3D organoids are grown using stem cells, which, with the right cocktail of nutrients and treatments, can become the organ of choice.

Future of Animal Testing in Research

Bioprinting, organoids, and organs-on-a-chip are all early-stage technologies with the potential for making in vitro research better predict the effects that a drug will have on humans.

Cytodiagnostics and Nanotechnology

Nano-biotechnology is aiding emergence of interface between life science and nanotechnology and has great prospects in healthcare solutions.

Recently, focus of nanoscience and nanotechnology research has gradually shifted from the development of high-quality nanomaterials and investigation of their properties to application side. Although biomedical science has been recognized as a field that can greatly benefit from nanotechnology, not all the nanomaterials are suitable for all healthcare applications. Some of the nanomaterial-based drugs, devices have already entered the market and others are on the verge of doing so.

Nanotechnology in medicine called nanomedicine involves applications of NPs currently under development, as well as longer ranges research that involves the use of manufactured nano-robots to make repairs at the cellular level. Future applications of nanomedicine will be based on the ability to build nanorobots. These nanorobots could be programmed to repair specific diseased cells, functioning in a similar way to antibodies in our natural healing processes. This way, nanomedicine offers great promise for the future, especially the mixing of diagnostic and therapeutic capabilities in healthcare. Nano surgery like laparoscopy is already being used for reproductive health problem detection, corrective surgery, tubal sterilization, chronic pelvic pain, etc. since past many years.

Biotech Solutions for Diagnostics, Treatment and Solving Food Problems in Space

It is anticipated by 2050, feeding nearly billion people will be a challenging task despite significant progress in crop breeding. For the past few decades productivity of agricultural crops have been enhanced *via* advanced plant breeding methods and crop management practices. Innovative biotechnological advances have aided immensely in enhanced agricultural crop production, breeding of new crop varieties, production of biofertilizers, biopesticides, disease diagnostics and conservation of crop genetic resources. The whole genome sequencing of crops and diagnostic molecular markers have potential to expedite plant breeding processes and would have a potential role in food and nutrition security.

Space synthetic biology branch of biotechnology is dedicated to engineering biological systems for space exploration, industry and science. Both public and private sectors are showing interest in designing organisms which can assist long-duration astronaut missions. The opportunities and challenges in this context are summarized in Box **1** along with possibilities that can benefit Earth.

Box:1: Grand challenges in space synthetic biology:

1. Resource utilization to:

(a) Ensure its functionality in extreme environments.

(b) Provide capacity to harness resources: wastes, volatiles, minerals.

(c) Produce stocks to manufacture cell-based biomaterials.

2. To manufacture:

(a) Construct adhesives to bind regolith, biocement and biopolymers

(b) Fuel for power and propulsion.

(c) Abiotic.

3. To provide life support by:

(a) Improving biological management of waste, and wastewater.

(b) Treatment, conditioning and recycling of air, water and solid wastes to create 'living' habitat.

(c) Production of nutritious food that is flavourful, texture rich.

(d) Provision of nutrients, and their recycling.

4. In Space medicine and human health to:

(a) Prevent disease and maintain human microbiome.

(b) Manufacture synthetic drugs not only for treatment of disease, radiation damage and effects of reduced gravity.

(c) Development of radiation-resistant, self- healing, protective clothing and personal shielding.

5. For Space cybernetics to:

cont.....

(a) *Develop device-level biological control systems:* biological sensors, actuators and controllers.

(b) *Design biological control systems* composed of biological parts, or which can partially integrate biological controllers and systems with abiotic sensors and actuator devises.

6. *In Terraforming or terraformation*:

A hypothetical process of modifying atmosphere, temperature, surface topography or ecology of a planet, moon, or other body similar to environment of Earth so as to make it habitable life like Earth. Para terraforming with few multi-functional species that complete carbon and nitrogen cycles.

We Need Biotechnology to Reach Mars

As space agencies are preparing for long-distance space travel and life on Mars, biotechnology would be of help to make spaceships and space stations that no longer dependent on Earth's constant supply.

In the long run, astronauts in space would be able to Bioprint their own tissues and organs as and when required. In 2019, Russian space agency sent space bioprinters to the ISS that are successful in 3D-printing human cartilage and mouse thyroid glands. NASA has also send one bioprinting factory to space station in 2021.It turns out that 3D-printing in space has some advantages since without restrictions of gravity, it is now possible to 3-D print tissues and organs from all sides at once, using magnetic and acoustic fields that keep the cells in place.

Growing Food in orbit: Astronaut Farmers

If food can be grown for astronauts in orbit, this will make space exploration and space environment more sustainable and accessible. NASA projects have sent and grown vegetables in space missions and studying how plants behave under 'stress of space life'. They have found that in space, genes are activated which prepare plants to respond to heat and flooding. Identification of these genes has allowed researchers to genetically engineer plants that can grow better in space conditions. Thus, to achieve the ultimate goal is being able to grow food on other planets and satellites many space research groups are putting in their efforts. In this context, China is already running tests for construction of a self-sustained 'Lunar Palace' on south pole of Moon, while NASA — and Elon Musk — has its eye on sending humans to Mars eventually. NASA's food scientists are researching crops that can be grown in flight. On Mars, astronauts fruits and veggies, and even staple crops like wheat can be grown. The final goal of growing crop in space is to be as independent as possible, and to be able to stay for a long time in space without depending on supplies from Earth so that there is no stopping humans from traveling farther into space. And biotechnology seems to be the solution needed to meet all these needs of long-term space missions.

Human Genome in a Smart Card

With falling costs of Gene sequencing following with advancements in technology over last decade, its cost will reduce even further in the following years. This means that personal genomics, therapeutics and diagnostics will be feasible in the near future. The biggest problem is storage of such large data and privacy of genomic data is also important since it can it contains privacy-sensitive data and can be used to identify an individual. Therefore, methods for privacy- preservation of genomic data should be developed and this could be possible in smart human cards under development by many research groups. Such smart cards would require methods for storing some parts of human genome needed for disease risk computation along with reference genome sequences and provision of filters to select genomic, exomic variations and they will be without risk of abuse of genome privacy of individuals.

Other details have already discussed in chapter 3.

Weapon Technology – Bioterrorism

Today humans face not only the threat of natural diseases. but also threats of biological weapons and bioterrorism, and with genetically engineered agents that may resist known therapies. The next generation biological weapons are organisms with altered characteristics.

More details have been discussed in chapter 3.

Wearable Technology

Now the era of wearable biotech enhancement has started and the future of wearables will move beyond digital technology; biotechnology will measure and improve the hormones, genomes, microbiomes, and more through "wearable laboratories" on human bodies.

Just as computers once occupied an entire room and now fit in the pockets, biotechnology is becoming faster, cheaper, smaller, and accessible to anyone. The era of "wearable biotechnology" will enhance human health and "wearable laboratories," and brainstorming new applications and directions are available with companies with futuristic applications.

Current wearable devices can sense an individual's physiological data. On the other hand, one-time use biosensors for detecting biochemical markers are currently available. Integration of biological sensing with wearable computing would pave way for the future of human health enhancement. The platforms range from purely organic bio-wearables to hybrid bio-digital wearables. They include a minimally obtrusive "wearable laboratory" for continuous real-time hormone detection through saliva, and a microfluidic chip for cultivating interactions with E. Coli bacteria. Lightweight, flexible substrates and textiles functionalized with freeze-dried, cell-free synthetic circuits, including CRISPR-based tools, that detect metabolites, chemicals and pathogen nucleic acid signatures are available.

Genetically engineered circuits, encoded in DNA or RNA, can be added to freeze-dried, cell-free (FDCF) reactions for activation by simple rehydration. Robust FDCF systems have already been developed for inexpensive paper-based nucleic acid diagnostics; sensitive programmable CRISPR-based nucleic acid sensors; on-demand production of antimicrobials, antibodies and enzymes; and low-cost educational kits for teaching.

Potential field applications for wFDCF sensors include warfighters and first responders operating in environments where a specific chemical or biological threat is suspected, and clinicians, health workers and researchers working in high-risk areas. For example, wFDCF-enabled coats and gowns in hospitals could provide alerts to prevent the spread of nosocomial infections. An additional promising application is patient-worn, sensor-enabled personal protective equipment, such as the SARS-CoV-2 face mask. It is expected that face mask with a lyophilized CRISPR sensor for wearable, non-invasive detection of SARS-CoV-2 at room temperature within 90 min, requiring no user intervention other than the press of a button will be a reality.

Wearable biosensors are garnering substantial interest due to their potential to provide continuous, real-time physiological information *via* dynamic, non-invasive measurements of biochemical markers in biofluids, such as sweat, tears, saliva and interstitial fluid.

It is likely that in the future, we will wear or ingest bio-digital technology to monitor and enhance our health and lifestyle.

Industry Solutions from Biotechnology – like Waterproof Cloth

Water- resistant fabrics are essential for everything from making rainwears to military tents. A MIT team has brought up a promising solution by using water repellent coating to natural fabrics *e.g.*, cotton and silk very effectively. Also, a new coating solution discovered by researchers at Simon Fraser University that can transform regular materials into waterproof surfaces. They expect that the product will be cheaper to produce, free of harmful fluorinated compounds, and effective on a variety of materials.

More details discussed in chapter 3 and 10.

Technologies for Molecular Sensing and its Role in Diagnostics and Treatment

The recent advances of molecular technologies and development of genomics aids in detection of pathogenic events at genome level. Also, structural and functional genomics approaches can explore disease-related genes and recognize their structural alterations or elucidation of gene function. These technologies and diagnostic applications of structural genomics along with mutation scanning and DNA chip technology are generating databases of disease-genes, genetic alterations *etc*. Also, functional genomics can explore the expression genetics (hybridization-, PCR- and sequence-based technologies), next generation sequencing *via* Bioinformatics and computational biology. Recent advances in microarray "chip" technology have allowed simultaneous parallel analysis of gene expression patterns of thousands of genes along with rapid discovery of single nucleotide polymorphisms (SNPs). Thus, biotechnology plays an important role in the development of diagnostic assays and may open new vistas in the field of disease management.

Biotechnology in Bioweapons – DNA Hacking, CRISPR, Futuristic Bioengineered Weapons

Already discussed in chapter 3 and 10.

Wearable Technology for DNA Damage due to Radiation – Markers of DNA Damage – MG, Dimers, Detection in Skin, Blood & Urine.

Already discussed in chapter 3 and 10.

Future of 3-D Printing of Nervous Tissue – Success Rates

Already discussed in chapter 3 and 10.

Tracking Food Poisoning

Most public health officials worldwide often fail to make any progress in preventing food poisoning from common pathogens. Incidents of contamination that involved fresh produce and processed foods, including peppers, lettuce, and peanuts, have led to mounting concerns about food safety. Food irradiation is a safe and effective tool, but it has been under-used and it also faces opposition from organic food lobby. But irradiation is not a panacea. Although it quite effectively kills the bacteria, it does not inactivate the potent toxins secreted by certain bacteria such as Staphylococcus aureus and Clostridium botulinum, and the approved doses are too low to kill most viruses. The toxins can cause serious illness or death even in the absence of live bacteria themselves.

Actually, various efforts to develop and evaluate food-safety practices should start at an even earlier stage than the farming of plants such as more aggressive use of new technology to make the plants themselves intrinsically safer. Exposure to Salmonella, E. coil, or other microorganisms at certain stages of the growing process may introduce them into the plant's vascular system. Sunlight and possibly photosynthesis itself may help pathogenic bacteria become internalized by the plants' cells, making them impervious to washing and the use of food sanitizers.

By inducing the production in vivo of "antisense" ribonucleic acid (RNA), recombinant DNA technology applied to plants offers the potential both to inhibit microorganisms' ability to grow within plant cells and to block the synthesis of the bacterial toxins.

Unfortunately for plant genetic engineers, recombinant DNA technology is regulated in an unscientific, excessive, and discriminatory way by USDA and EPA. Regardless of the risk of the product, the technology is subjected to hugely expensive and dilatory regulatory requirements. Instead of revising regulation to reflect scientific consensus and the vast experience with recombinant DNA-modified plants and foods derived from them, regulators appear to be inclined to increase the stringency of regulation.

Creating Human in Lab

Scientists have now created living entities resembling human embryos in their labs and two such new experiments are the most complete such "model embryos" developed to date.

Scientists have started creating structures resembling the human embryos by using chemical signals to coax cells into forming themselves into entities resembling very primitive human embryos. Scientists have developed most sophisticated laboratory model of the human body and created a system of miniaturized organs to be used to detect harmful and adverse effects of drugs before they are prescribed to patients.

Defense Threat Reduction Agency (DTRA), has built a system built from many human cell types, tissues representing human organs in human body such as the heart, liver and lungs. Each of these miniature organs are tiny 3D tissue-like structures about one millionth size of adult human organ and system can be used to mimic tissues/organs and can be used as a testing and predicting platform.

Wake Forest Institute for Regenerative Medicine (WFIRM) 's miniature organ model has already been able to measure toxicity in many drugs approved for human use that were later pulled from the market when it was discovered that these drugs could actually be quite harmful to people. Another hallmark feature of WFIRM's human organ tissue system is the blood circulatory system. To date, more than 15 tissue and organ products/technologies developed by WFIRM scientists, including muscle, bladder and vaginal organs, have already been tested in humans in clinical trials.

Tiny samples of human tissue cells are isolated and engineered into miniature versions of the human organ. They can contain blood vessel cells, immune system cells, and even fibroblasts, the cells in the connective tissue. Each of these organs, also known as organ tissue equivalents, performs the same functions that they do in the human body. For example, the heart beats about 60 times each minute, the lung breaths the air from the surrounding environment, and the liver breaks down toxic compounds into harmless waste products.

Programmable Biohybrids

Significant efforts exist to develop living/non-living composite materials— known as *biohybrids*—that can support and control the functionality of biological agents.

Biohybrids are a fusion of digital fabrication technology and biology that explores new relationships between organism and machine.

One day *microbial cyborgs i.e.*, bacteria combined with electronic devices could be useful in fuel cells, biosensors and bioreactors. The scientists have to develop materials that both nurture the microbes, as well as efficiently and controllably harvest the electricity or other resources they make. Now, researchers have developed one such material that enabled them to create a programmable "biohybrid" system that conducts electrons from electricity-producing (exoelectrogenic) bacteria.. They added a porous hydrogel of carbon nanotubes and silica nanoparticles (woven together by DNA strands), exoelectrogenic bacteria, liquid culture medium. This material conducted the electrons produced by bacteria to an electrode and the bacteria grew well and completely penetrating the material. For cut off the electricity, an enzyme that snipped DNA strands was added that caused disassembly of the material. The nanocomposite material that supported exoelectrogen growth and conducted electricity in a controlled way to yield a *programmable biohybrid materials system.*

The Hybrid Living Material (HLM) approach for developing fabrication platform to produce biohybrid materials of wearable scale, self-supporting 3D structure, and programmable biological surfaces that are replicable and customizable, thereby unlocking paths to apply industrial modelling and fabrication methods toward the design of living materials.

Engineered Living Materials (ELMs)

Engineered living materials combine the desired properties of both synthetic soft matter and living biological cells/tissues and are emerging to the forefront of interdisciplinary research which involves synthetic biology, materials science, device engineering, and robotics.

ELMs-Based Structures for Actuation

Actuator is a device that can respond to a control signal by converting an energy source into mechanical motion and are used in soft robotics, biomedicine, and biomimicry. Certain types of biological cells such as cardiomyocytes and muscle cells, undergo rhythmic contractions, which can be used as the energy source for actuation. These devices can be used to study drug responses, contractile development of human stem cell-derived laminar cardiac tissues and has opened new avenues in the fabrication of living cells inside the sensors as functional soft actuators.

Thus, HLM approach produces biohybrid materials of wearable-scale, self-supporting 3D structure, and programmable biological surfaces that are replicable and customizable, thereby unlocking paths to apply industrial modelling and fabrication methods toward the design of living materials.

CONCLUSION

Molecular biology offers powerful tools for diagnosing and combating human diseases. Many important genes are conserved from species to species and genes identified in model species have been related to human genes termed homologs. Biomarkers are proteins produced by diseased tissue or their production is increased when tissue is diseased. Detection of genes or gene expression patterns also provide important biomarkers for early detection and diagnosis and monitoring of disease and microarray offer promising results. Mutations in specific genes also result in many genetic diseases and require more sophisticated techniques for their detection in both foetuses and adults. Different proteins, *e.g.*, insulin, human GH have been produced using recombinant DNA technology and are used for human diseases.

EXERCISE

1. Short notes:

i. Single nucleotide polymorphisms (SNPs)

ii. Exome sequencing

iii. Genome editing

iv. ART assisted reproductive technology

2. Discuss briefly:

i. Personalized medicine & targeted cancer therapy

ii. CARs

iii. Tregs cell therapy

iv. Nature nanomachines

3. What are Nanobots

4. Describe nano cubes, nanotubes based drug delivery systems

5. Discuss future of DNA bioengineering

6. Short notes:

i. DNA origami

ii. Designer drugs

iii. Gene therapy

iv. Biomimicry

7. Discuss role of biotechnology in tracking evolution

8. Discuss role of biotechnology in tracking ancestry

9. Discuss Antisense RNA technology & RNAi

10. Describe bio-printing, 3-D & 4-D printing

11. Short notes:

i. Microfluidics

ii. Virtual cell, in-silico modelling

iii. Regenerative medicine and organ transplantation

iv. Astro-biotechnology

12. Discuss bioterrorism, Battlefield medicine, and role of biotechnology in bioweapons

13. Discuss implications of creating new life

14. What is DNA biohacking

15. Discuss CRISPR and its ethical issues

16. Discuss ethical issues of creating designer babies

17. Describe extra-terrestrial life and disease

18. Short notes:

i. Genetic biosensor

ii. Wearable biosensors

iii. Microbial cell factories

iv. Biotechnology – colours

19. Explain cytodiagnostics

20. Discuss role of biotechnology in tracking food poisoning

21. Discuss programmable biohybrids

CONFLICT OF INTEREST

No potential conflict of interest is declared by the author. It is also declared the complete work is an individual effort by the author and there was no financial/ administrative/ academic support availed from any individual/ institution /organization.

BIBLIOGRAPHY

[1] Wilson K, Hofmann A, Walker JM, Clokie S, editors. Wilson and Walker's principles and techniques of biochemistry and molecular biology. Cambridge university press; 2018 Apr 19.
[2] Karp G. Cell and Molecular Biology. John Wiley & Sons Incorporated; 2007.
[3] Hartl DL, Jones EW, Hartl DL, Jones EW. Genetics: principles and analysis. 1998.
[4] Molecular Cloning: A Laboratory Manual : Joseph Sambrook And David Russell.
[5] Primrose SB. Principles of gene manipulation and genomics by Sandy B Primrose and Richard Twyman.
[6] Molecular Biotechnology: Principles and applications of recombinant DNA.

SUBJECT INDEX

A

B

C

D

E

F

G

H

I

P

R

S

T

V

W

Y

Z

Made in the USA
Las Vegas, NV
15 November 2026

bb264bac-4f59-4b51-adb8-d2a616b6d986R02